50 YEARS A NATUROPATH

Dr Xandria Williams PhD ND

50 YEARS A NATUROPATH

Xandria Williams PhD ND

ISBN: 978-0-9568552-4-4

This book is published by Xtra Health Publications in conjunction with Writersworld Limited, and is produced entirely in the UK. It is available to order from most bookshops in the United Kingdom, and is also globally available via UK-based Internet book retailers, and from the author at xandria@xandriawilliams.co.uk or tel: 44 (0)20-7824-8153.

Copy edited by Sue Croft

Cover design by Jag Lall

WRITERSWORLD
2 Bear Close Flats, Bear Close, Woodstock
Oxfordshire, OX20 1JX, UK
☎ 01993 812500
☎ +44 1993 812500

www.writersworld.co.uk

The text pages of this book are produced via an independent certification process that ensures the trees from which the paper is produced come from well managed sources that exclude the risk of using illegally logged timber while leaving options to use post-consumer recycled paper as well.

Dedication

My love and thanks to Aunt can readily be imagined once you have read this book. They will doubtless be expressed directly when she and I meet up, sometime in the future.

Acknowledgements

In general:

I owe personal thanks to my literary agent, Sarah Menguc, for her support and warm friendship throughout several decades, and for steering so many of my books through their development stage and into fruition, both in Australia and the UK, and in countries farther afield.

Huge thanks and appreciation are due to Sue Croft, copy editor, whose support, patience, and assistance had a huge part in bringing this book to fruition as I have struggled for a full year adversely affected by near fatal covid.

Over the span of the fifty years described here there are of course, more people than I can count who deserve thanks for their contributions: friends, colleagues, students, and those we variously called patients, or with the changing fashion, clients. Many are alluded to on these pages and all live on in my memory and heart.

Anton, who will know who he is, has been a guide through it all and, has, I believe, triggered the key points that you will find in these pages. Without these key points what has been a wonderful and amazing life could well have been very different. I have been blessed and very fortunate

Key points:

Aged about 12 when divorced parents met up for one more day by an amazing coincident and enabled Aunt to find me.

Aged 17 when my choice of university was affected by a teacher's comment "of course there is Imperial College but you would not get in there": a challenge to which I immediately responded.

Aged 20 when my choice of career as a forensic chemist was diverted to that of geochemist by a chance interruption during my interview.

At about 28, in Perth, Western Australia, when I was introduced to Mr Kress, Anthroposophy, and a view of us as spirits, temporarily living in a physical body. This is a view that has quietly underlain my life, and provided me with much sure ground on which to travel.

My determination not to marry, or be owned or controlled by anyone, as I was in my childhood, and which has given me the freedom to follow my career in so many changing directions.

The many factors, often small in themselves, that enabled me to forge ahead as one of the very few women in a male-dominated world during my early career years.

In relation to Cancer:

Cancer has been the focus of the past decades of my career as a medical biochemist and naturopath, and these people merit a special mention for making this an exciting time for me.

Dr John Beard, embryologist, for the trophoblastic theory, and understanding the concept and the use of pancreatic enzymes;

Dr Otto Warburg for his elucidation of the ultimate cause of cancer, the metabolic and biochemical approach, building on and developing the normal and healthy function of the mitochondria;

Dr William Kelley and his development of an extensive, integrated, and very practical protocol;

Dr Joanna Budwig, for the importance of flaxseed oil and the oxygenation of the mitochondria;

Frank Wiewal, founder of People Against Cancer, and Lothar Hirneise of *Chemotherapy Heals Cancer and the World is Flat,* both of whom knew Dr Johana Budwig well. We met up in London and America and they passed on to me their enthusiasm for, and understanding of, her work;

Dr Waltraut Fryda, for focusing on the dangers of stress and the consequences of adrenal exhaustion;

Dr Nicholas Gonzalez, building on the work of both Dr Beard and Dr Kelley, for his supreme efforts to have this approach accepted by the (drug) medical profession

Dr Thomas N Seyfried, for his book *Cancer as a Metabolic Disease*, that unrolls and explains the ideas of Dr Otto Warburg, and shows the deeply rooted biochemical underpinnings, the ones that Warburg had anticipated even though that biochemistry had not been fully known at the time.

In relation to a metabolic approach to cancer:

These people were, I think, key in developing this metabolic, biochemical approach to cancer. I could include many others:

Dr E Schandl of American Metabolic Laboratories for his CA profile (the 'CA1 profile' to us) for giving us a test that can help to indicate the start of the cancer process possibly five or even ten years before the tumour can be detected by any other means;

Dr Olga Galkina, Medical Biochemist, for her laboratory, her analytical services, skills, and support, enabling us to test and monitor the health and the cancer development of each of our clients within what we have labelled our 'CA2 Profile'.

Such a list of acknowledgements is, of course, potentially endless. It includes clients, students, colleagues, assistants, and members of my Open House Coffee Club Community, and more friends than I can count. I remain deeply grateful to them all.

I am now in my early eighties and somewhat directed by the changes and restrictions enforced on me by the effects of over a year of battling with major and life-threatening covid. My focus is turning to psychotherapy, the mind-body-spirit connection, and what some people like to think of as quantum healing. I look forward to this phase with enthusiasm. As ever, it is a joy to me that at the end of each day and the start of the next, I can focus on the people that I hope I have helped, and will continue to help.

xandria@xandriawilliams.co.uk

education@xandriawilliams.co.uk

Tel: (+44) 020-7824-8153)

Mob: (+44) 07474 108 208

Contents

Chapter 1

CHILDHOOD

M y first eighteen years were ones of endurance. Then I escaped… to Imperial and life, to Aunt and affection, and to the most amazing career I could ever have imagined. Yet increasingly, over time, I have come to recognise how much I learnt from my awful childhood, how much strength I gained from it, and how grateful I am for such a tough beginning.

Although this is essentially a biography of my professional, not my private life, I feel it is important (and have been encouraged in this by close friends) to start from the very beginning and lay the foundation. So here we go.

As I said, I *endured* my first eighteen years: I don't ever recall 'happy'. There were times when things were tolerable, but even these were shadowed by fears of imminent upset. I escaped, of course, but into myself; there was nowhere else to go. I twice tried running away and even started a third attempt, but after that I gave up.

My male ancestor was of "the ancient Welsh family of Penrose Castle" (then Brechan Castle), according to the family bible of the day. He went to Ireland as "Captain of a Troop of Horse", with William of Orange and fought in the Battle of the Boyne in 1690. His reward was a property of several hundred acres in County Kildare, on which he built Williamstown House, where my grandfather, a younger son, grew up. This grandfather became a doctor and then a surgeon in the British army, mostly stationed in Burma (now Myanmar) and farther east.

Father was Anglo-Irish and I was born in Dublin. In 1940, at four months of age, I was taken from there to Colerain in Northern Ireland when Father volunteered into the British army. This was a family tradition.

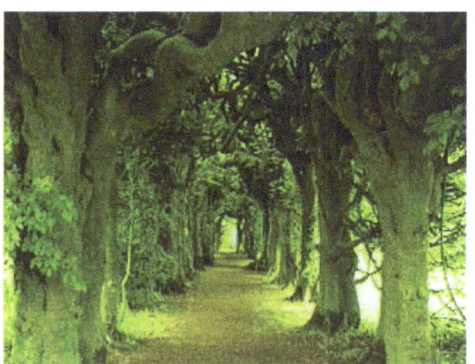

Driveway arch at Williamstown House, 1940

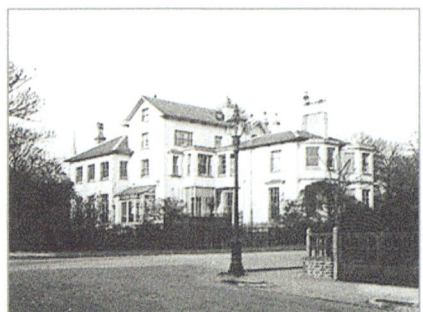

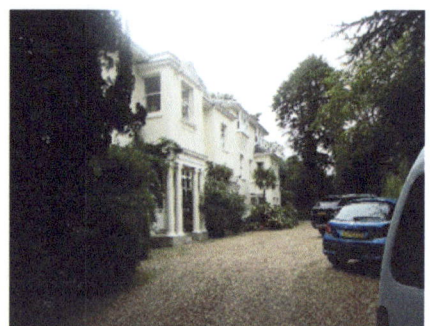

This was the home of my grandparents on the female side when I was a child, and yes, it was the whole house! I chose to visit it many decades later – it is situated in Blackheath in south London – and it looks somewhat similar now, but is divided into five flats and deprived of the many acres in which it sat. These at the time included a lake with an island, and paddocks for the horses and gymkanas.

My maternal grandfather was a chemist. I could choose to make a story, as a medical biochemist, of being the granddaughter of a doctor and a chemist, but I knew little of this history when I started to shape my own career.

Once Father went overseas, Mother took me back to Scotland and her family.

My earliest memory is from 1942 when I was two years and three days old. Brother had just been born and I was sitting on the floor in the nursing home.

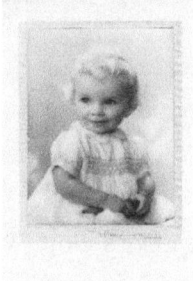 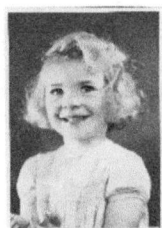

Sometime later I have another memory of standing beside a very long pair of legs clad in khaki uniform. It was presumably Father on compassionate leave from the army where he was in the tank division in North Africa.

In 1944, when I was four years old, Female Parent was incarcerated in a mental hospital as an extreme manic depressive. I don't recall who looked after Brother, aged eighteen months, and me.

In 1945, at five years old, I was in Edinburgh. Female Parent was again incarcerated and Aunt (Father's sister), was called over from Ireland to look after Brother and me. I learnt to read in my second school and was thrilled with the discovery. I vividly recall Aunt teaching me large numbers.

After the war, in about 1946, Father got a job with Unilevers in New Zealand. At the time, all passenger ships were required for the repatriation of the troops returning home, and so he travelled there ahead of us. A few months later we were due to get a train from Edinburgh to Southampton and subsequently board a boat for Sydney. With airflights a thing of the future, we had no other option.

The winter of 1946/47 was very bad with huge drifts of heavy snow blocking almost all roads and trainlines. In those days, trains that were scheduled to reach a port at a certain time when a ship could be sailing, were called boat-trains, and with a choice of two we were eventually able to book a passage on the earliest one. That was fortunate. As it turned out, we were on the last boat-train to get through the snow from Edinburgh to Southampton for days. We could so easily have missed the boat that was to take us to Australia, a journey of four weeks, via the Suez Canal and various stops including Alexandria, Port Said, Aden, Bombay, Colombo and Madras, as they were then called. We were accompanied by our English nanny, presumably because either Father or our maternal grandmother did not trust us to the sole care of Female Parent.

I spent six months in Sydney, at another school, while we waited for a boat to Wellington, New Zealand, to join Father. We eventually got berths on the very small boat that normally only covered the New Zealand North-South Island run, a trip of only a few hours, and were tossed round like a tub in the rapids for four days as a result.

In 1947 I first went to a co-ed school in Eastbourne, near Wellington, a mile from Muratai where we lived. I hated it, but I do not recall why. I ran home progressively earlier on each of the first five days. As a result, I was taken from that school and sent to another one. This was a girls' school in Lower Hutt. It had one advantage; I was able to ride on the bus with Father to get there. I was one of three who were the youngest in the school and all three lower classes were in the one room, so it was somewhat overwhelming.

Meanwhile, there was a lot of parental fighting and little happiness, although I do recall two fun occasions with Father. At eight I was on the move again. My parents had split up and divorce lay ahead. Amidst considerable adult fighting, decisions were made. Nanny left us, and austere, Victorian, strait-laced maternal Grandmother arrived, presumably to take Brother and me back to the UK. This time we sailed via the Panama Canal. I loved that boat trip and was even allowed to hand round the cakes to the other passengers at teatime.

Back in England, we first rented a house in Eastbourne on the south coast. Confused by the two Eastbournes, I ran away from home three times (East, West, and inland) trying to find Father, but it was always the wrong Eastbourne (my geography at that age wasn't very good and I forgot about the oceans we had crossed). I was first sent to a day school, and then to a boarding school when Female Parent was again incarcerated as insane (the terminology used at that time).

We moved north, back to Edinburgh. I suspect this was because Grandmother had family there and wanted support, and because Female Parent was again behaving very oddly. On one such occasion I was really afraid and ran to the neighbours for help. They must have called doctors and taken Female Parent into care. In fact, she was certified and given electric shock therapy, for which she never forgave me. I was sent off to live with a strange elderly couple. I assume they were distant relatives of maternal Grandmother as we were told to call them aunt and uncle. We had had no contact with Father's side of the family since leaving New Zealand: Female Parent's instructions to the lawyers about Brother and me were "no communication, and no contact details to be shared with them".

Yet another start at yet another school. This was a local day school, after which came a boarding school in Shropshire.

Back row 4th from left. Definitely not happy

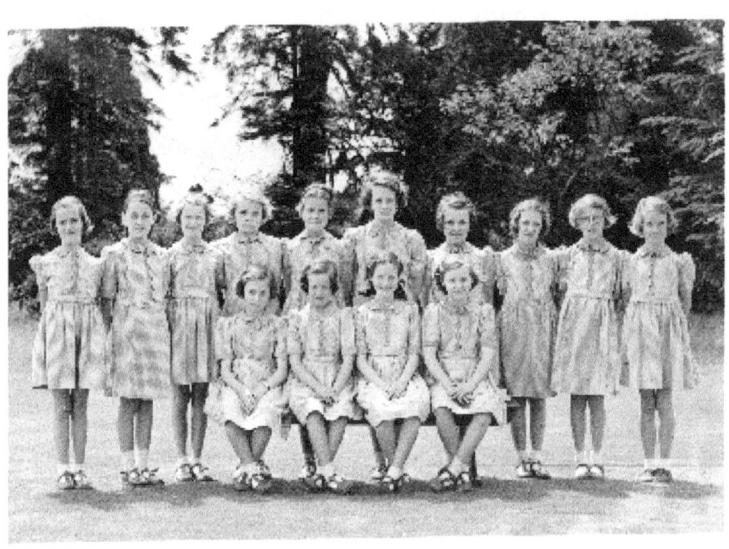

Discipline at that school was strict. We made our own bed every morning, then stood to attention at the foot until our handiwork was passed by matron. This habit has stuck with me ever since. Even now I am almost incapable of leaving my bedroom for the day until I have fully made the bed and tidied the room. I visited this building fifty years later when it had been returned to a family home. It was a beautiful and elegant building in extensive grounds, some of which were formal and others open fields.

I was back in Edinburgh for one spring holiday during which Female Parent was released from the mental home on a one-day exit. I wanted her to stay at home, of course, and tried to persuade her not to go back that evening. "I can't stay. It is all your fault I am in there in the first place", I was told, and sent back to school as she left. The guilt was heavy.

Post-war rationing was still on and we queued for sweets each day after the evening meal. One morning for breakfast we were given stewed dates and custard. The 'skin' bits on the dates made me retch and I refused to eat it – I couldn't get it down. The dining hall was the huge entrance hall to this lovely country house. Corridors led off it to various classrooms and a gallery ran around it on the first floor. Lots of people walked through it all day, peering down at me from above, or at me between classes. I sat there, miserable and embarrassed, but unable to eat the food without retching. I wasn't allowed to say a word. The matrons took it in turn to sit beside me as they did their mending, and tried to get me to eat up so we could both leave. Students and staff arrived for lunch. I continued to sit. I was oh so hungry, but each time I put a spoonful to my mouth I started to retch. I was still not allowed to say a word. In the afternoon, groups came and went to various classes. Evening supper was served. Then it was time for the day's sweet ration – three toffees or their equivalent. One toffee equalled five Smarties; two small pieces of chocolate equalled half an inch of a 'Crunchie' bar. Rationing was tight, as well as the discipline. I hated to miss my sweets. With one rush I gobbled the revolting dates and custard and forced them down, determined to claim my sweets, only to vomit it all up over the matron's lap and her mending. I was never made to eat stewed dates or figs again, with or without custard.

Back in Edinburgh, I recall when Female Parent announced she'd had a letter from Father, via the lawyers, who had passed it on. My hopes soared. Then she read it out: "Please tell the children I do not wish to communicate with them. I have found someone else and am happily remarried. I have a son [a newly adopted baby, though I wasn't told that at the time] who I love much better than them. Do not let them write to me." Thus, the end of hope. Many decades later, after she died and I went through her papers, I found the letter. In essence that was the truth of his message, though not quite so harshly put.

Aged nine, I remember a summer term in Shropshire. It must have been a reasonably alright time as I have no bad memories – at least at the emotional level. Most of the girls had toys. I collected 'interesting' bits of wood, stones, or moss, and built a story around them, but I don't think anyone was fooled.

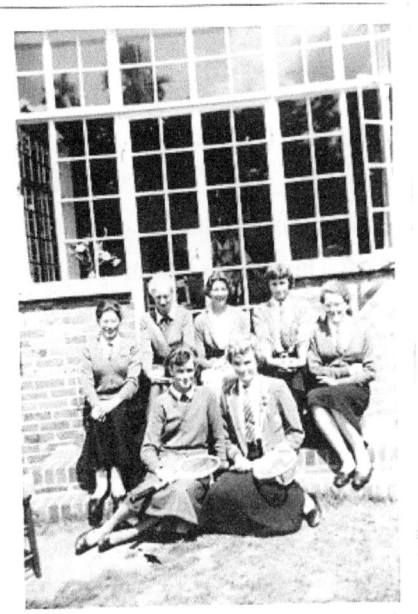

I recall being left in this large country house over various holiday times, when all the other kids had gone home. I don't think I was lonely, just pleased to have peace. Sports were my greatest pleasure.

I was head of the rounders team, with the photo to prove it, and a variety of other teams as well. It was a pattern that was to continue. I have photos of me heading up various sports teams throughout the years. I always looked the most glum and solemn-faced child there. There is not a smile to be seen on my face in any of them.

The next letter from Grandmother told me we were 'going home'–but where to? I was already reconciled to losing the one friend I had made in Edinburgh and had learnt not to make such connections. I was told by letter which train to catch and at what station (Crewe) to get off and change to another. I'm not sure why, but I landed up in the guard's van, sitting on a pile of sacks, presumably mail sacks, and recall one of the guards talking to me. After a sudden stop, the rain, or roof water cascaded down into the guard's mail van and I was soaked. I knew Strict Grandmother would not be pleased, and she wasn't. Then the four of us, Grandmother, Female Parent, Brother and I, were on a second or third train from Waterloo, heading for Guildford. It was a nice house but had only three bedrooms so I had to share with Female Parent. Disaster.

In 1951, I went to Tormead Day School for Girls in Guildford for one year – I was eleven and this was already my 11th school. Female Parent and Grandmother were constantly fighting: I was the meat in the sandwich. Grandmother, aged about sixty, would lie on her bed and shout to me "Tell your mother…", which, of course I did. Then Female Parent, lying or sobbing in her bedroom, would respond "Tell your grandmother…" and so it would go. Downstairs it would be face to face. I was never sure which was worse. In this constantly fraught environment, it was too embarrassing and unpredictable to take school 'friends' home, so I didn't make friends.

Then Female Parent and Grandmother split up; Grandmother had had enough and bought a flat in Queensgate in London. Female Parent, Brother and I moved to a smaller house in Guildford, but it had only two bedrooms, so I still had to share with Female Parent. Her unpredictable moods made sleep difficult.

One day Female Parent went up to London, which was unusual, and I don't recall the reason. The three of us usually went up only once or twice a year without any real purpose for going that I can recall. That day Female Parent returned to say that, by an amazing coincidence, she had bumped into Father at Paddington Underground station. This was the second of his five days in London on his only business trip from New Zealand, where he still worked for Unilevers. Did we want to see him? Certainly I did! My world lit up, though Brother was less sure. Two years younger than me, with fewer memories of Father, he was placid and less disturbed than I was by Female Parent. The meeting was arranged for Father's fourth day. I was in pieces. Couldn't he come back? Couldn't we all live together again? He was married … well, couldn't she come too? Of course she couldn't.

An unknown adult took Brother and me up to London and made sure we met Father. The morning was spent at Madam Tussauds, the afternoon at London Zoo. I couldn't think beyond the day. We had tea in the Cumberland Hotel where Female Parent joined us. Agony. It was the beginning of the end of this amazing day, one I soon realised would never be repeated. I was even more distressed when I realised that Brother got to go to the Men's room with Father and I was consigned to the Ladies' room with Her. I was inconsolable on the train back to Guildford but knew I couldn't risk showing it.

Aunt, Father's sister, living in London, had wanted to find us from the time we returned to England. However, as Female Parent had decreed, from the time of the divorce, and through the lawyers, there was to be no contact, this had not been possible. This contact had now been made. Aunt had previously done everything she could think of, during the years since the divorce, to find us. Now, following our day with Father, she had contact details and she made tentative moves to reach out to us. She was to become a major part of the rest of my life and the single most important person in it, for over forty-five years, but at the start and for the next seven years until I left home, I remained closed off, both to her and Paternal Grandmother. Based on my experience to date, I never knew when they would turn disproving, or worse.

My overall memories of these early years are totally devoid of happy times. I was not shown any love or affection. There was never any warm touch or word of praise or indication of affection or approval.

Consequently, I became very much a loner, simply wanting peace and to be left alone. My constant thought was that if I did everything right and did nothing wrong, we might all have peace. I think I enjoyed studying. At any rate there are no bad memories around it. I assume I enjoyed sports and gymnastics. I certainly played a lot of it and captained many of the teams. In fact, I was generally school games captain.

Female Parent had no friends. That was apparently my fault – I was an impediment. The only adults I ever spoke with were the shop keepers and the teachers. Odd though it seems to me now, I knew nothing of other families, of married couples, of men, and how they behaved, of people earning an income, having a career, relationships. My life seemed to shuttle between traumatic home and introverted school studying. I knew my ongoing mantra was "You can trust books, not people". The more I write these memories down the stranger they seem. At the time, I just trudged on, grasping what brief pleasures I could from my studies and sports, a snatched half hour of stolen peace (nothing religious about it) in the local High Church, stolen from my shopping duties. I endured the rest, thoroughly introverted. Someone at some time said I resembled a hedgehog, forever rolled up into a protective ball.

I sat for the Eleven-plus exam. I don't think I knew what it was although I knew it was essential to pass, so I practised endlessly, desperate not to fail, afraid of the consequences if I did. By this time I was focused totally inward, and just relieved to get through each day without major turmoil, or worse. I aimed always to do what was expected, to avoid making waves, to avoid trouble. There were no good days. There were a few, a very rare few, that were not an emotional disaster.

It seems I had passed the exam and had won one of the two County Major Scholarships given by the Surrey Education Board, to a boarding school place. I don't recall any excitement about this. It simply happened, and I stolidly went along with events as they unfolded, just glad there was no furore or failure. The place I had won was at a school elsewhere, but it was decided that I could transfer this to Tormead, as it was already my eleventh school. I would board there, even though it was only a mile from home. That was all I really cared about. Because of my scholarship's criteria, Female Parent couldn't keep me as a day girl, although she tried. Perhaps they realised how unstable life was at home. Brother was also boarding, but somewhere else, of course. Boarding sounded like a wonderful reprieve from home, but then I learnt that *She* had insisted on me being a weekly border. That meant three nights a week at home.

I had by then apparently become even more silent and introverted. Anything I liked, wanted, or enjoyed, was forbidden, given away, or destroyed, so I learnt not to show any feelings. My daily promise to myself was "I won't let anything matter to me to-day", for then I knew I couldn't be hurt, or not so much. By now I knew I was a "horrid" child and could not expect to be liked, certainly not by Her family, made up of distant twin sisters, their husbands, and four cousins.

"Look what I've done for you, see what you've cost me." How I hated her refrain. She clearly didn't like me very much, but perhaps she felt she had reason. After the separation, and back in the second Eastbourne, it seems all I had done was cry and say "I want my Daddy". I remembered one or two fun times with him, even if not much affection, in New Zealand, but none from her, ever, then or later. I don't recall any words of warmth, or ever receiving a touch or indications of affection or approval. In addition, she blamed me for triggering her incarceration each time when I had had to tell some other adult, neighbour, or whoever, that "Mummy is going mad again". She complained, for a while, that if it wasn't for me she could have married again. Who would take her on? I assume the few people she did meet steered clear of her erratic behaviour. So we had no visitors at the house. I made few friends at school. It was too easy to get hurt if I showed I cared, and too embarrassing to invite them home.

Eventually I had had enough. I hated being beholden to her. One day, after a trip to the cinema when she complained at the cost of taking me, I said, "Alright, tell me how much you are willing to spend on me and I will manage on that." I was eleven.

She replied, "£30 a year. And that's for everything."

She made it very clear that she would provide food inside the house, bed and board; after that it was up to me – clothes, books, hobbies, fun, everything was to come out of my £30. With a very imperfect idea of how far that money would stretch, I agreed; I would have agreed to absolutely anything to have some autonomy. £30 for the year then was worth about £800 now, or £16 a week, for *everything*. I soon learnt, when she was ill again and I had to manage our finances, that it was only a very small percentage of our total family income of £600 a year, but I didn't care, it was worth it! I was determined to make it work, and I did, for the next six years. I never once asked for anything more. It was a small victory. In any case, I had few hobbies outside study, sport, and escape. I did join a local tennis club and spent as much time there as I could to get away for a few hours.

There was another advantage to this strict financial regime. I no longer had to go to the cinema when they (Female Parent and Brother) did. I hated their film choices, too much tension and suspense, too frightening. I had more than my fair share of that at home.

The responsibility of this regimen also gave me excellent lessons in budgeting and 'living within my means', lessons that have stood me in good stead throughout my life.

My first term as a school border was a relief. I shared with other girls of course in various small dormitories, but there was no "sturm und drang", no holding my breath hoping I wouldn't do something to trigger off an outburst. Peace and solitude. Within the school environment, where the staff didn't suddenly flare into an out-of-control manic phase, or dissolve into attention-demanding depression, I could easily isolate myself from the others and stay within myself. I enjoyed the studying. I had already learnt that I could not trust people, aka Female Parent, Father, Grandmother; they let you down. Books were a different matter – you could trust books, and I immersed myself in them. I also continued to immerse myself in sports, where I could let out some of my bottled-up frustration and miseries.

I was less good academically, coming about halfway up the class of twenty-eight, and in particular not much good at literature, art, or languages. I wasn't offered the chance to learn German, which I regret, but the time was needed for maths, which I enjoyed. I failed French, fluffing the oral test by replying "Très bien, merci", when asked "Comment vous appelez-vous?" I claimed nerves rather than ignorance, but my French didn't go much further on paper either. In comparison, numbers were easy. I didn't understand how people could get them wrong; they simply fell into place.

As the school was only a mile away, I cycled there each Monday morning. One of the worst times each week was cycling home on a Friday afternoon, as late as possible, and on tenterhooks as to the mood She would be in when I got there. Would She be sobbing and ranting, or super manic? How much of the week-end could I get through without exciting an outburst? For I still believed, wrongly of course, that if I could just do everything right, things would be manageable. It was probably against this background that at school I was always at pains to obey the rules and do whatever was expected of me, so long as I could just figure out what it was.

Head down and tail up, I do not recall being aware of what one might loosely call school politics, and so I was surprised when I was one of the first three girls in my class to be made a prefect. Perhaps because I was so quiet, yet so diligently trying to do the right thing and not cause trouble, as had become my habit at home, they felt I could be relied on.

Occasional trips to London usually involved brief meetings with Aunt and Paternal Grandmother, now that they had found us. We met for a stilted afternoon tea. Female Parent would be either over-gushing, or heavily complaining. I would be embarrassed or apprehensive. Aunt was to say years later that never once in those years did she see me smile. She thought she could save Brother, emotionally, but suspected that I was too damaged.

I used to soothe myself to sleep each night by escaping into a dream world. I would play out imaginary scenarios where Female Parent disappeared. I didn't wish her dead, just 'not there', so I was never sure, in the scenarios I created, why she had disappeared. In my self-created dream, Brother and I were alone. Kind people took us in, almost always with Aunt as a leading figure, even though I wasn't yet at all confident about her either. One of the girls at school was adopted. I asked what that meant, and learnt about 'orphans': no parents, no grandparents. I so envied her. I wasn't clear in my mind as to just what her home life was like, but I was sure it was preferable to mine. I wished I was an orphan, even though I had no clear idea as to what the alternative would be either, perhaps like boarding school.

Escape. How I dreamed of it. But I could think of no practical way out. Female Parent had control, of us if not of herself. I was essentially straightforward, and no match for her exaggerations and manipulative pretences; these frustrated and infuriated me. To me, facts were facts, truth was truth. I endured, and did my best to cope. Brother was more relaxed. He let it all run over him, like water off a duck's back. He was also two years younger than me and didn't play a leading role in coping with the turmoils. He couldn't be blamed for having her incarcerated, and, of course, always had his own bedroom to which he could retreat.

At school, my first favourite subject, aged five, had been arithmetic. A few years later it was maths. A year or two on I discovered 'science', which I thought wonderful, so logical and predictable. Science I could understand. A year or two later again, 'science' was subdivided into physics, chemistry, and biology. Chemistry, the subject that was to be the love of my life from then on, was an especial revelation. Since paternal Grandfather had been a doctor, and maternal grandfather an organic chemist, it could be said that my grandfathers, though I never knew neither of them, framed my career.

At Tormead school, science teaching was basic, but I was fortunate in that the headmistress was a mathematician, so I was soon one of a group of four that could study specialised pure and applied mathematics with her.

Female Parent continued to be focused on her unhappiness and needs and her periodic but unpredictable swings between mania and ranting depression. Her passes through normalcy were so brief they were barely noticed. I endured, and did my best to cope. As ever, I struggled not to show vulnerability or hurt, which could have been the basis for more trouble. Striving always to get everything right and avoid more emotional turmoil, I was full of guilt-laden self-reproaches when I had not managed something correctly. I seemed always to be tormented by the thought that 'If only I had done so and so, we might have had peace'. I grew ever more silent and withdrawn.

When not boarding, from the age of about twelve I essentially 'ran' the house, under Her shouted directions. The shopping, of course, fell to me. My route to the shops and back enabled me to pass through the grounds of Guildford's Holy Trinity Church, a beautiful and peaceful building which was very High Church in its liturgical practices. If I was lucky and timed it correctly, I could pass by during a time when the choir was singing and the incense swinging. I dived deeply into the beauty, or more importantly, the peace and calm of the music, at least for as long as I dared to stay.

From about the age of fifteen, I worked in the holidays to earn some much-needed money. Some of the later holidays I worked in chemical laboratories. Two summers were spent working at Distillers Ltd. One year the work was focused on developing yeasts. In the second, probably 1956 the focus was on growing micro-organisms with the aim of producing the newest vitamin, vitamin B12, the discovery of which led later to two Nobel prizes being awarded in 1964. This work involved me in silver soldering the containers in which the organisms were incubated, a skill in which I took great pride.

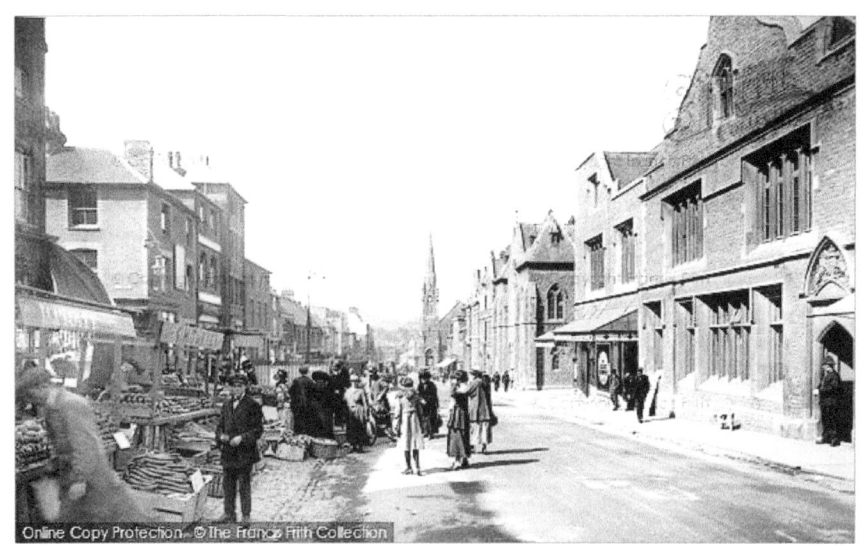

North Street where, at that time, the weekly market was held

Towards the end of 'O' Levels the subject of my future came up. *She* wanted me to leave school, get a job and support her. However, at a three-way discussion with the school authorities I learnt that my scholarship meant I was destined for 'A' levels and a degree course at university, so I was lucky. *She* was told I had to stay at school, still as a boarder, for two more years. I was so thankful! I could relax, knowing I had this further two-year reprieve from living at home with Her.

I settled in to two years of 'A' level study in chemistry and physics, both at the then Guildford Technical College, and pure and applied mathematics with the school's headmistress. I took pleasure in these subjects; they meant facts, reality, security, logic, and a complete absence of unstable, unreliable, and potentially harmful emotions.

School had required that during each holiday we should read four non-fiction books and write a short summary of them. The local library was free, and one of my oases of calm to which I could occasionally escape. One of the books I had picked, seemingly at random, though underscoring my future path, was a biography of Bernard Spilsbury, the noted forensic pathologist. I loved it, and the window onto the world that it showed me. From then on, I had hopes of becoming a forensic chemist, even though a future more than three years ahead seemed impossibly far away. I was, after all, used to living day by day, just trying to make it through, one at a time. I liked the idea of doing analytical chemistry, finding out 'the truth' of what had happened, and in a future scenario being able to pronounce confidently on it in a court of law. My world then was both very insular and very much black and white. 'Truth' was, I thought, an achievable goal. I liked the idea of being able to pronounce on the 'facts' in court, backed up by science and devoid of emotions.

Towards the end of 'A' levels, the subject of 'which University?' came up. I had no idea. School had no careers advisor. Female Parent declined to be involved. I only knew that I wanted to study chemistry. I applied, like some of the others in my technical college class, to University College, Kings College, and Queen Mary College, all in London, these being the only ones I knew about. Walking along a corridor at the Technical College one day, the head of the science department passed me and casually asked what I had applied for. I told him. "Oh yes, that's fine, you're focusing on chemistry, aren't you," and he was about to pass on. "Yes, is there anywhere else I should apply?" I asked. "Oh well, there's Imperial College, but you'd never get in there". That did it. On an instinct, I wrote off for the application to Imperial and sat all the appropriate exams. When their acceptances came through it was an easy decision: I chose Imperial. In my senior school years I had felt sorry, each summer, for the girls who were leaving. Boarding at school had been my haven and I could not imagine wanting anything outside it. But that summer my thoughts turned to Imperial and I could see a future ahead, although a mixed one.

One of my rare pleasures and escapes had been joining the Girl Guides (free). In addition to the weekly meetings, this involved going to camps at Whitsun weekends. I loved these, not so much for the individual people, but for the sense of group belonging. I also enjoyed all the rules and knowing exactly what I was expected to do; it provided a measure of security, just as I enjoyed school for its protective and stable cocoon. And I particularly enjoyed the camping.

In 1957 there was a Baden Powell Centenary International Girl Guides camp in Windsor Great Park. I was amazed to find that I had been selected to get one of the treasured places, and even more that I had been chosen as the lead and speaker of the three Guides who were, on behalf of the International Girl Guides Association, to present a camping set to the Queen, destined for Prince Charles and Princess Ann who were children at the time. I have no idea how this came about.

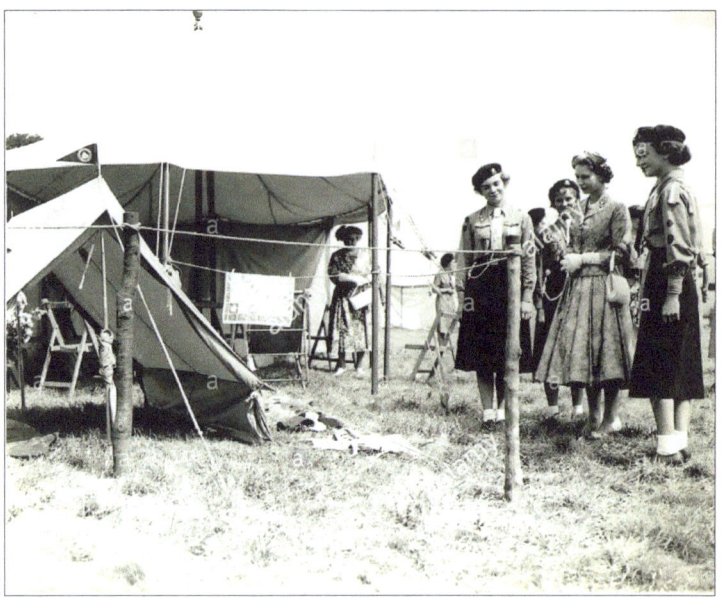

I am on the Queen's right-hand side.

Aunt and Paternal Grandmother came as my support group, so that although Female Parent was there, I could avoid having much to do with her and didn't need to fear having to cope with her if she became outrageous, or decided to lambast me.

As I had worked during all my school holidays, I had accumulated a small, and, I had thought, well hidden savings nest. Even paying

Female Parent for my board, as she required for the final two years at school, I had managed to save something. This went into a Post Office savings account which She had arranged and which I had signed. What I didn't realise was that she had also put herself on it as a signatory. I understood none of such legal matters. When I was ready to go up to Imperial, I was shocked to find it alarmingly empty. Perhaps she thought it would mean I had to remain living with her and not go to university. But I was not to be deterred.

It was supposed I would continue to live in Guildford and commute to South Kensington for the five days a week required for my studies. It's fortunate that I didn't, I doubt I would have got much studying done. Fortunately, Maternal Grandmother intervened and I found myself occupying the spare room in her flat in Hyde Park Gate, two doors up from Winston Churchill and the friendly policemen who guarded that house day and night. It was also a few hundred yards from Imperial and convenient for lectures. It was a somewhat uncomfortable atmosphere in the evenings but a lot better than home had been.

I had made it. I had managed to endure my childhood, to survive without any life-affirming warmth, approval, or affection. Were there any good points? Yes indeed: winning a scholarship at eleven that led to boarding school and an escape from home; the connection that enabled the link to be made with Aunt; learning to budget my money; discovering chemistry and the pleasures of study; a headmistress dedicated to mathematics; lots of sports; the trigger that made me apply for Imperial; learning not to expect anyone to do anything for me and thus being self-sufficient from an early age. It was all much easier than risking making friends or being vulnerable. These traits have served me in good stead ever since. Expect nothing from people. It was easier to immerse myself in books, I liked it and did it assiduously whenever I could steal the time.

I assume my social skills were zero by this point. Certainly, my awareness of the outer world, how 'normal' families lived, behaved, and interacted, how male adults behaved, was non-existent. In fact, as

I write this, I realise I have no idea what a family house or home feels like from within, or how it functions. It seems to me I lived in a permanent war zone of potential and unpredictable hazards.

Chapter 2

Imperial College and First Degree

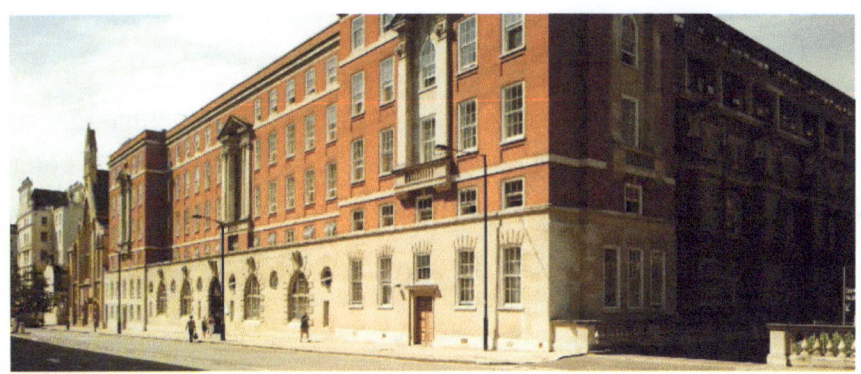

With my lack of awareness of how the 'normal' world functioned and my zero social skills and limited communication about anything other than my studies, I must have been one of the most naive and unworldly freshers ever to get to university. Looking back to the younger me as I wandered around the campus when I started at Imperial, I realise I had very little idea of what was going on.

I stood in the Freshman crowd at Imperial College, then called IC, and subsequently simply 'Imperial', the September of 1958, listening to the Rector's opening speech to us students who made up the new intake for that year, as he explained our future and his hopes for us. We were told that only two per cent of people got university places. Not only that but we were at one of the top three universities in the country. How had I managed that? I had no confidence in my abilities, having received very little praise or encouragement and only doing what I thought of as averagely well at school.

I had a financial scholarship on which I could live – just. Forty pounds a term. It seems the financial scholarship was easier to get than the place at IC and so the former was never in much doubt. All I had to do now was manage to stay there for the next three years. I just hoped I could survive the exams and avoid being thrown out for failing – which happened to twenty-five percent of the class each year, as we were told by the Rector. I found this thought terrifying as I had no confidence in my ability to achieve all the required goals. All I wanted was to stay there for ever.

In this strange new world, then, on Freshers Day, not fully understanding the purpose of it, I followed my inclinations and somehow managed to join hockey, squash, and tennis clubs. I bought the books I was told I needed for my course, figured out the timetable, and got started.

I gradually relaxed into the life I was going to love. I thrived in the impersonal, academic, and seemingly organised atmosphere. It was probably fortunate that I did not chase after a social life, which I considered to be dangerous excursions into treacherous waters. Instead, I spent a lot of the evenings studying. Certainly, I talked to very few people.

At that time, in 1958, IC consisted solely of three colleges, all situated between Exhibition Road and Queensgate, and from Beit Hall, our Student Union Building in the north, south to the Science Museum. Walking south from Beit Hall we passed the building of the Royal School of Mines, which held less than a thousand students, very few of who were female; Then there was the City and Guild Engineering building. This housed 1500 students of which only one was a woman; and, finally, the Royal College of Science with about 1,000 students of whom less than ninety were female, and of which I was one. Altogether 3,000 students of whom something approaching a hundred were women, or so I was led to believe at the time. My own year, studying chemistry, consisted of sixty students, six of us women,

In spite of my girls' boarding school experience and restricted upbringing, I managed, as far as I can recall, to mix into a liberal and overwhelmingly male environment with little trouble, probably because I didn't consider them to be a different sex, merely different people. They were just other humans to be negotiated. Or possibly it was because everywhere I looked, almost everyone was male, and I forgot I was different. This was to be good training for the ten years, post-graduation, that lay ahead, when I was to work in the totally male-oriented geological and mining world.

Cautiously I enjoyed the first half of the first term. The lectures each morning, from ten to one were interesting. The laboratory work each afternoon, from two to five, was like being in a special and almost sanctified place where I had peace and could focus totally on the care needed for the experiment I had been given.

Most evenings I studied, determined as I was to pass the exams and keep my place. But when conservative social possibilities were offered, I generally accepted them. I was rarely short of a boyfriend when one was needed, though I was not in the least interested in anything serious. I never thought of it, and had absolutely no intention of marrying. I considered marriage, if I thought of it at all, to be a terrifying situation to be avoided at all costs. After the previous eighteen years I had a horror of anyone having control of me, or even a say in my life. Even the possibility of it did not appear in my mental horizon, though this was, admittedly limited. In those days, at eighteen, marriage seemed like something belonging to a far distant future. I seemed to live day by day, as I had done for the previous eighteen years, just hoping to get by. Even so, gradually I found pockets of time that I did enjoy – but not too much, just in case it was taken away from me.

There was one social excitement, and it took me totally unawares. Each of the three colleges had a 'mascot', a vehicle from the past. The miners had a coal-fired steam roller, the engineers a 1920s (or there-abouts) car named, I think, Clementine, and we at RCS had Jezebel, an early twentieth century fire engine. One of the first student meetings of the first term included the election of the Queen of Jezebel. As usual I sat solemnly silent in the lecture theatre chosen for the student meeting.

I was simply going with the crowd, waiting to see what was going to happen and feeling sure it had nothing to do with me. An election proceeded, and I was suddenly declared to be Queen of Jezebel, and being crowned with an ornate, if cardboard, crown. It was all a bit of a laugh, but it did lead to many unusual episodes during that year, as I performed the various duties expected of me. This included polishing Jezebel!

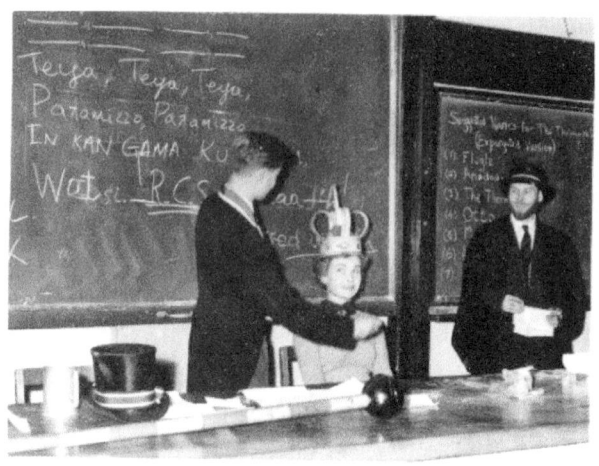

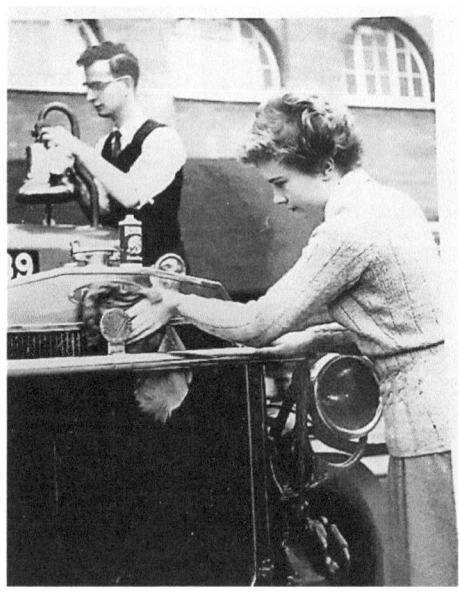

I soon managed to get a room in Queen Alexandra House, next to both the Albert Hall and Imperial's Union building, and moved out of Grandmother's flat. Great improvement. I moved part way through the first term. Here at last was a home of my own and freedom. Alexandra House, as I understood it at the time, had been funded by a man whose aim had been to provide a place for female students in the group of buildings bounded by Exhibition Road to the east, and Queensgate to the west. It included the three colleges of Imperial, including the Royal College of Science in which I was enrolled, plus the Royal College of Art and the Royal School of Music. The idea, apparently, was that this would integrate the three groups of women and their skills. In this it failed totally. At the time, QAH was in fact filled with music students, plus one student from the Arts College. The remaining room was empty, kept for a science student so they could fulfil their charter. When I applied, I was a shoe-in and just what they needed to satisfy this unfulfilled requirement for a science student.

Time schedules and visitors time at Queen Alexander House were much more restricted than in Beit Hall at IC, and the wise IC women students, looking for greater freedoms, shunned it. But it suited me perfectly. What more did I need? Quiet, safety in the form of reliable tranquillity, peace, time to study, and limited social pressure.

However, a few weeks into the term family problems reared their head and seriously interrupted my studies. I was no longer at school. I wasn't a child. This time I was an adult. This time I was supposed to cope, fully. 'She', in the form of Parent, yet again, was in a mental hospital. I had to cope. Somehow I managed it, though it did have a disastrous effect on my first-term study record. For two or three afternoons a week I would go down to Aunt in Sloane Gardens. Aunt – boy, was I glad I had discovered her – or her me! I was to be forever grateful for the connection that had been made by the chance meeting of Parents on the Underground a few years earlier. I had liked Aunt from our first meeting. For some reason I almost trusted her, and I didn't give trust easily, if at all, but we were just beginning to become friends. She would drive me down to the hospital where I would spend an hour or two 'coping'. This involved collecting up the disastrous letters that Parent, in her usual manic mode, had been writing: hiring theatres, buying houses, hiring lawyers, publicists, and more. Each afternoon I destroyed the letters, tore up the cheques, cancelled the arrangements, and talked with the nurses. Then it was back to Sloane Square and dinner with Aunt, Uncle (by marriage), and Paternal Grandmother (a delight, and great fun, as only a sanguine temperament can be).

I was getting to know Aunt. Aunt was getting to know an eighteen-year-old niece who, apparently, looked and sounded like the brother she adored. In retrospect, many decades later, I figured out that she, with no child of her own, was probably as wary of losing me as I was of doing the wrong thing and losing her. She was to tell me later that she and paternal grandmother figured they had me for the three years of my degree, after which I would almost certainly move on with my life. I would probably marry, and go where that took me. Aunt had wanted children desperately, but after several miscarriages had been forced to give up and stop trying. I was to become the daughter she had never had. I gradually got to know her, to trust her just a tiny bit. We said afterwards that it was a good time for us to have met – we had no daughter-parent issues to resolve. We could meet as friends, and grow together ever better, as really good friends, albeit I was the wounded one, and she was enormously caring and generous. Gradually, over the three years, it dawned on me that here were two people, Aunt and Grandmother, who seemed to quite like me. It was a novel experience. It was also one I was wary of trusting and I kept waiting for something to go wrong.

At some point, possibly in my second term, after being invited down to her flat for dinner once or twice a week, it had somehow been six weeks since I had seen or heard from her. I forget why. I do recall thinking "well that's all right, I can cope, I can manage without her. I did before, I can do it again". I was fiercely determined not to let anything matter to me sufficiently, such that I could get hurt. I would not let myself feel. Then suddenly out of the blue she phoned, dinner was on again, would I like to call in. Perhaps she too was uncertain, not wanting to crowd me. Gradually the relationship grew, and I soaked it up, but always warily.

As new students we had been told, though only after our arrival, that we were the elite, since we were at IC, and as such we were expected to do the London University degree in two years instead of the more usual three. Terrifying. We were also told by the lecturer on thermodynamics that "because your degree is done in two years, your first term exams are especially important, almost like the usual end of first year exams. You are expected to do well". I thought of the 25% failure rate the Rector had predicted, and my lost afternoons coping with Parent, and I quailed. He went on to say "When your first term results are posted, look at the results of the whole class. Those in the bottom ten per cent of the list will remain in the bottom, and probably fail. The top ten percent will remain at the top and probably get Firsts or IIAs. Then take the middle 80% of the list, turn it upside down, and put it back. That will be your end result. Even though I have told you this, it will still be the outcome."

At the end of the first term I was clearly in the bottom 10%, though at the top of it, and I quaked. I had worked my heart out, despite distractions with Parent and the lack of early studying opportunities while living with maternal grandmother. I had stayed back in the college library most evenings, whenever I could, but clearly the turmoil with Parent had taken its toll. Perhaps it was this that spurred me on to studying even harder for the next three years, although I did manage some social life. However, I need not have worried. The lecturer's words were prophetic, and I was to be propelled to the top of the middle 80%, and get a IIA degree three years later.

One of my 'escapes' as a child had been to read detective novels that I garnered from the local library while out shopping. I also read biographies – they were required to be on the reading list I presented at the end of each term while I was still at school. Even now I was still under the spell of Bernard Spilsbury whose autobiography I had picked up on one such library foray. This forensic chemist continued to inspire me while at IC, and a career as a forensic chemistry became my goal. I could imagine myself working quietly and steadily in an analytical laboratory. This was further helped by my love of the quiet and focused time we spent in the laboratory in the afternoons.

At the end of the first year we would drop Maths and Physics, somewhat to my relief, so the second year was devoted entirely to chemistry. At the start of my third year it would be time for me to choose a specialty within chemistry. I had already given a lot of thought as to whether I chose organic chemistry or analytical chemistry. It was probably going to be a 49:51% split between the two. In thinking this through, I wasn't thinking ahead or making long-term plans; a year still seemed a very long time.

In fact, I don't think I have ever made long-term plans. Somehow, interesting, appealing, and appropriate opportunities have frequently come my way and dictated my path through life, especially through my career. I loved organic chemistry and had I chosen that, my ancillary subject would have been biochemistry. I might then indeed have gone on to become a forensic chemist, probably stayed in England and followed a somewhat predictable path. Instead, I chose the one with the most immediate appeal, and analytical chemistry won. The ancillary for this was geology, and as a result I became a geochemist, subsequently travelling the world – a total of twenty-seven times, in fact, between the UK and the Antipodes. But that was in the future, and at this point a forensic career was still in my mind.

I had joined the college's chemical society, which I think was optional, and my forensic career aspiration was known to the organiser. When a forensic chemist came to give a talk to the society one evening, I was invited to join the core group and the lecturer at the top table in

Hall for dinner. He regaled us with professional anecdotes throughout the meal, and I lapped them up … until he was in full flow about someone who had had all five fingers chopped off. He was telling us how he had had them laid out on a dish on his work bench in the laboratory, ready for examination. Just at that moment the waitress presented each of us with a plate of five anchovies, lying parallel, on a single piece of toast. I'm not sure any of us enjoyed that dish.

I loved my three years at Imperial. Like 'Oxbridge' we had our own boat race, the three colleges competing on the Thames. In my first year, while still Queen of Jezebel, I was on the embankment with a crowd of RCS science students, all unsuspecting. Across a culvert was a crowd of City & Guilds engineering students. Suddenly, there was a cry of "Queen of Jezebel, go get her!" and I was grabbed and dragged across to their side of the culvert. Next thing I knew, a couple of flat topped (inspectors?) police were in front of me. "Are you in trouble, miss, can we help you?" I was appalled, I was having far too much fun. "No, no thank you, I'm fine". They melted away and the triumphant engineers loaded me onto Clementine, their antique open-topped car, and with much hilarity drove back to Imperial. A victory photo and then party at the City & Guilds building followed. Great fun.

There was an amazing perk to be appreciated as a result of living surrounded by music students. Queen Alexandra House was given a block of free seats in the Albert Hall on the slopes (M as I recall) just to the left of the cellos, for *every* evening performance. A treat. I wasn't, of course, well versed in classical music, but I came to enjoy it, especially the peace of it. The evening meal followed student hours and was at seven o'clock. This gave us plenty of time to eat and then go across to the Albert Hall by eight. Concerned about my studies, I became selective and would generally choose to go in for the first or the second half of the program. I got used to hearing the discussion of those sitting next to me. "Did you hear the falter on that demisemiquaver?" What did you think of the modulation at the start of the crescendo…?" It dawned on me that I was possibly the only person totally enjoying the music for its own sake, the other students all being there to study.

I was fortunate in having my financial scholarship of forty pounds a term on which to live. It could have been possible, but I was even more lucky as Aunt doubled that. With my inbuilt determination to live within my means and be reliant on no one (somehow Aunt didn't count) honed to a fine skill during my school years by my financial restriction to £30 a year for everything beyond my bed and board, I managed. I considered this to be 'plenty', even though I now also had to pay for rent and food. During the school years, I had learnt to spend as little as possible, and to want little. I didn't see why I needed more than two or three changes of clothes and I had learnt to sew most of them, although this was a habit I dropped soon after leaving school. I had learnt to make most of my own outfits by mixing and matching, and dying things that became faded. I don't recall thinking much about money, it didn't seem important. I didn't like waste as I had learnt to be careful, and it was second nature to me to spend as little as possible. Money, somehow, was irrelevant.

In those years, there was a row of shops along the south side of, and presumably over, the tracks at South Kensington Underground station. The Rice Bowl was a favourite restaurant, and just affordable for us students. Their vegetable chop suey was a vast pile of rice and vegetables costing two shillings and ninepence, and was too big a meal for most people to finish. I had no trouble. My grant stretched to about three shillings and sixpence a day for food. This scored a couple of sardine sandwiches at twopence ha'penny each from the Union snack bar for lunch, and a threepenny bar of chocolate that stood in for either breakfast or an afternoon snack, depending on the time I got up each morning. I cooked most of my evening meals myself. An occasional splurge was at the Rice Bowl. We all did much the same and loved the style of Chinese that we could afford – in fact it was the only style we knew, although slightly wealthier students would have beef or chicken chop suey for the vast sum of three shillings and sixpence.

I joined the squash club, a new sport to me, and was soon playing in the IC team and won my purple colours (Oxbridge had blues so we had purples). This was not such an amazing achievement as there were so few women at IC to choose from. I did the same with tennis.

I also joined the editorial group focused round *Felix*, the IC magazine, but mostly as a gopher and for the fun of it rather than as a writer or a political thinker.

I had managed, by the start of the third term and with Aunt's top-up, to have sufficient money saved to buy a somewhat elderly and second-hand Lambretta scooter. It didn't let me down, although it did have a habit of stalling. This made making right-hand turns a time of apprehension. For many weeks, at the start I travelled round London making only left-hand turns and so proceeding in a series of anticlockwise loops.

Then it was exam time. At the end of the first year, the half-way mark of our basic degree, the pressure was heavy. Current boyfriend was in his final year, heading for a physics degree. We studied together. After we had each eaten, in our separate abodes, his in Beit Hall, we would come together in my room in Queen Alexandra House and spend the evening studying, with occasional coffee breaks. At ten, when visitors had to leave – one of the restrictions that kept ICWA women from wanting to live there, but not one that had bothered me – he would leave, and I would settle down to a further two hours of revision. I needed no whip to persuade me. I was going to do everything I could not to fail and have to leave Imperial. Though I don't recall that I thought much about 'what would happen if…', I guess at some level there was some inner confidence, however small.

Then came the summer holidays. For the first two weeks I collapsed in a blur of exhaustion, finding only sufficient energy to drag myself to the dining room for lunch and dinner, having slept through breakfast, to watch Wimbledon until dusk stopped play, then back to bed. Two weeks later I was ready for some fun.

Six of us, three couples, had arranged to holiday together, first for a week's sailing round the Norfolk Broads, then for a week on canal boats. Three couples on three boats. Sexual freedom had barely arrived. One couple slept on one boat, and we thought them very daring. For the rest of us it was the two men to one boat and two women to the third, but we sailed one couple to each boat during the day. We might have raced, but after the high tension of first-year exams, I think we were mostly content to drift.

I was to get myself to the Broads on my newly acquired Lambretta. To achieve this, I had to master the right-hand turns without the machine stalling. Having done no more than a few miles round my part of London, getting to the Broads on my own – the others going there directly – was daunting. However, I managed it, there and back, and felt suitably proud.

For the rest of the summer, I worked. IC was very good at organising appropriate summer jobs for the students, and I had one in an analytical laboratory on the edge of London, first analysing phosphate levels in brewing yeasts, then learning to do silver soldering. Vitamin B 12 had not long been discovered, and the goal was to feed microorganisms with a suitably nourishing broth to persuade them to produce large amounts of the vitamin. To this end, each day a number of large glass autoclave jars were filled with a variety of different brews, about which, in my low status as undergraduate student, I knew little. The top was clamped on, various pipes attached, the whole thing secured with silver solder and then autoclaved. It was a proud day when I was told I could do the silver soldering on my own – and warned that it would be a disaster if one of the solders failed and that part of the experiment was ruined. Nearly sixty years later, as I write, that sounds strange, but it is the best I can recall. I know I enjoyed the work.

Second year. The boyfriend of the summer had graduated and gone to work in Holland for Phillips. We second-year chemistry students were now, as promised, spared the weekly hour or two of maths and physics, the ancillary subjects of our first year, and I could focus almost entirely on chemistry. Wonderful.

However, there was one minor academic challenge. To complete our degree, we had to translate chemical papers from two languages out of three, Russian, French, and German, into English. This being the time before individual computers and easy translations, some linguistic skills in the major languages of science, as they were then deemed to be, was thought to be essential. I don't recall anyone trying to struggle with Russian, so that left us with French and German. The exam lasted for two hours and could be sat every six months, autumn and spring, until passed. Both papers were given out at the start, one paper had to be handed in at the end of one hour, and the second at the end of the second hour. You could use a dictionary but obviously this took time and you risked failing to finish.

I had studied French at school and even though I had failed, I had not done too badly. I had not done any German at all. Fortunately, German is a relatively scientific language in the sense that many of the chemical words are similar to the English equivalents. Wasserstoff, the stuff of water, being hydrogen, for example. And the symbols of the elements, relating to their Latin name, natrium, Na for sodium, Kalium, K, for potassium. 'Was is das?', sounds sufficiently like 'what is that'. So we had a clear strategy, based on the fact that both papers were handed out at the start. For the first ten minutes I dutifully scribbled my rough attempt at translating the French paper, handed it in at the end of the hour, expecting, and in fact planning to fail. I then spent an hour and fifty minutes, with the fevered help of my dictionary of scientific German, working on the German paper, which I fortunately passed. Six months later, sitting to translate the French paper in one hour did not seem too difficult.

I was one of the lucky ones – why was I always so lucky? I just took it in my stride at the time, but on reflection I do wonder at my good luck, a vast change from my first eighteen years. The room in Queen Alexandra House had been wonderful, so close to the IC Union that I could take part in all sorts of student activities, including a number of sports teams, without taking too much time out of my studies. Now, at the start of my second year, I was to be given one of the eighteen or so rooms available for women, actually in Imperial's Beit Hall. How I loved it. I spent many nights beforehand dreaming of how I would arrange the furniture in my own room, and impatient to get started. Here there were no time limits, no restrictions on visitors. There was the very real feeling of being fully a part of the 'authentic IC community. I loved the room, the furniture, and the ease of it. A shared kitchen and bathroom continued to feel 'normal' and a great improvement on the communal life at boarding school.

I continued to play squash, tennis, and hockey for the college, even adding hockey to my 'colours'. Some time that autumn a group of IC women were put together to go to Delft and compete with women at the University there. Funds were, presumably, limited, and the maximum number of students allowed in the team, was thirteen, including the captain (but not the coach). I was going to be busy. Being on the teams for hockey, rounders, tennis, squash, table tennis, gymnastics (floor work, climbing ropes, and vaulting), swimming (breast stroke, back and crawl – no butterfly in those days – and relay), athletics (100 yards, 220 yards and relay – no metric in those days, strictly British Imperial measurements), I was busy, to say the least.

One of the amazing additions to my list was badminton. I had never ever played this sport, but it seemed that all but one of the colleges badminton players had no second skills so could not be included in our team of thirteen. I was given some rapid teaching of the rules and aims and, supported and instructed by our one qualified badminton player, went for it. I barely knew what I was doing but I was determined not to let the shuttle cock land on our side of the net and flew at everything in sight, whacking it full force in the direction of the opponents. My partner must have been good because we won our match, a fact which I was assured of afterwards by her explanation of the scoring system.

I forget how we got to Delft, there being no Channel Tunnel at that time, and flying being a relatively rare and expensive luxury. I imagine it was by train, ferry, and then another train. We were meet at Delft station by our opponents, on bicycles. I was horrified when I was told to sit on the back carrier of her bike, and no, not facing forward and sitting astride her back carrier, but sitting sideways facing the pavement. I then had to balance my (luckily small) suitcase on my lap and put on top of that the tools of my trade, hockey stick, squash, badminton and tennis rackets. All that was bad enough. But we then set off, over bumpy and irregular cobbles and within inches of the edge of the canal, with little or nothing to stop a possible ducking. I was glad to arrive, dry and in one piece. It was a thrilling week. I was, of course, still largely introverted and serious, but there were enjoyable evenings sitting with hands round the colourful bowls they used in which to serve the endless coffees. One organised trip took us to Rotterdam for an afternoon. It was yet another piece of luck that I somehow took in my stride, unsurprised at whatever came my way. I was not an outward thinker.

Students at IC were mainly men: I was a woman. Students often whooped it up all year and then 'swotted like mad' for the weeks prior to the exams. I studied hard all year long. Students usually had a lively social life. I had one or two close friends whose company I enjoyed, but generally kept at arm's length from fear of being vulnerable. I generally had a not-very-serious boyfriend, but was not particularly involved emotionally. Students mostly drank alcohol and often got drunk. I didn't drink alcohol.

By the March of my second year I was going out with an exceedingly popular and gregarious chap who was president of the wine tasting society. I had never had so much as a drop of alcohol, electing to drink orange juice on such occasions. There had, of course, been no alcohol in the houses in which I had grown up. Faced with the wine tasting society's annual dinner, and partnered by one of the most popular guys, who was also a wine connoisseur and head of the society, my friends insisted that I simply had to drink wine, and that, no, I absolutely could not ask for orange juice. I knew nothing about the effect of alcohol, certainly not in any detail. I am not even aware of seeing students under the influence. I was strictly a head down tail up introvert and hadn't given it much thought. This, however, was clearly my time to start drinking.

'Hall' in IC was a large, long, slim room, along the north side of the quadrangle. The dinner invitees filled a U shape of tables at the far end of the room, away from the door. The evening started in the Common Room with three types of sherry, and a discussion to which I listened with interest but little understanding. We then moved into Hall and throughout the long, but highly enjoyable evening, were served soup, entre, a fish dish, a meat dish, a dessert, a savoury, and cheese, with, of course, a different wine at each course. I imagine the meal was excellent, but I soon began to suspect that the many different courses were there largely to give us a reason to try a different wine. Fortunately, the servings were appropriately small, but I had a good appetite. The glasses were also small, with plenty of room in which the bouquet could collect and then be appreciated. I drank them all, seeing no reason not to. As far as I could tell I was feeling no effect. There were more talks, which I found interesting, and then we rose to go back to the Common Room for coffee, port, brandy, or liqueurs. As I stood up I recalled that if you were drunk you could not walk in a straight line, this being the test the police used then to determine whether or not a driver was driving under the influence. As luck would have it, the floor consisted of long, lengthwise wooden planks, so I aimed to walk to the door along a single plank line. This accomplished with no apparent difficulty, I decided I could not be drunk and settled down for coffee and port. It was a wonderful evening, not like anything I had ever previously experienced – good company, a proud place at the head table with an interesting partner, although the relationship was not to last long despite my accomplishment of the evening, which he recognised.

A few days after this dinner, my partner of the night, introduced me to his friend, DZ, and the latter and I became great friends. Some weeks into our relationship he invited me to the May Ball. Balls were an important part of our calendar and there seem to have been a number of them each year, but this one was special. Aunt, inevitably and wonderfully, was determined to make the most of them for me, and, a week ahead of each one she would insist that I lunched with them in her flat in Sloane Square and follow this with a shopping spell in Peter Jones. This was to buy the dress, the shoes, the gloves, and the matching stole, all obligatory. Aunt was a trained beautician, I think as much for a hobby as anything, though she did help some private clients. So, towards evening prior to the ball, she would invite me down to their flat, ensure that my makeup was perfect, and that the colours matched the dress – also obligatory, as far as I can recall, in those days. The male partner of the day, and I can bring to mind at least five in those years, would turn up bringing the (again obligatory) orchid to be pinned to the dress, and plied with drinks, after which the two of us would be dispatched into a taxi and sent to the ball.

The exception was this May Ball, since DZ had his own car, one of the very first batch of the iconic Mini cars to roll off the rack. Down at Virginia Waters, where Imperial had its biological station, much used in the summer term, we danced the night away, or almost. Shortly before the end I found I was being proposed to by this lovely man, and, too surprised to say anything else, I simply said yes. I don't think I had any real thoughts of what that involved, or what it could mean. It just seemed like the correct answer to give. I liked him enormously. Did I love him? I assumed so. And of course, I was heartened and soothingly nurtured that he thought that much of me. After my first eighteen years it was almost enough just to be liked. Back at Imperial that night we

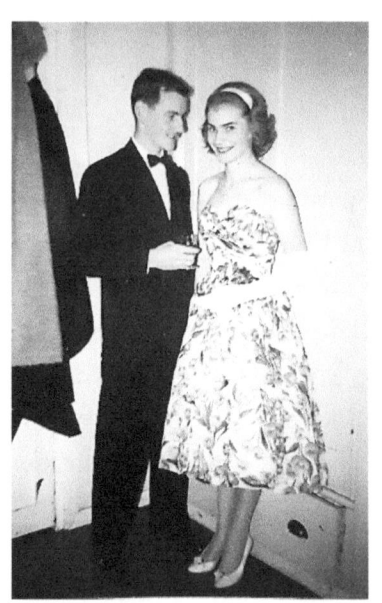

went to our respective rooms in Beit Hall, me on the third (and only female) floor, and he on the fourth (one of three male floors). This was only 1960 and virginity was still important, certainly to my mind.

This was the third term of my second year and the final year of our basic Bachelor's degree. Final exams loomed and suddenly there was the fear of this critical hurdle. I was as always convinced, at least outwardly, that I would fail or do badly, I never wanted to raise my expectations and never assumed I would pass, or do well enough, and always studied until my brain was too dazed for more. Aunt was wonderful. Towards the end of the term, I would revise during most of the day in my own room, then go down to her flat for dinner, which they had around eight, and chat with her and paternal grandmother. Aunt's husband was such a quiet introvert that I barely recall his presence, and certainly do not remember talking with him. He occupied his time building model aeroplanes and designing the radio control, for which he was much respected. They retired at around ten and I was left free to study in their sitting room until I dropped, and then go to sleep on the sofa. In this way I put in long hours of study. I would start after dinner, telling myself I only needed to revise for one hour. That didn't seem too daunting, but of course, and as subconsciously planned, one hour became just one more, then another, until I normally stayed at it until around four in the morning. In their small flat this must have been an enormous inconvenience to them, but they insisted, and I was grateful. I was unused to any form of caring or support and this I found precious beyond measure. I would surface around ten the next morning, have breakfast with Aunt and Grandmother, then scooter back to IC and study some more. Revision for hours at length was always boring, but at least this routine broke it up and made it possible.

In this way I got to the end of my second year.

DZ was an Australian geologist. He had come over to the UK at the Royal School of Mines to do his PhD, and was at the end of the second year of this. He had, or so we thought, a third year to go. As such we would both finish our three years at IC at the same time. In a year's time, I suppose it was assumed that he and I would go to Australia, presumably married, and set up life there. At the time Canberra was on a path of new, rapid, and enforced growth. The population was growing faster than the housing, and it was suggested to me that we should buy and live in a caravan, albeit a large one with two bedrooms. The idea appealed to me, but a year was a very long time in those days and at that age, and I really could not see even as far as, never mind beyond, this third and final year that was coming up. In the meantime, there was the summer vacation to look ahead to.

This year the summer break was no solo trip on my easy-stalling Lambretta. It was four of us carefully shoe-horned into our beloved Mini. DZ was very firm. We were allowed a small – very small – suitcase each. A sleeping bag each, plus two tiny ridge tents, that covered our sleeping needs. This was all stowed in the tiny boot or on the roof-rack. A beauty box, (a prerequisite in those days) was permitted for each of us women and these were stowed under the legs of the front passenger. Fortunately, this tiny vehicle had remarkably capacious pockets beside all four seats. The back pockets took our primus stove and cooking materials in one, and food in the other. Camera equipment, much bulkier then than now, went inside the passenger door pocket, and maps and other paperwork went beside the driver. We set off in high spirits and were soon thankful that we had not been allowed more luggage. It was not uncomfortable, but it was certainly tight.

DZ had worked the trip out, almost to the hour. Two weeks were planned; the stops were planned; the camping grounds were planned. We were not rushed, but there was no loitering. We had a fixed schedule, to reach Copenhagen two weeks later. I was grateful for his input and happy to leave it all to him. As he was the owner of the car, the other couple accepted his right to do this.

We drove down to the south coast and the four of us and our laden Mini flew over the Channel to Le Touquet. The next stop was Paris, camping in Fontainebleau, then threading our way down through France to Nice and Marseille. Somehow in those days we could afford to eat one meal a day in a restaurant, even on our student funds. I recall a wonderful evening going through the French Alps, with the river flowing on our right and parallel to the road. We pulled off and set up our tents in the area marked 'camping' cut on a piece of driftwood attached to a tree. It was on a narrow wedge of gravel between the river and the road. The owner of the house and restaurant on the upper side of the road came down and took our dinner order, for there was no village nearby to go to for food. Once ready, we climbed back up, crossed the road and into the farmhouse. We were offered one massive bowl full of gleaming whitebait, then melt-in-the mouth Vienna schnitzel and homegrown tossed salad, followed by fresh homegrown fruit and cheese and biscuits. A meal, and a view, fit for royalty.

Along the coast we headed east into Italy for Genoa and Milan where I had been looking forward to Italian pasta. Perhaps we should have been prepared. As an appalling inexperienced cook, one of my standard meals was based on spaghetti bolognaise. I made this by boiling up a plateful of simple pasta. The sauce consisted of a generous serving of minced meat which I fried, and a packet of dehydrated mixed vegetable soup. I made this up into a thick paste by adding only one cup of water, then mixing in the meat. I served the lot on a relatively small pile of spaghetti and covering it with grated cheese, Cheddar of course. Cooking facilities were limited, and shared, at college. But we enjoyed it. It was certainly better than the version I had been served as a kid by the Parent. This latter usually consisted simply of a plate of boiled white pasta, a large amount of Echo margarine (the cheapest one could buy) and a small amount of grated cheese. I was no sort of a cook. I had had, of course, to cook endless other meals at home, as a child, but they were simple, and often directed simply by shouted commands from Parent in her bedroom. I had made no effort to actually learn. All I cared about then was getting through each activity in such a way as to avoid a ruction, and in no way was cooking about to become a hobby or interest. So, pasta in Italy was one of our aims. Beautifully cooked pasta with a variety of delicate sauces.

This was high summer. It was hot. It was Italy, and we were surrounded by Italians. I, knowing no better, was wearing shorts. After several pinches on the bum, I grabbed the tablecloth and wrapped it round me.

We then turned north, through Switzerland, where we met up with Aunt and Uncle in Zurich for half a day. Uncle took his hobby, the building, designing, making, and flying of his model aeroplanes very seriously, and this was a major event. I think we went through Austria after that, but maybe not. We did drive through the beautiful Hartz mountains, and on to Frankfurt.

I loved Chinese Food, as cooked at our Rice Bowl restaurant in South Kensington, and so did DZ. By the time we reached Frankfurt we were more than ready for just such a Chinese meal. We had been advised that this was the point on our trip where we had the best chance of getting a good Chinese meal. I had imagined it would be like the meals I was used to in our Rice Bowl restaurant. Inside, sitting down and perusing the menu, we were in for a shock. The place was elegant; that should have warned us as prices were ridiculous and the portions small, nothing like our beloved Rice Bowl. But the food was delicious. It was a very new experience,

I loved Luxemburg. In fact, I loved everywhere we went, visiting wonderful scenery and quaint villages rather than big cities and works of art. DZ had an amazing camera for those days, a reflex Asahi Pentax, on which he took countless slides. He had done that through all his years in the Australian bush, and they became my introduction to his country.

Some days later as we drove further north, we were all hungry. With the necessity of changing currencies at each border, we were reluctant to buy more Deutch marks when close to the Dutch border and agreed to do without breakfast until we crossed it. The other woman in the quartet was South African. She was sure, for whatever reason, that she could manage the Dutch language and buy us some food at the first village we came to. Asking for bread, as she thought, and indicating the size of a loaf with her hands, she then asked for cheese, indicating a much smaller amount, and came back to us in triumph, only to find that we had a huge slab of cheese and a loaf not much bigger than a couple of buns. Never mind, it filled us up.

We split up in Copenhagen and left the other couple. DZ and I went on our way together. We explored the city, finishing up in the Tivoli Gardens. This was to be our last night together as he was due at a conference nearby and I had to go back to London for the summer job that Imperial had organised for me. I still avoided most alcohol and so had been drinking fizzy grapefruit juice during the evening Our behaviour was constrained in those days, and no woman ever initiated any move. I was simply hoping at least for a worthwhile goodnight-goodbye kiss at my hotel bedroom door, before the evening was out, particularly as we would be separating for at least two or more weeks. But the fizz had given me hiccoughs and I was mortified by this lost opportunity at the hotel when we went back to collect my luggage, for I was flying out that night on a last flight, to London. Being separated for two whole weeks seemed unbearable as I hugged him, watched him depart, and headed for my plane. Then I was told there would be an hour's delay… but it was too late to call him back. Then another delay. Finally, I phoned the hotel and told him. It must have been the airport hotel for he was back in fifteen minutes and we talked for another half hour, although this was through a barrier, as I had gone through

Customs. The flight was called, but I told him not to leave until my plane had actually taken off. This was just as well as the flight was again delayed. This time I checked out through Customs and we had another hour together, and the desired hug. Then again, I went back out through Customs. My passport, after that night, was stamped in and out of Denmark several times!

Back in London, and in my college rooms, and with almost no sleep, I headed for Hammersmith hospital where Imperial had organised my holiday job. In fact, this should have been a job in America as it was Imperial's policy to find an overseas job for us students in our second summer vacation. However, that plan foundered, because Parent withheld approval, and my passport. So, Hammersmith it was, and very interesting it turned out to be.

I was to work in an analytical laboratory associated with a cyclotron where various isotopes were being made. One of them was radioactive arsenic which was being used to locate brain tumours. This was an experimental procedure and only being given, as I understood, to people who were thought likely to die anyway within twenty-four hours. Another project involved radioactive iron, though I do not recall what that was used for.

One day there was great excitement. A technician walking along the round corridor that circumvented the cyclotron had had a Geiger counter in his hand and it had accidentally been left switched on. It suddenly sounded way off scale. It transpired that at around 10.30 that morning someone had been transporting a 'hot' (radioactive) iodine target along the corridor and some of the iodine must have escaped and fallen on the floor. The discovery was made shortly before 4.00pm. As a 'gopher' student I had been running along that corridor many times during those preceding hours. One of my jobs at the end of each day was to collect up the wrist, waist, and lapel radiation badges from each staff member, including my own, and read and record the results. On some days one or two of the staff would have levels above the daily limit of safe tolerance. When I reported this, I was generally assured that the levels would be averaged out and almost certainly fall below the threshold over the month. As a raw student, and hoping for some excitement, I was disappointed at this lack of interest or response.

On this occasion, several people had high levels of radioactivity and my levels were particularly high. No one seemed concerned! When I enquired about this, they pointed out to me that I would only be there for a few more weeks and, averaged out over the year, my exposure would therefore be low. Unaware of the dangers of radiation at that time I was more excited by the drama of the story I could tell, than about fears for my health. Little did I know what the long-term results of this would be.

Somehow and sometime, possibly before the start of the final year, DZ and I took our beloved Mini and drove up through England, Edinburgh, where I had lived as a kid for a year, along the banks of Loch Lomond, out to Ardnamurchan Point, then down through the Lake District and so back to London. Travel to the other side of the world was a lot more difficult then than now, and at least twice if not three times as expensive. DZ was aware that he was unlikely to be back in the UK again. He also felt he should make sure I saw all I could before leaving my home country.

I hadn't driven in Europe, but in England, both before and after our European trip, DZ had taught me to drive and, with the required L plates on, I had shared the driving with him for hundreds of miles. It was therefore time I took my driving test. I had used Parent's Guildford address for the paperwork and DZ and I duly turned up on the testing day. I took to the wheel, the examiner issued instructions, and it all seemed to go very well, as it should have done given the length of experience I had had. At the end of the test, the examiner sat in the car, wrote me out my licence, signed it and gave it to me. To my surprise she then got out and proceeded to walk back to the main road, cross it, and continue back to the office. Nonplussed, I sat there for a few minutes, wondering what to do when there ws no one in the car with me. Unsure, I got out of the car and walked back myself. I was meet by a seriously worried DZ. He had seen the examiner walk back alone. Where was I? Had I crashed his Mini? Was there a problem? Why had I not driven back? I explained that I had always had someone with me before when driving. I simply hadn't realised I was now a fully competent and entitled solo driver!

In our third year each student had to choose the branch of chemistry in which they wished to specialise. I was not going to choose physical chemistry with the attendant additional mathematics. Inorganic chemistry did not appeal to me either. I tossed up between organic chemistry, which I enjoyed and found intriguing, and analytical chemistry. Organic chemistry would have included studies in biochemistry as the ancillary. However, I still had a career in forensic chemistry in mind and so I chose analytical chemistry.

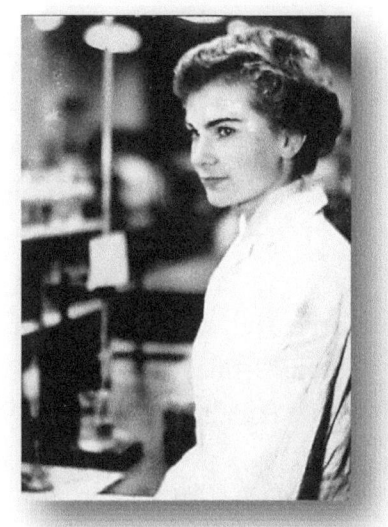

As a result, I had geology as the additional subject. I would have preferred biochemistry and it didn't make much sense as I still planned on being a forensic chemist, but there seemed to be no choice. I was, though, intrigued, as I would be learning something of DZ's subject.

One other student, PY, also chose analytical chemistry. On the appointed day, at the start of this final year, we both turned up in Professor Theobald's study. He sat there, resplendent in three-piece suit adorned with fob watch and other indications of a bygone age and enquired, "And what are you going to be, what career have you chosen, Miss Williams?"

"I want to be a forensic chemist."

A knock came on his door. The visitor's query was dealt with.

"What did you say, Miss Williams, that you wanted to be?"

"A geochemist."

I was probably the most surprised person in the room. Why had I said that? But the professor was such an authoritative person that I did not want to look like the idiot I was being and admit my mistake. But perhaps it wasn't a mistake? Perhaps it was my sub-conscious talking. Be that as it may, my topic was set. I was to write a dissertation on geochemical mineral prospecting or exploration, and train up in rock and soil analysis.

For my second year I had scored a room in Beit Hall which was without doubt *the* place to have a room. For the start of my third year I shared a flat with two of the other women in my year, just a short distance away across Queensgate. Each evening I would have the meal prepared on the exact dot of 6.30 DZ would arrive, we would eat, and then both hot foot it back to his laboratory in the School of Mines, where we would work on our individual theses. It was a great help having him to talk over my subject with, and to help with general guidelines as to how to arrange the dissertation.

DZ was under considerable time pressure to complete his thesis, but we assumed he had the year. However, just before Christmas he received a letter from Canberra. He was to return to Australia by March. Dismay. He had still to finish his thesis and his time was even shorter than he had thought. Would we get married here, in London, in a rush, with no honeymoon, but with Aunt and Paternal Grandmother in attendance? I would clearly have to stay in London and finish my degree. Or would I, still single, go out later, join him and get married there? There was no quick solution, but the longer we waited before deciding, the less time there would be to arrange the wedding.

His time was now seriously threatened and so I helped by typing up his thesis. In those days it was done on waxed stencils. You had to hit the keys with significant and uniform strength, so that each letter was cut through, and the depth of the cut was similar for all the keys. The pages were then inked, the back removed, and the stencil could be used to make six copies. It was hard and slow work. One mistake meant you had to stop, use a filler, line the page up again, retype that letter, and hope you had hit the same spot. More than one or two mistakes in a page usually meant retyping each page. The worst pages were the references, where so many names had unique spellings.

Procrastination over our possible wedding plans ensured that, in the end, there was insufficient time to marry, and he returned to Australia. After he had gone my life settled back to the introverted single life of my earlier time at Imperial. I found I liked it. Strangely, I didn't seem to miss him much. Perhaps I was not really ready for marriage. Aunt was to tell me later that she had told him that if we didn't marry before he left, she didn't think I would go out there and marry him. He hadn't believed her, but as in so many things, she was proved right. I eventually wrote to him and called the whole thing off. I was sad for him, but I think also a bit relieved for myself. I was definitely turned off by the idea that anyone would have a say in my life, or have any sort of control or rights over me as they had in the past, and this fear now rose to the surface, adding to my decision.

That Easter, my third at Imperial, was taken up with geological field work down in Devon, in combination with those who had chosen inorganic chemistry as their speciality.

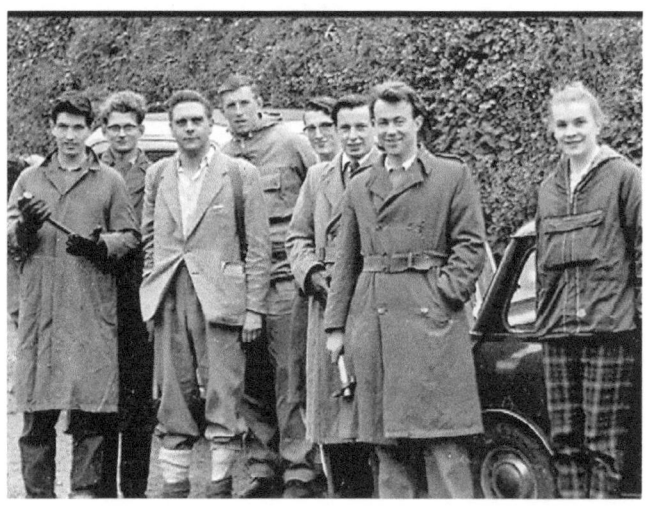

During this term I joined a group of car enthusiasts, of the racing kind. I spent week-ends at Brand's Hatch, Goodwood, or similar places involved in motor rallying or timed sprints – never actually racing. A friend had a Mini, and another an MGTF, both of which I drove, as and when allowed – and loved it.

And so I completed my degree I won a IIA, which took me beyond my wildest expectations. I had survived eighteen years of traumatic childhood, met Aunt, had a wonderful three years at Imperial, nearly been married but escaped, and was left wondering – what next?

Chapter 3

From Imperial to New Zealand

What next? I had a IIA Honours BSc degree from IC, arguably one of the top three universities in the UK, an ARCS (Associate of the Royal College of Science) for my third and research year, and an excellent report from Professor Theobald. It was time to wonder, what next? I had, of course, been considering this since I ended my engagement. The obvious options were in applied geochemistry or further research. I had an offer to work in Ghana in the geochemistry section of their Geological Survey. That was exciting, and definitely tempting. I discussed it with a friend who had been there, but eventually declined it. The alternative was to enrol for a higher degree.

My engagement was over, I was single again and free to make my own decisions. I had a missing parent – Father, left behind in New Zealand when the Parents divorced. In addition, he was Aunt's much-loved brother It was a no-brainer. I would go and search him out. Although she said little, she had always spoken favourably of him and I could tell that she was keen for me to go there. As was becoming a long-term habit, I was keen to please her. I would try to go to New Zealand. My decision made, I sent off applications for doing research, aiming at a PhD, in geochemical mineral exploration and related studies, to universities in New Zealand and Australia.

Having anticipated, while I was engaged to DZ, a move to Australia, my mind was already focused in that direction. Any one of those universities would take me very much closer to the missing Parent, and I might get to meet, even come to know him. Additionally, both were countries with wide open spaces, ideal for my form of geochemical exploration, and both were part of the Commonwealth with English as a first language. The universities were all keen to have overseas input, and, I hoped, particularly input from Imperial which had a strong geochemical research focus in its Royal School of Mines.

I had three positive responses to my applications, two from Australian universities and one from Otago University in New Zealand's South Island. Going to Otago would mean I would be living in the same country as Father, even if on the 'other' island. JR, in the chemistry department there, but funded by the New Zealand Geological Survey, replied to my application. He offered three possibilities for my thesis: research into the New Zealand coal industry (which I later discovered was his almost total interest); research into two major clay minerals (in the geological sense), heulandite and clinoptilolite and their inter-relationship; and last but not least, geochemical mineral prospecting and exploration.

I replied, making it clear that the only one in which I had any interest at all was geochemical exploration. For this, he was able to get funding from the New Zealand Geological Survey. As a result, I was promised a good graduate employee income, significantly more than a research student grant. All this was settled in the summer of 1961, when I was twenty. I expected to start in February 1962, which was their autumn and the start of their academic year. However, they asked that I arrive by the end of November. This I arranged.

A sea trip was provided, so I booked, and paid for, my passage, cancelled my room at college, packed up and was ready to go. Oh to be so free! My entire worldly goods went into one trunk in the hold and one suitcase in my cabin. I spent the last evening at Aunt's house, where I stayed the night. We planned the ways in which we would keep in touch. She gave me a portable radio with long-wave, and I dreamed of listening to programmes from the ship's upper deck at the same time that she listened to them in London. Not possible, of course, but it was nice to dream. The next morning, I was driven to Southampton by the current boyfriend who kept insisting we could turn round and go back to London any time I changed my mind. I didn't.

I spent four relaxing weeks on board ship – air travel not yet being established as the usual mode of travel, and certainly not for people moving their entire worldly goods with them, even though mine were limited. I spent much of the trip as part of a loose two-couple quartet, one of whom, JS, was to remain a friend for many years, if a somewhat distant one geographically, as he lived in Sydney. Life on board was a delight. I had been to New Zealand by boat before, of course, aged about seven. We had gone out through the Suez Canal and on the way back through the Panama Canal. This time the boat would go round South Africa, with memorable stops at Madeira (eating bananas and drinking the local wine on the upper deck as we sailed out of Funchal harbour), Cape Town, and Durban. At both of these latter two I met up with distant relatives of maternal Grandmother.

'Sun, sea, and sand'? Not quite. No sand, of course, but after the weather of the UK, it was delightful.

Life on board was very social. The twins, who drove the taxi, spoken of later, can be seen in the background.

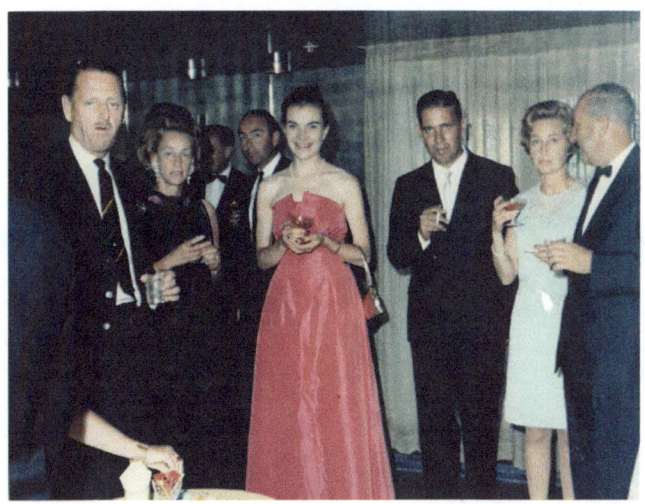

After, too, the pressures of completing my degree, the relaxation was wonderful, and any chance of becoming bored was removed by my introduction to bridge. I came to love this game, and played it eagerly whenever other social opportunities were limited, such as on other sea voyages, or later, when living in Fiji and social life was limited. At the end of the trip I spent two days being shown the sights of Sydney by JS, and then flew on to New Zealand.

I had written to Parent, arranged to meet up with him on my arrival, and been invited to stay. He and his second wife met me in Auckland, their most convenient city. They had a large, camping, caravanning park built round a wide bay off Lake Rotoiti, eleven miles from Rotorua.

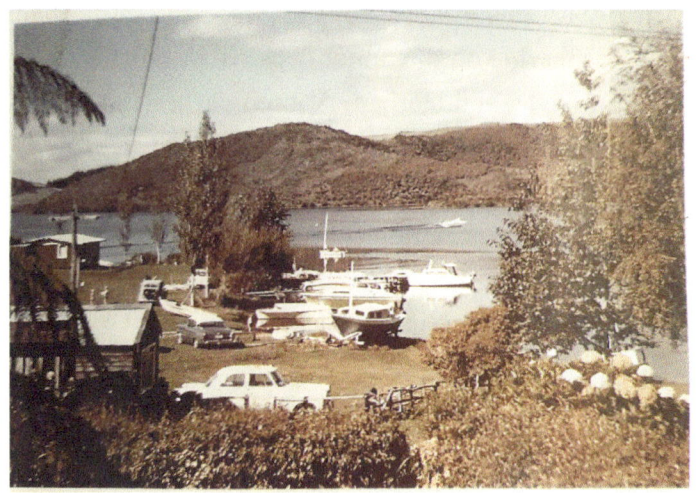

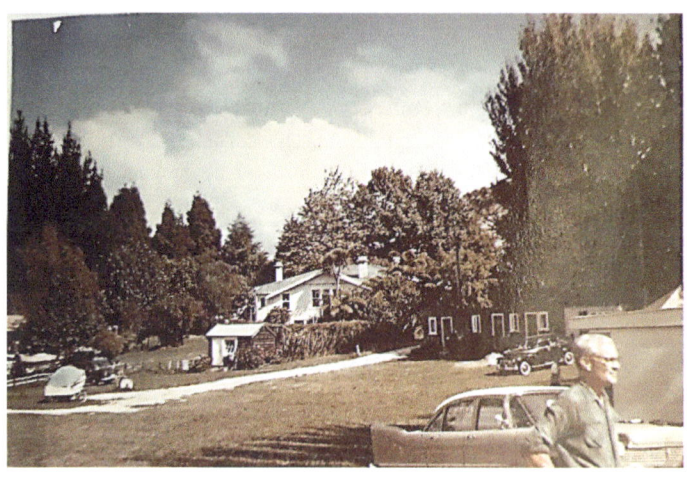

They also had a dozen cabins where people could stay, and a large house for themselves. They offered their clients fishing, a range of water sports, exotic scenery, volcanic activity, hot pools, geysers, and more.

It started well. Parent turned out to be warm, funny, witty, and a great raconteur, though I was later to learn that many of his stories owed much to his imagination. There was also a half-brother by adoption. He was many years younger than me and clearly nothing to do with the "two children that I have and love more than you" which he had apparently written, according to female parent, a year after our return to England in 1949. More from his imagination? But I gave it no thought, wrapped up as I was in the pleasure of meeting up with him. Knowing he was Aunt's sister, and loving her as I did, I was anticipating an equally warm relationship with him. It should have been. I was to stay with them for six weeks and had not anticipated any problems, I was, after all, his daughter, wasn't I?

Gradually things settled down. However, I was clearly not the flavour of the month. His wife was certainly jealous and as a result he was on edge. I tried to make up for this in the only way I knew how – by being more helpful, doing more for him and them such as painting the roof – a horrid job in summer heat, but corrugated iron roofs do have to be painted regularly. It seems I did not do it well enough. Eventually he suggested that I stop trying to do work for him and spend more time with his wife so that she didn't feel left out.

Should I consider her a step-mother? I knew so little of normal family life that I had no yardstick. She certainly didn't feel like a step-mother, but then, as I had just turned twenty-one, that was perhaps not surprising. I was, at one point, upbraided for sitting in 'her' chair on one side of the fireplace. "You can sit on the sofa, but obviously the two chairs are where we each sit, like any normal family." To which I nearly replied that I had had no experience of living in, or even visiting, a 'normal family', but I bit my tongue. Just as some years later when I was to meet him again and he asked why I didn't call him 'Dad', I bit my tongue on the nearly automatic response, "but you never were, or acted like a dad to me in anything you did". To me it just didn't fit. Nor did it honour the reality of our relationship. But that is for later.

After we had left New Zealand in 1949, it appears that he had moved in to stay with JH, his friend and colleague at Unilever where he worked. JH had two sisters, the vivacious and popular one, and the quiet one. Father had married the quiet one. According to Aunt he had been distraught at losing me, aged nine, finding me more to his temperament than Brother aged seven, who was quiet. So was she, the quiet one, jealous? Did she fear that his attention would turn to me and away from the son they had adopted? It seemed so.

Be that as it may, I had fulfilled my plan and met up with the missing parent. It had not been a great success. I suspect I was more of a bother to him and a complication to his life than a pleasure. I'm not sure what I had expected. I'm very sure I had not had huge hopes, I had learnt to expect little and was, in any case, pretty self-sufficient, so I was not unduly upset at the way the meeting up had unfolded. As usual, I took events in my stride, and accepted the outcome. I was sad, but nevertheless relieved when the six weeks were up and I could go on down to Dunedin, to my waiting place in the Geological Survey where there was a laboratory and research degree waiting for me at Otago University. As so often before, I reminded myself that you could trust books, studies, and science, but not people.

A year or so later, while in Dunedin, I learnt that Gran, paternal grandmother had died, back in London. I only knew her for the three years that I was at Imperial. Even in that short time I soon realised that she was a woman of strong will, feisty, grey-haired, beautiful, with a wicked sense of humour, overlain by a lot of light-hearted joking and optimism. Sadly, she was confined to a wheelchair by crippling and painful arthritis.

She had been born on a Tuesday, met her future husband on a Tuesday, been engaged on a Tuesday, and married on a Tuesday. In fact she had been married three times, each time it was on a Tuesday and each time it was to the same man! Grandfather, a surgeon in the British army in 'the East' had come back to England on his three months' leave with the express purpose of finding a wife during this time. This was not an uncommon course of action in those days. They met, became engaged and went through a registry office marriage ceremony in England. By then his leave was up and he sailed back to Burma that same day. The haste was due to his conviction that Great Grandmother would stop the process if it wasn't formalised before he left. When Grandmother arrived in Rangoon, they went through another ceremony, this time for the sake of propriety. However, Gran was determined to have the 'real deal'. This included the white dress, bridesmaids, best man, and so forth, and this was accomplished, again on a Tuesday, a month or so later.

I never asked after which wedding day the marriage was consummated – one didn't. But I do know that she had three children, one of them my father, and that they were all born on Tuesdays. Sadly, the eldest died soon after birth, and also on a Tuesday.

Aunt told me the story, by audio tape, which was the way we communicated when I was away from London. Back in London, Gran was clearly failing one Thursday and their doctor was convinced that she might have only a day or two left and that he would be needed over the weekend. He announced that he would forego his regular golf week-end, so as to be available when needed. Aunt assured him that Gran would live past the week-end and insisted that he went off to golf as usual. He was finally persuaded, but returned early, on the Sunday evening, fully expecting to find Gran had passed. She hadn't. Apparently, she was quiet on the Monday, and typically, even joked a bit. During that Monday night Aunt woke up and went in to see Gran. Gran was awake. "What time is it?" she asked, to which Aunt replied, "It's twelve thirty-five". After a small pause Gran said, "Ah, so that means it's Tuesday". "Yes." With that, holding Aunt's hand, Gran stopped breathing.

Chapter 4

Otago

A rriving in Dunedin by plane, I was met by JR and his wife and taken to the accommodation that had been arranged for me. As luck would have it, on the day of my arrival, a space in a share flat was becoming available and I could stay there if I wished. I was driven to it and left alone to explore the town. This was interesting, but not rewarding as the shops were all closed by then, it being five o'clock.

The next day I meet up with JR again, my supposed PhD supervisor, in his office in the chemistry department. In Otago University the chemistry and geology departments were next door to each other in one of the long, thin, older buildings. Access on the upper floor of the combined building was a long corridor above some spacious lecture theatres. Fittingly, from my point of view, this corridor connected the Chemistry and Geology departments. Where it opened out there were two rooms. One was for electronic equipment shared by both departments, and the other was to become my office and laboratory, symbolically set between the two departments.

The first day, sitting in his office, I learnt the worst. JR made it clear that he would prefer me to switch my chosen topic to coal chemistry. I reminded him that I had already declined that when we first communicated by mail, having no interest in it and no experience or knowledge of it. He then explained that he had no interest in, or experience of, any form of geochemical exploration, a statement that took me by surprise as that had been my stated aim for research towards a PhD. It had also been the reason that the Geological Survey had been willing to pay my salary and expenses while there.

His compromise suggestion was that I study mineral chemistry of heulandite and clinoptilolite, two related rock minerals in which he had a secondary interest. Unfortunately, I had none. This was not a good start. However, I am, by nature an optimist and I hoped some positive outcome could be engineered. In any case, I had little choice but to stick it out. I had paid my fare here, had no money left and no alternative options. I wanted to do research and I wanted my next degree. I certainly did not have the confidence to make an overt fuss. In retrospect, it seemed clear that he needed a research student for his own academic purposes, had not had one for a while and saw my application as an opportunity.

At noon that day I went to the docks to identify and collect my trunk and organise its transport to my new apartment. There was no time for lunch. Back to the Chemistry department. JR introduced me to CP, another graduate, who had arrived from England a month earlier. He informed me that we had both been invited out that evening to the home of someone else from the Chemistry department, who was going to the UK for study and research. He had apparently taken several hundred photos (colour slides in those days) of all aspects of New Zealand and the life at Otago. He wanted an opinion of them from us, as new arrivals who knew little or nothing of the country. That sounded fun. What time? We were to arrive at 6.30 pm and CP would collect me. I was used to dinner at eight with Aunt back in London, so this seemed decidedly early. However, I agreed.

We arrived, we talked, the four of us sitting around in their sitting room. We talked some more. We sat – and again, we talked. I hoped for a drink, a sherry perhaps, but no. We talked some more. I looked at CP, who shrugged his shoulders. We continued to talk. As time went by, I got progressively hungrier. My stomach rumbled, protesting that I had given it nothing to work on at lunch time either and, as was my habit then, I had not had breakfast.

Finally, our host said that he thought the light would soon be OK for the viewing, dusk falling at around eight-thirty. What, no dinner? Not even a drink or a nibble? This was when I discovered that the usual time then for dinner in New Zealand was six o'clock, and oh yes, I should call it 'tea', not dinner. CP and I watched the slides with diminishing interest. Each time the host's hand went out for another cassette of slides, my heart sank further. Finally, at close to eleven o'clock, he said that was all and hoped we had enjoyed it. Oh, and would we like some coffee? Yes please! I tried not to shout, just crossed my fingers. With the coffee came some generous slices of thick chocolate cake. Phew. I loved it. Would I like another slice? Definitely, it was wonderful. But my stomach was not even half satisfied. Could I have another slice? I risked being thought greedy and rushed on to explain that I simply loved chocolate cake (not true), that this was the best chocolate cake I had ever had (definitely not true either), and that I would forever remember this wonderful evening (if not for the reasons he thought). CP drove me back to my flat, but I was all too aware that I had had no time to shop, the cupboards were bare, and the closing time for shops had been 5.00pm. There was no hope of food until the morning.

The next day I learnt that JR was going on holiday and would be away until the end of January, that being the norm, apparently, for the summer vacation in New Zealand academic circles. Most of the other academics, in both departments, were also going to be away. I wondered why I had been asked to arrive in November.

But all was not lost. I made a few friends. Then the woman who had vacated 'my' room in the flat, came back for her wedding in the church across the road. I was invited to the wedding lunch, which was to be held in the flat. I met her brother, who ran the family sheep 'station' in outback Otago. The evening was all very interesting, even if I did feel a bit like a fish out of water. One of the chemistry students had invited me out for 'tea' that evening and I had accepted, thinking that the wedding lunch would be over by late afternoon. It wasn't. In fact, even when I got back after my evening out, at least half the guests were still there. It was apparently a true New Zealand shindig. All the related wives, from all parts of the country, had obviously been preparing the feast for days – good hearty country fare it was. Another insight into New Zealand life. I think the final guests, including the bride and groom, finally left around two in the morning. But by golly, a dozen or more of them, again including the bride and groom, were back by nine the next morning. Unbelievable. They all helped with the tidying up. Then I realised that the bride and groom were leaving for England that evening, and this was also the great family farewell and send off.

Things quietened down after that. People dispersed. I was introduced to no one new, the university staff all having departed on the long summer holiday. I had no research project to start on and insufficient confidence or experience to start anything on my own. My room was drab and uninteresting, so I bought paint and wallpaper and brightened it up. I meet one or two people. I studied heulandite and clinoptilolite and found them also to be drab and uninteresting. The Geological Survey offices were closed for the holiday, so there was no hope there. I had no car, so I walked, went swimming, and explored the city further. The bride's brother and family took pity on me and very kindly invited me to stay for a few days over Christmas.

My first experience of a sheep station was illuminating. It was certainly a very different way of life to anything to be found anywhere in the UK countryside. We drove for what seemed like hours through sand and dust, between low-lying scrub and sub-tropical and foreign-looking skimpy trees. It was a 'jolly' Christmas and very different to Christmas in England, even making allowances for the season, which in this hemisphere was summer.

Soon I was back to Dunedin and the flat. The department was still closed, so no help there. It was time to explore the beaches. However, I then committed what was apparently an unforgivable sin and left sand on the bathroom floor of the flat. When the flat owner returned and found sand on the floor, she suggested I might like to find my own flat? I would, and did. A lovely woman took over my room and offered to pay for the wallpapering I had done. "Oh no, that's alright," I demurred politely, fully expecting the English response of "No, really, you must let me". I had certainly improved the room considerably, and at some cost. Instead she said, "Oh, thank you". Another step forward in my understanding of NZ habits. A pity. I could well have done with the money, not having been paid yet.

I needed transport. I couldn't buy a car as at that time overseas currency was hard to come by in New Zealand. Buying a new car (necessarily imported as none were made in NZ) was only possible if I could show that my money covered the full purchase price and had all come from outside NZ. It had, but it was nothing like the full price of my chosen Mini, or any other car. For this reason, few other people could afford new cars either and so the price of second-hand cars already in the country was high, often even more than the full new price. I bought a Lambretta scooter again.

Things settled down after that. I found myself a delightful, if small, flat. At work I was somewhat betwixt and between, being signed up for the chemistry department at the university but employed by the NZ Geological Survey and attached to their Dunedin office. I eventually visited the Geological Survey office and received a warm if uncertain welcome. No one seemed to know quite what to do with me since I was allegedly going to be doing research with JR in the chemistry department of the University.

A solution came in the form of the Geological Survey's senior and economic geologist, BW, who saved the day. Logically, he was the one I was most likely to work with, although he had not been expecting that and was not experienced in managing a research student. He suggested I join him and BR, his field assistant, and we would go on a trip to one of the areas where he was doing field work. Could I be ready to leave in a few days? Indeed I could. I set to and made a model of the basics of a small testing kit, one that could be carried through the day as I collected samples, and set up in the evening as I ran the tests.

This was another new experience. We loaded up the 4-wheel drive and the three of us set off, destination Queenstown. At that time, Queenstown was very much a small town. We had rooms in a basic but pleasant motel. I set up my lab in mine. I had organised the field pack and designed it so that at least stream and river water samples could be analysed at each collection spot. Soil and sediment samples would be analysed back at the motel with further check analyses in the Otago laboratory. We explored the town and found there were precisely three places to eat – the Chinese restaurant, a fish and chip takeaway, or an exceedingly dull and unimaginative hotel on the edge of Lake Wakatipu. The three of us looked at the Chinese and settled for self-catering in BR's room.

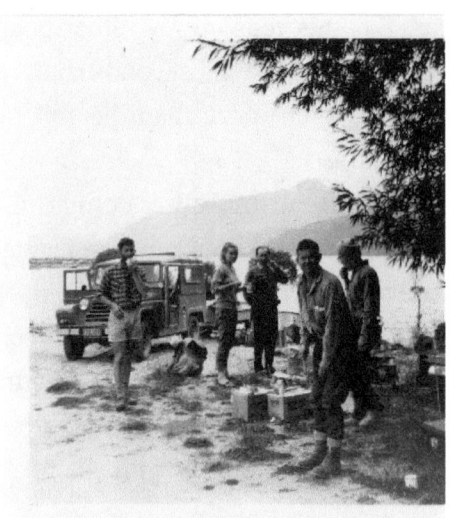

Next morning it was time to set out. My only field work to that date had been along the beach during my third year at IC as part of the geology ancillary course. That had been a walk in the park. Under instruction I had purchased the prescribed rugged boots. Initially thinking them to be on the heavy, clunky side, I soon realised how essential they were in this terrain, as was the invaluable ankle support they provided.

We drove the few miles along the edge of Lake Wakatipu, to Moke Creek, and then crossed the creek itself several times as it zig-zagged through the cuts in the schist rock ridges. Then it was pack-on-the-back and hiking upwards. We had to climb up steep hillsides of tussocky grass for about a thousand feet. As a city dweller and inexperienced walker, I had assumed the skyline was the 'top' and just hoped my breath would last until I got there. I was rather dismayed to find that after a short drop there was another equally high ridge to climb farther ahead. BW noticed my look of dismay, but I quickly endeavoured to turned it into a gasp of pretend delight at the view – or so I hoped. I was determined not to be beaten. I needed to make a niche in this new and unplanned situation and the logical place would be in the economic section of the Geological Survey with the support of this senior economic geologist. Later he was to tell me that he thought at the time "OK, if field work is not for her, she can stick to the laboratory".

In fact, I was very lucky that he had even been open-minded enough (for those days) to include me, a woman, in the field trip. I was delighted when it turned out to be the first of many, and the three of us spent many months in the following three years, doing field work throughout the South Island with occasional trips to the North Island.

Mineral exploration was to involve soil, river water, river sediment, and vegetation analysis. There was no clear project in mind at the time, as my arrival within the Survey had not been anticipated. BR, however, understood my dilemma with JR, and his failed promise, and was beginning to formulate a plan. He suggested that I study any small outcrops of minerals such as nickel, zinc, or copper, and explore their possible presence, even in trace amounts, throughout the local soils and rocks. He was definitely an applied geologist and not a research or university geologist, and it was not much of a plan. But it did seem that it might resolve the dilemma in which I found myself. I would do this in parallel with, and hopefully in support of much of his economic geology.

So we started to look at the trace elements of many of the rock formations in which he worked. There were various small copper deposits in the area, also shows of nickel. These could be used to work in combination with the general geological mapping. Even better, we might find small deposits of copper. A major part of Central Otago had been worked over by swarms of gold seekers in the 'gold rushes' of the previous century, and the geology intrigued me. Unfortunately, BW was not a research scientist and had never supported a research student and this was to turn out to be a significant disadvantage by the time I completed my thesis – but at least it led to three years of great fun.

The area involving the large numbers of creeks flowing into Moke Creek, was to become one of my major sampling areas. For nearly two years I sampled all the creeks in the area every four weeks, come high summer or low winter. Every fourth weekend I would collect samples on one of the two days and on the other I would either water ski on Lake Wakatipu or, in winter snow, I would ski on Coronet Peak. Having proven myself and my bush walking determination to BW, he saw no reason why I could not be involved in field work just like the rest of his staff, and thus I was set to take my place fully in the male-dominated world of geological exploration. I was very lucky.

I studied other areas along the Routeburn River that flowed into the northern tip of Lake Wakatipu, and up and around the Shotover River, all in Otago.

I worked in the Longwood Range in Southland province. I worked with Lime & Marble company in Nelson, looking at nickel in their areas. As part of this I drove down the northwest coast of the Alps until the road stopped. I also had reason to drive up the southwest side of the Alps as far as the Hast Pass, which was as far as that road went. The two roads didn't meet at that time, though since then it has connected with the one coming down from the north.

A memorable trip involved the three of us using the Survey dinghy to carry us and our gear to the mouth of Milford Sound off the west coast of Fiordland, where we camped for one night in Anita Bay. By prior arrangement, a cray-fishing boat picked us up and carried us a further eleven miles south to Poison Bay. There was no other way to travel. A couple of years earlier it had taken BW and GG, another geologist, both good mountain climbers, eleven days in their attempt to reach Poison Bay by climbing over the mountains that plunged down into the fjord and sea, but without success. There were amazing deposits of New Zealand greenstone there that we were to study and map.

The first night camped in Poison Bay, we gorged over the large sack of crayfish we had been given. These were the six-inch ones, just a tad too short to be harvested and sold legitimately. A few days later we wished we had saved even one. The fishing boat that was due to return and collect us did not arrive as planned. Our supply of rabbit and venison was limited, less by the long-range shooting skills of the two geologists than by the difficulty of reaching the kill spot even when they did score. Perhaps I should have been worried by this delay as the only way out of where we were was by this boat that was supposed to be collecting us, but I only remember the excitement and the pleasure of the trip. We were definitely hungry when the boat finally made it back through roughish weather. We were then taken back to Anita Bay, our dinghy, Milford Sound, and any food we could find!

Another field area involved a copper deposit that had been dug up by a farmer near Parakao and Pupuke, this time in the northern tip of the North Island. The deposits were not all that interesting, but seeing the northern part of the North Island was exciting. It is not tropical, but was approaching that, and to my English eyes, the vegetation was fascinating.

On another trip I went back to Lime & Marble near Nelson, this time with GG as well as BW. BW, GH, and I had been walking, camping and climbing, as well as, of course, sampling (me) and economic mapping (them). The weather had been cold and damp and it was a treat to spend one night in the home of a delightful couple who farmed the area. Dinner included two lamb chops each. Sitting round a table is very different to sitting around a camp fire. GH did not seem to realise this. Finishing one chop he flung the bone over his shoulder. Thankfully it flew out of the open window. BW and I had both observed this and grimaced at each other. Luckily our hosts had not noticed. As the evening grew cooler, they closed the window. I looked at BW and nodded, wondering what GH would do with his second bone. I needn't have been concerned, as BW must have kicked the appropriate leg under the table, nodded at GH and indicated the closed window. To my startled gaze, GW indicated his acceptance of the situation, looked around, saw the lit fire and sent his bone in that direction. I was glad we only had two bones to deal with or goodness knows where the third one might have gone.

GH was almost the epitome of a taciturn misogynist, with zero social skills. On the second night before our return to Dunedin, we stayed in a small hotel. At the end of the evening I stood up to go to my room and was mildly surprised when GH followed. Early for him, I thought, the guys often stayed on in the bar drinking. We climbed the stairs. At the fork at the top I said "Goodnight, GH" and was then surprised when he followed me down the corridor. The same thing happened at the fork in the corridor. "Goodnight, GH" I said again, and I started to open the door to my room. I was startled when it became obvious that he was planning to enter it too. I said another very firm "goodnight". He stood still, looking somewhat disconcerted and uncertain until I had firmly closed and locked the door on him. Yes, definitely no social skills.

When I left London and came to New Zealand, the biggest wrench had been leaving Aunt. We had solved this, at least partially, by long-distance talking. Aunt's leaving present to me, in addition to the portable radio, had been a portable typewriter. She had also bought one for herself. Our mutual promise was a weekly, or better, flow of letters. However, this was hard work and not as intimate or heart-warming as I wanted. After a few months, Aunt bought a tape recorder and suggested I did the same. This was no neat and compact present-day wonder. Looking back, it was large, cumbersome, and not very flexible. About the size of full LP record player, it took reel to reel tapes. These could be eight inches in diameter, as I recall, but neither of us could talk for that long, so we settled on small disks less than ten centimeters in diameter. Thrilled with my purchase I rushed home, figured out how to operate it, set up the tape, plugged in the microphone and switched on. Silence. Nothing happened. Words did not come. What was I to say to a silent room? I tried writing up what I would say. Too stilted. Disaster. Then a tape arrived from Aunt. Hearing her voice brought her presence into the room and I found that if I stopped her tape, inserted mine and started talking immediately, I could get the hang of it.

For a while this was a necessary approach – I had to hear her voice first. Then it became second nature. Whenever I had something to say or to share with her, I would start the tape and talk away. In that way we were to stay very close, both emotionally and in touch with each other's lives, through all the thirty-five years that we lived too far away from each other to make frequent visits. We would each send tapes, sometimes weekly, sometimes at longer intervals. Fortunately, as the years went by, the equipment improved until we were using small hand-held, battery-operated tape recorders, and could make the tapes wherever we were.

Life in New Zealand continued like this for three years, during which time I travelled much of the country and built up a three-year stretch of active field work on my CV, which was to stand me in good stead in each of my subsequent jobs. Socially, life was also great fun. I had a few proposals, but I was determined to remain single. I had long since vowed, after my struggles of the first eighteen years, that I would never again be owned or controlled by anyone. The moment a boyfriend got serious or proposed, I withdrew from the relationship and fled in fright. In later years a good friend likened me somewhat to a hedgehog, withdrawing into itself at the slightest hint of danger. I could not argue with that.

I had one particularly good friend, JB, a woman who was a dedicated occupational therapist. Like me, she was British and fairly newly arrived in NZ. Not content with all the field work I did, I would willingly satisfy her wish to see more of the countryside at the weekends, and the two of us would go off touring. By this time, I had bought a Mini station wagon, thanks to a small legacy from Grandmother, and we travelled in style. In this way I covered the more settled parts of the country, where the land had been farmed too much to be a good hunting ground for interesting rock structures or mineral enrichments.

At the end of my three years, I was due to submit my thesis and consider my future options. One offer would have involved continuing to work for the New Zealand Geological Survey, but based in their head office in Lower Hut, near Wellington at the southern end of the North Island. Another offered possibility was to take up a position with the UK Overseas Geological Survey in the then crown colony of Fiji. The third was to go back to England and, with luck, find a way to focus my career on research. I chose Fiji.

The job opportunity interested me enormously. I had already developed an enthusiasm for learning more about the peoples of the South Pacific. While camping out on field trips in the various parts of New Zealand, we had entertained ourselves with music from the islands – BW's delightful guitar playing on a steel guitar, my somewhat poor-quality attempts with a ukulele, and field assistant BV on spoons. In between, BW would regale us with stories of his trips to the Cook Islands (administered by New Zealand) and the Antarctic. Most of BW's guitar playing focused on Mauri and Polynesian music and so inevitably BV and I had fallen in with that and I had learnt to love it.

Then the time came. I had written up my thesis, had it printed, and presented. One external examiner was in America and one local one was in New Zealand. I faced them, along with JR, who was still officially my supervisor although he had had no hand in my work, and had offered no help or guidance since the first couple of months. There had been a somewhat prickly three-way discussion when I had enlisted BW's help to sort out the mess caused by JR's near insistence that I study coal geology. BW had been a delightful geologist to work with, but had no background in academia and no real idea how to direct my research or structure a thesis. JR glowered at me throughout my viva and asked what I considered to be several asinine questions that were tricky and rarely pertinent. None the less, I thought the presentation had gone fairly well, but of course had no way to assess or compare it with others. I knew it would be a few weeks before I received the result and that by then I would be back in London.

I packed up my flat, sold the Mini and faced the final week. The current boyfriend and I had not, of course, been living together. That was definitely *not* done in those days. But since I had had to vacate my flat a week before departing to enable packing, cleaners, and removalists to do what had to be done, we had arranged (very quietly!) that I would stay with him in his flat. This was very daring. Also very exciting. And somehow, I managed to forget that at the end of the week I would be leaving him. There was a small chance that his accounting firm could transfer him to Fiji, but I don't think either of us fully believed that. And in any case, at the age of twenty-three I was still a long way from contemplating a settled relationship. Far from it? It wasn't even on my radar.

I flew up to Auckland and met up with Parent – I knew I might never come back to New Zealand, in which case it was unlikely I would ever see him again. We stayed overnight in a motel with one bedroom and a sofa bed in the sitting room. Unused to family living, I thought little of it, and took it for granted. Parent made some quasi-humourless remark about the propriety of spending the night in a unit with a young blond which took me by surprise. He was a parent after all. But then, I wasn't too sure about what fathers did. I hadn't had one.

He did make one attempt at parenting though. Perhaps he felt it was his duty. "I don't know whether or not you are a virgin (I was twenty-three), if you are, I'm ashamed of you – but if you get caught I will disown you." As parenting went, it didn't amount to much. Maternal Parent's attempt some years before had been no better. In my late teens she had instructed me "don't let men touch you 'down there'" with a hand at waist level, pointing downwards. The rest I worked out for myself.

And so I left New Zealand, armed with an anticipated Ph D, three years of memories of a marvellous time, especially the exciting field work and the wonderful friends I had made, but stripped of one fantasy in the form of Male Parent.

Having chosen Fiji for my next destination, I had to return to London for the formal interview for the job. In preparation for my time in Fiji I was required to spend a week at Farnham Castle in Surrey, learning how to cope with "life working with the locals, and my role in the Colonies". It was probably one of the last bastions or remnants of historical 'Colonial thinking' in that area.

I planned my return trip to London. All my previous crossings of the globe had been by sea. This one was going to be by air. At this time such a trip, about twelve thousand miles and twelve time zones, was taken in four-hour stages. This meant there was just time to get settled on the plane, have a pre-meal drink, eat the meal, relax and read for a bit, and finally get ready for landing. It was permitted to break the journey at each landing point, and this I planned to do, staying over for one or two nights each time. On account of this I had planned my route most carefully. I made a brief stop in Fiji, my future destination, but only stopped in Nandi, on the west coast of the main island.

As a child, when going to New Zealand I had had the luck to stop off at Pitcairn Island en route, a place visited by only a very lucky few.

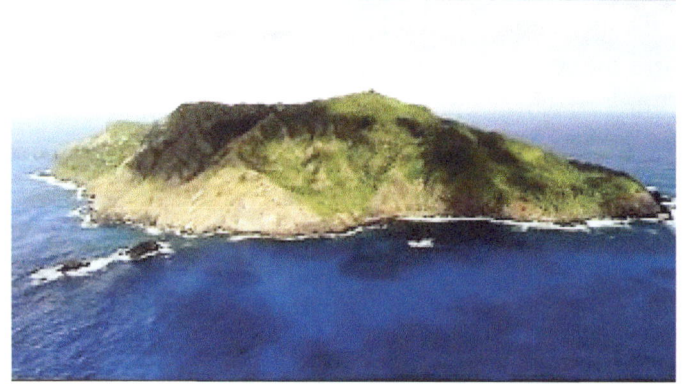

This memory intensified my fascination with the South Pacific islands, their peoples and cultures. It was further invigorated by my next stop on this trip – Hawaii, where I planned a slightly longer stay, partly so I could hear more of the Polynesian music that I had come to love. It also further stimulated my interest in both Polynesia and in geology.

Confusingly, the capital, Honolulu, where I stayed, is on Oahu, one of the smaller islands. It was very touristy, very American, but after the quiet of small-town Dunedin, it was also exciting. I then flew to the larger island of Hawaii and went to the rim of the Kilauea volcano, which was active at the time, to explore.

After that it was on to San Francisco where I had a delightful couple of days, and then it was New York, in tribute to Aunt. She had loved New York and spoke nostalgically of 'Greenwich Village'. Sad to say I found it disappointing. And so, back to London and Aunt. Wonderful. They had moved out of Sloane Square by then, bought a flat in Clapham, where I was invited to stay, and an enchanting cottage in the New Forest where we spent my few weekends.

During that time I received the devastating news that my proposed PhD thesis had been accorded the status of MSc. I was shocked, it was not what I had expected, and it took some getting over. Soon afterwards, however, I received a letter from the external examiner, Dr Hawkes of the US Geological Survey, congratulating me on my PhD. I replied, explaining the down-turn, and in his reply he expressed his surprise; he had thought it a good thesis. All of this salved my bruised soul, at least somewhat. Discussing it with BW sometime later, I learnt that he, and some others in the Dunedin Survey, put it down to sour grapes on the part of JR in return for my refusal to work on coal chemistry with him. But who knows?

Chapter 5

Fiji

After a couple of months it was time to get ready for my journey to Fiji. That autumn in England was cold. Farnham Castle seemed even colder. But the week I spent, not in the ruins but in the amazing hotel nearby, was great fun. Most of the others in the group were going out to be District Commissioners in various far-flung parts. I was, apparently, an interesting oddity being an academic, a lone female, and heading for the South Pacific. It all added to the fun.

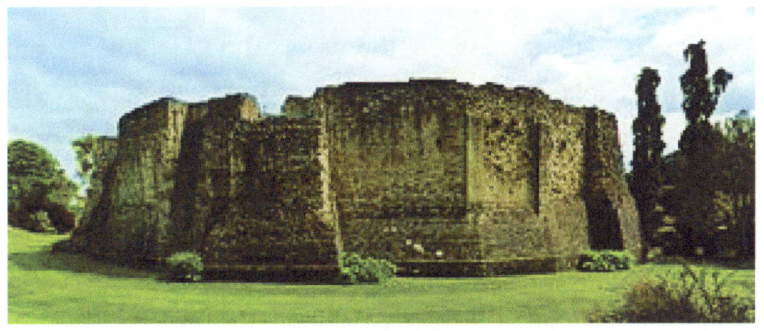

https://www.farnhamcastle.com/gallery

When it came to packing to leave the UK yet again, it took discipline and blind belief to travel wearing the coolest clothes tolerable for a cold departure from London, and pack only the coolest of summer clothes. The rest of my wardrobe I left behind in Aunt's garage. When we landed in Nadi (pronounced Nandi), Fiji's international airport, I was glad I had. It was hot, to me unimaginably hot, though at least it was dry heat. In Nadi we changed to a smaller plane for the flight across the main island to Suva, and greater humidity. I had read up on the Fijian climate and knew to expect the average daytime temperature in Suva to be between 75°F and nearly 90°F in the wet season from January to March, dropping to around

80°F from May to October. Night-time temperatures dropped only very slightly, from 73°F to 68°F. My cool temperate living to date had not prepared me for what this was going to be like in practice.

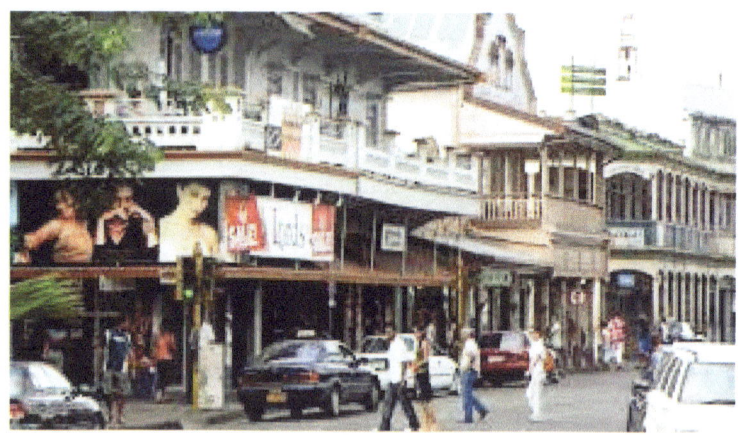

I was met at the airport by the wife of the Geological Survey's Director, who explained that the Director was busy. She drove me to the government apartment that had been organized for me. Here I could shed my very British stockings and court shoes and swap them for bare feet in sling-back sandals.

I was then taken to the Geological Survey offices to meet the Director and then the geologists. It turned out to be a very hierarchical structure, British Civil Service style, and the Director clearly planned to keep his distance. Fortunately, the geologists were a friendly crowd. I had been assigned a large laboratory plus the only air-conditioned office other than that of the Director himself. I was pleased to find that this was not for my personal benefit (as a woman perhaps? Heaven forbid, that would have been a bad start), but for the atomic absorption spectrophotometer. This was a delicate creature and would hardly have withstood the full blast of the Fijian climate. The office did, however, make me very popular in tea and lunch breaks as the geologists arrived to cool off.

I was assigned two Fijian women as laboratory assistants. A house girl had been arranged for me for the cleaning of my apartment, and a field crew had been selected as my support field assistants. The latter consisted of a 'Talking Chief'. It was explained to me that he would be my line of communication with the locals (Fijian or Indian) when I was doing fieldwork and that he would speak for me during the various ceremonies that would be required each time I passed through a village, even if that was only on my way to collect samples. I would also be accompanied by my house girl on these trips as it would, of course, be quite unseemly for me to travel with only men for company. All this the Director explained for me in somewhat strangled voice. He was clearly unhappy at my role in a male-only environment but was acting under instructions.

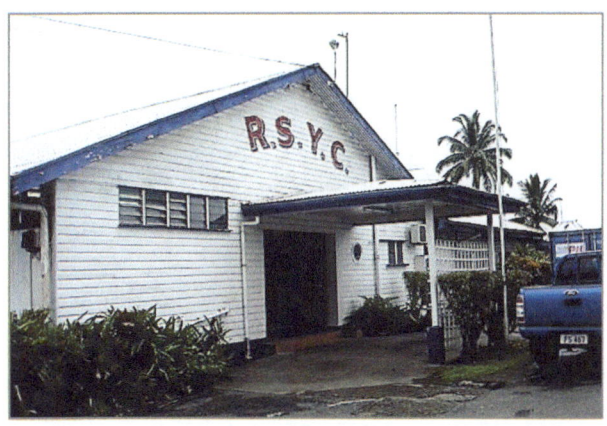

The next day I was introduced to what was to turn out to be the social hub of my life in Fiji, the Royal Suva Yacht Club. I had happily anticipated a chance for some real sailing, which I had enjoyed in both the UK and New Zealand, but that seemed to be a side issue. The main focus of the club was the extensive bar, lounge, and pool area where people met, mixed, mingled, and drank. In that climate, drinking was a constant activity, and inevitably it could involve a lot of alcohol, though I retained my disinclination to consume very much.

Being inherently British, conservative, and a traditionalist, that first evening I asked the wandering Fijian waiter for a glass of sherry, only to be somewhat taken aback when he asked if I wanted ice in it. Ice? In sherry? Clearly education was needed here. But I was soon put right and came to realize that it was *my* education that needed improvement. The climate dictated the ice and turned a warm drink suitable to cold climate lounges and drawing rooms into a refreshing alternative suitable to the dehydrating tropics. I was to spend many happy hours here, mixing and getting to know people, both those that lived in Fiji, and occasionally some of the tourists that flowed in and out of Suva on 'boat days'.

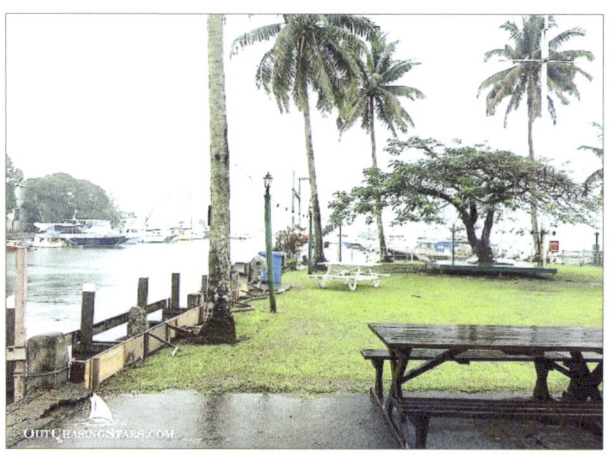

I quickly bought a car as it was the only way to get about. I was told that a Morris 1000 was the most practical for the roads. I bought one that had had only one owner and, in what was clearly a well-oiled rotating plan, was told that this could be sold back to the garage at an appropriate price when my contract in Fiji was finished. I was glad to have that possibility settled in advance.

I settled in and loved it. My first job was to equip and stock the laboratory which, when I arrived, was essentially an empty room with nothing but work benches, open shelves, a lead-lined fume cupboard at one end, and several sinks. Great. I was to prepare a list of all I would need. This would be airmailed (this being long before the days of the internet) to London and the items dispatched by sea. I set to.

Most of my list was accepted, understandably so, since none of them, including the Director, had any idea as to what I would be doing or need. However, there were some surprising crossings out and requests for a rewrite. I had come face to face with Civil Service bureaucracy. 'Test tubes' was to be rewritten as 'tubes, test' and similar transpositions of noun and adjective occurred throughout the list of equipment items. I felt a bit sorry for the chemical supply companies in England when they received this, but assumed they would understand, laugh, and pack what I needed. However, when it came to the list of chemicals I required, I stuck my heels in. Transferring 'hydrochloric acid' to acid, hydrochloric' might just have worked, but how was I to transpose 'sodium meta bisulphate' or 'hydroxylamine hydrochloride. I was pretty sure these and similar verbal contortions would only ensure that there were gaps in my supplies and therefore long delays before I had a fully operating laboratory. I bearded the lion's den, faced up to the Director, explained, and won the day.

My flat was furnished with standard government supplies: 1 bed, double; 1 table, dressing; 6 chairs, dining; 1 pan, frying, and so it went. I was required to sign them all off. After a quick trip into the few shops in Suva's main street for the necessary extras and a supply of food stuff, I was fully 'housed'. Getting used to the heat took a little longer, but I loved it, the more so once I had bought several of the locally correct 'shift' dresses. These were little more than simple tunics without sleeves or collars; cool, comfortable, and practical.

Having done all I could to order what I needed, it was time to get acquainted with the local roads. DS, a tough Ozzie field hand, oversaw the vehicles, and was quick to whisk me off for a day's exploring. I learnt later that he took me over the roughest roads he could find, which were plenty, to check whether or not I could drive his beloved heavy four-wheel drive Land Rovers in that terrain. However, I was used to them and simply enjoyed the experience, rather to his surprise. Then it was back to the office, more planning, field trips, and some small amount of sample collecting at local sites of interest until my laboratory supplies arrived and I could get to work properly.

Before leaving England, I had been given the names of various people who I should look up once I arrived in Fiji. They were variously friends or colleagues of my Australian or English friends. This relatively quiet spell at work made this the obvious time to do so. I soon realized there were hierarchies even here. Fairly early on I was invited to dinner at Government House, as were all English arrivals. However, your place at the tables depended on your status within the colony. Government officials ranked at the top, followed by professionals who worked merely with their heads. As a geochemist who, they assumed, grubbed around in the soil like the geologists, I came somewhat lower down on the list. The seating for dinner clearly reflected this. During a lull in the chatter, gossip, and stories, I felt it was my time to contribute.

"You know the story about two little babies in hospital?" I began. "One was a little boy baby and one was a little girl baby. The little boy baby turned to the cot with the little girl baby and asked, 'Are you a little girl baby or a little boy baby?' 'I don't know,' she replied, 'how do you tell?'" At this point the table became disconcertingly quiet, but I continued regardless. "'I'll tell you', said the little boy baby. He picked up his blankets and threw them down to the bottom of his bed. 'Look,' he said pointing down towards his feet, 'blue booties'." The laughter that followed was part amusement combined with a large amount of relief. Whatever did they expect me to say?

Two or three weeks later it was my turn to entertain the people who had offered me both friendship and introductions after my arrival. My six chairs, dining, plus another four chairs, casual, allowed me to have a dinner party for ten. Food preparation was simple with the luxury of my own dedicated house girl. The food was no problem: a cold avocado consommé, chicken casserole, followed by my specialty, a light and creamy cheesecake. The choice of wine presented a difficulty. In desperation I went to the local wine shop and faced up to racks of Australian wines about which I knew little. I resorted to the strategy of asking the shopkeeper, an Indian, which were the most popular wines. I was assured that top of the list was Barroso Pearl, a cool white. I bought, I chilled, I served, I toasted, I sipped, I blushed, and apologized. The best that could be said was that it was slightly better than flat lemonade. I explained my lack of knowledge of southern hemisphere wines, and thankfully was forgiven.

This was 1965. At this time Fiji was very much a British crown colony. I believe that the British, plus a few Australians and New Zealanders, made up something like five percent of the population. Of the rest, slightly more than fifty percent were Fijians. These lived mainly in rural areas and worked in labouring and other physical jobs that required their great strength. Slightly less than fifty percent were Indians, who worked in shops and offices. True to this division the Geological Survey office staff were largely Indian, and the field crews were almost entirely Fijian. I loved this too and enjoyed learning from all the groups.

Great excitement. My laboratory shipments arrived from England, all on the one boat, which was a small miracle. Why not from Australia, much closer? No, that would never do. "The colonies buy from England." I set up the lab and was ready for true field work and sample collecting.

At that time gold was the third income source for the colony, following tourism and sugar. Viti Levu is the largest island of the 353 that make up the country – I never did discover how large a cluster of rocks had to be before it could be called an island. On the north side of Viti Levu was a five-mile-diameter caldera, remnant of a long-inactive volcano. It was full of, and surrounded by six-foot-high sugar cane, which was to make soil sampling difficult. Along one edge of this caldera were the small township of Tavua, the workings of the gold mine, and the settlement of Vatukoula, ('gold rock' in Fijian). Emperor Mines had been established in the 1930s.

My job on this project was to set up multiple short sample lines 'radially parallel' along and around the caldera rim, looking for geochemical signs of a further gold deposit. The aim was to test the soil for selenium, a trace mineral commonly associated with gold. Selenium is much more active and mobile than gold and, it was thought, could be used as a marker or trace element indicator for gold deposits. I learnt years later that it had subsequently, unusually, and much to everyone's surprise, been found that tellurium had turned out to be a better indicator element. However, by then I was well on my way to my next assignment.

The days started early, in the relative cool of the early morning, but within no time we were all hot and dripping with sweat. Jeans were essential, as were long-sleeved shirts – to protect us from the sugar canes as much as from the sun. In fact, on average, there were only about six hours of direct sunshine in the day, as much of the time it was hidden by clouds. Trying to lay a grid by sound led inevitably to some very straggling lines, but we did the best we could, spacing the lines one or two hundred feet apart with samples sites every twenty-five feet along each line. The muscles of the Fijian crew were called into action for both digging and collecting, and then carrying the soil samples. At the end of the day, we would pile into the Land Rovers and drive back to the hotel, situated close to the mine offices. First stop was always the bar, no matter how hot and sweaty you were. The first lemonade shandy, my drink of choice, didn't even hit the sides and seemed to disappear almost without swallowing. Then it was shower, tidy, plot the samples sites and head back to the bar. The guys slept in the miners' huts, but I and SM, my inevitable Fijian female assistant, stayed in the hotel, me in a small room and she, somewhat to my disgust but apparently with her full approval, with the hotel staff.

I joined the mine and survey staff for dinner and seemed to fit in well enough. There was, of course, a lot of ribald humour, but I had learnt to take this in my stride and, I hope, give as good as I got. I certainly remember it, and almost all my stay in Fiji was a very happy time.

After a few weeks it was back to Suva to sort the samples and teach the two Fijian laboratory 'girls' how to analyze them. The process was very simple. It started with a hydrochloric acid extraction, which was followed by extraction of the selenium into an organic solvent. The density of the resultant colour of the selenium solvent complex was then measured on the spectrophotometer. There was much embarrassed giggling when I asked the women if they liked the work, but I gathered they did and were rather proud of their new and unusual skill.

Back in town, social life was very simple. The wives were in Fiji because of their husbands. They all had house staff, no jobs, and nothing much to do, so they played mahjong most of the day. The working day stopped around five, and getting home usually took less than ten minutes. The population of the whole of Fiji at that time was only 460,000 and the urban population less than a third of that, spread around numerous small towns and villages. Suva was not large back then. As a result, the pre-dinner drinks and meal were unfashionably early. By eight o'clock most of us were grouped round bridge tables with glasses of gin and tonic at our elbows. There was little choice and nothing much else to do. I do not recall a cinema. There were only two places to eat – the 'Grand Hotel' of course, which was uncomfortably formal and stuffy, and the steamy Chinese café which was hot and noisy. I mostly made my own meal and then joined whichever group of bridge players I was invited into. Luckily, I had rediscovered my love of the game, especially when it was combined with a great deal of chatter.

Having settled my team in Suva into their roles, it was time for more field work, this time on the west of Viti Levu, not far from Nadi. The coast road was little more than a dirt track that turned and twisted as it followed the stream-cut coastline. I was working on a manganese deposit but had the luxury of staying in Sky Lodge hotel. At that time there were three comfortable hotels set round the international airport. Back then the planes flew more slowly and had a reduced fuel capacity compared to today. As a result, the length of each segment of the flight was much shorter than today when you can go almost the whole way without stopping and certainly with no more than one stop. The hotels were filled with tourists and air crews, all breaking the long haul from either Sydney or Auckland to America or other points north. Of these,

Sky Lodge was where most of the aircrews stayed and was the most relaxed and fun. I stayed there too with DS, the vehicle manager, and any geologists.

The social area of the hotel was mostly the bar with some lounge seating around the edge, and a restaurant off to one side. This meant that I would come in from a day's hot and sweaty field work, stagger into the bar-lounge, tip at least one large cold shandy down my throat, head for my room along one of the open-air corridors, clean up, return to the bar, perch on a stool, and see who was there to chat to.

On one of my early visits, I got into conversation with a chap who worked at a local cigarette factory, either Rothmans or Marlboro, I think. He did his best to convert me to cigarette smoking, offering me an endless supply of free cigarettes. I accepted his offer but with no intention of taking up smoking. What I had quickly realized was that if I turned up at the bar, ordered a drink, and sat there looking around with nothing to do, I could be asking for trouble. There was a preponderance of predatory male flight crews looking for fun. It was much easier to have a cigarette in my hand and something to play with while I looked around and decided who I felt comfortable talking to, than be left staring into empty space. I duly puffed in and blew out, making sure none of it got far beyond my lips. The rest of the cigarettes he gave me I took back to Suva, and then passed on to smoking friends. He must have wondered that I never got sufficiently hooked to be converted into a paying customer.

The Fijian islands are mainly volcanic. Much of their coastline is surrounded by a stretch of flat-lying coral, underlain by a platform of coral only a few feet below the surface and extending possibly a hundred yards or more out into the ocean. One of our senior and best Fijian assistants, JL, had to be watched on the night of the full moon. If he was camped within a short distance of the sea, such that the moon was reflected along this low-lying surface, JL, with eyes tightly closed and arms outstretched, would walk straight out along the moon's path, with no apparent awareness of what he was doing or the danger he was welcoming. He had to be restrained or brought back.

Back on the east coast and Suva, there was laboratory work to be done and smaller field projects, one of which involved exploring the geochemistry associated with the manganese nodule on the west coast. The work remained varied and unpredictable.

There was also bridge to be played and a social life to be enjoyed, though precious few single males for company. The government was the major employer of the 'European' population, and most of these were married. This was followed by the 'bank boys', mostly young men who were sent out from banks based in New Zealand or Australia. They came to work in Suva for a year or two of fun and excitement. Several young Australian and New Zealand school teachers came too, but mostly lived in designated hostels rather than setting up home for themselves, as I had, and they were the ones who mostly complained of the lack of social life in the form of young men. I was definitely an oddity and fell into no particular group, but was happy to keep mixing with the general government staff, all the way from top officials, through clerical levels, to us 'grubby' geologists.

My working time in Suva was largely taken up with sorting, analyzing, and reporting on all the samples I had collected while in the field. There were also discussions with the geologists as our various disciplines cross-fertilized.

Then came the rainy season. Annual rainfall was 115 inches. This was somewhat spread out through the year, but most of it fell between December and March. We were on the edge of the monsoon belt, however, and the showers were generally brief and heavy and so quickly over. I was warned that from December to March it would be too hot and too humid for any sort of socializing. I doubted this, it seemed unlikely, but I was soon to learn the truth. It was so hot we all sweated like stuck pigs, and so humid that the sweat simply didn't evaporate. All I could do, each day of those three months of the wet season, was go to work and be thankful for my wonderful air-conditioned office and the need to keep my spectrophotometer cool, drive home, lie on my bed, take intermittent cold showers and wait for morning. Activity was not an option. Both entertaining and socializing would have been intolerable. In time this season passed, however, and life returned to normal, in so far as living in Fiji could be termed 'normal'.

I took a great interest in the various Pacific islands and races – the Melanesians, Polynesians, and Micronesians – and scoured the local library for books on them, both fiction and nonfiction. I was fascinated by the whole history of the area, and this fascination was to continue for some years, even after I left the islands.

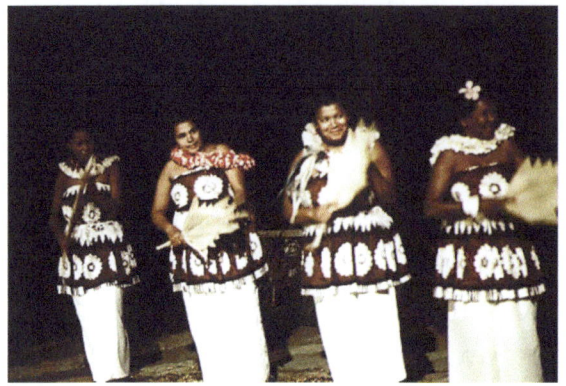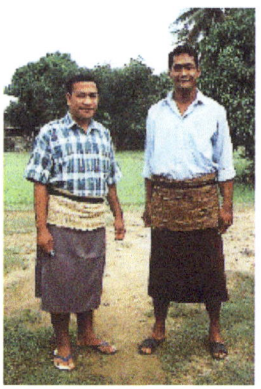

formal Fijian costume   informal Fijian wear

During this time, the local shipyard had been building a boat for the Geological Survey. It was to be used for fieldwork between the islands. Because I was the only woman on the professional staff, I was asked to launch it. I was delighted to oblige but saddened that there was to be no champagne. Instead, I was to use yangonna, a peppery drink made from crushed and pulverized roots and stems of piper methysticum, a plant common in most of the Pacific islands. The roots and stems were pounded, mixed with water and made into a non-alcoholic beverage known generally as yangonna on Fiji and kava kava in most of Polynesia.

On the appointed day I chose a long shift dress. This was 1965 and slacks were unacceptable except when I was actually in the field. I was anticipating the heights or gymnastics that might be asked of me as I slung the appropriate liquid at the prow of our small boat. The ship-yard was large, as much of the local travel was done by sea and most people were boat owners of some sort. It was crowded with both the Fijian boat builders and Indian office workers, all come to observe the fun, happy to have a bit of a break and to see what this spectacle might produce. I was shown a tall and somewhat unsteady looking ladder propped against the side of the boat, and given a half coconut shell full of yangonna.

I was schooled as to what to say. As far as I can recall, it was, or sounded like "I name this boat ndau ni vatu, may god bless all who sail in her". Knowing Fijian pronunciation, it was probably something close to that. I accepted the coconut shell I was given, laden with the libation, and started to climb the ladder that was leaning against the hull, only to find that, even perched on the highest step on which I dared to balance, I was below the deck of the boat. It seems no one had thought of this. Nor had they thought of the breeze, albeit light, that was blowing from the direction of the boat to me. I was glad that I had opted to wear a long straight shift and not a short or gathered one. With no other option I used a strong overarm toss hoping most of the yangonna would go over the boat, and ducking slightly as some was blown back my way. Ignoring this, I managed to announce in clear tones "I name this ship ndau ni vatu, may God bless all who sail in her" as instructed. There was a short silence, then a collective sigh, and finally clapping and cheers. I clambered down carefully, joined our staff and enquired about the slight silence and then the sigh. It seems that what I said did have the correct pronunciation. Had I failed in this, and said "I name this ship *nda* ni vatu..." etc. I would have been naming it 'Master of Gallstones' instead of 'Master of Rocks'. I could see why that would have made for some leg-pulling, and I am glad I got it right and it did not go down as a piece of geological hilarity.

The boat was quickly put into use. I was scheduled to work on the Yasawa islands, a chain of about twenty volcanic islands arcing round the north west of Viti Levu. It was a simple boat with two low bunks such that two people lay with their feet to the prow and just enough room between them for a small door that led to 'the heads'. This was for the sole use of Serima, my house girl, and me, though privacy was limited as you had to back into it in a squatting position and pull the door to before you could use it. The men used a sling over the aft end of the boat. The engine room was to the rear and there was a small space between it and the bunks for cooking on an open Primus stove.

In addition to SM, there was my Rotuman- talking chief-come-field assistant, the boat's captain, and his off-sider. We met up in Lautoka on the west coast where I was introduced to the local District Commissioner. The Yasawas have since become very modernized with large hotels and a strong tourist pull, but back then the only way to get there was either on our own boat or that used by the District Commissioner. There were certainly no hotels, and no buildings other than the beautiful Fijian huts made in the traditional style. I was told that the islanders almost never left these small islands and had almost certainly seen no other white person than the DC, and certainly not a white woman before. That I was leading this small expedition was going to startle them even more than the sight of me.

We set off, reached the first island and then established the pattern that was to be followed for the next few weeks. The crew man would row the Rotuman and me so that we could land on the island. The two of us would then start walking round the coastal shore of the island. Each time we came to a stream running down off the volcanic peaks, I was to collect river and sediment samples. This sounds simple, but the fact that most river mouths, however small, were occupied by dense mangroves complicated this to a certain extent. The fact that mangrove crabs roamed up and down the mangrove stems made you careful where you put your hands as you hauled yourself through the mangrove 'trees'. Hot, wet, muddy, and sticky, we would then emerge onto the further bank, collecting samples at suitable points, and soon afterwards, repeat the whole process.

The crewman and the dinghy stayed off the island at the edge of the underwater coral shelf, fishing, though usually throwing the fish back. When those of us on the land deemed it was time for lunch, we would wave to him. He would collect up his fishing haul and row back to the boat where SM would cook the very fresh fish in coconut milk. Then we would be collected and taken back to the boat in perfect time for the meal. I doubt I have ever had better lunches, certainly not while doing field work.

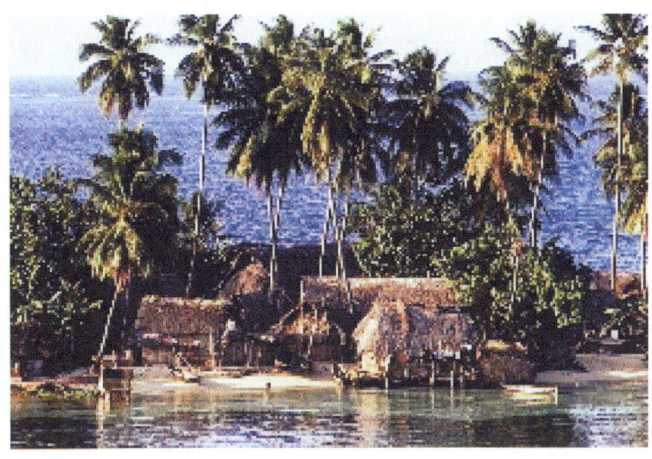

Progress was slow, as frequently there was a small village, or at least a collection of huts, at the mouth of each river of any size. When this happened, we had to follow the expected procedure. Our arrival, after all, was a major and significant event for them. We would gather, the Rotuman, SM (who occasionally accompanied me) and I, and sit politely on the floor facing the local Fijian chief and some of his elders. Yangonna would be prepared, the local Fijian chief would give a speech of welcome, and in return my talking chief would make a speech on my behalf. Yangona would be passed to each of us in coconut shells. The completion of this indicated that we each respected the other in their respective homes, the visitors and the hosts becoming 'one people' with a common purpose.

SM, if she was present, would feel it her duty to be protective of me and to drink the yangonna for me, something she hated, and that women generally did not do. I assured her there was no need, that I could both drink the peppery liquid and, equally important, stand up afterwards. If I had some difficulty, it was usually from the cramp of sitting cross-legged for so long, nothing to do with the drink, although it was supposed to have some intoxicating effect. I did feel that, as leader of our group and the first white woman that many if not all of them had seen, I had a duty to perform correctly.

I was, however, thankful for SM's offer come the evening meal. Some nights we were spared the boat (uncomfortable and unstable) and would be invited to stay in the village chief's bure (pronounced mbure) or hut. Dinner would then be shared. It generally consisted of freshwater eels that were abundant in the rivers, and a nameless green aquatic plant, somewhat akin to a freshwater spinach, but not nearly so tasty. SM loved them both and was perfectly happy to eat my share as well, for which I was very grateful.

I was used to fieldwork, I was used to being in strange or new parts of the world, I was used to fending for myself. It took one incident to remind me that SM was not. Her life had been entirely focused within a large and protective family that was firmly based in Suva and always on the main island of Fiji. One night we were offered the chief's house. This, as usual on these islands, consisted of only the one 'room' or space. SM and I being in it meant that the Chief and his family had moved out elsewhere. This was normal Fijian hospitality and I accepted it as such. Anything else would have been seen as insulting. The lighting was by a paraffin lamp and this was placed between the two sleeping 'beds' and beside a small window with curtains on each side. There was an old iron bedstead with iron springs, which I ignored since it promised no comfort whatsoever, and was possibly only a status symbol. The walls were hung with several photos (or newspaper cuttings) of Queen Victoria, also a common sighting. SM insisted she wanted the lamp left on through the night, a symptom of her apprehension. I agreed. An hour or two later we were suddenly woken from sleep by a crash, and I opened my eyes to darkness and my ears to SM's scream. I responded with "Don't worry, it's all right, just the curtain blowing the lamp over" and thoughtlessly went straight back to sleep. On waking I discovered that Serima had been truly terrified and had lain awake for the rest of the night fully expecting goodness knows what. When I talked this through with her the next morning and asked her reasons, she said "Men, they do strange things to women". Clearly, the time had come for me to stress my authority: "Don't worry. No one will hurt you when I am here. I am white woman, I am English, I am head of this expedition. No one will hurt you with me here." It may not have been politically correct (not then a current concept), but it certainly worked. "Oh thank you, marama" she said, and relaxed visibly, a state that continued for the rest of our time working together.

Many more field trips followed in the months ahead.

I thoroughly enjoyed my time in Fiji. I enjoyed the field work and exploring the islands. I enjoyed the people I worked with. I loved the climate, though perhaps not the wet season, and thoroughly enjoyed the social life and the relaxed living style. I was particularly interested in learning all I could about the south pacific islands and their different histories and cultures: Micronesian, as my Rotuman field assistant claimed to be, Melanesian (Fijians) and Polynesian (such as those from Tahiti). However, I was aware that my time there would soon be coming to an end, by pre-ordained design. Fiji was heading for independence and the change from colonial rule to local rule.

My next job was to train my successors. Indian geologists would take over the geochemical-related field work and sample collecting. A new member of staff would take on the analytical laboratory work. I was introduced to the man they had chosen, and this presented problems from the start. I did my best, but there seemed to be no way I could establish a co-operative and positive relationship or handover. I put this down to the fact that he was male and I was female. He was well into his forties and I was only twenty-six. He was local (Indian) and I was not from Fiji. I had two degrees in chemistry at that stage, and he had none, only some school science. He was hell bent from the start on proving that he knew more than I, that he did not need to be trained, and that he had better ways of doing the analytical testing than my ways.

For a while he watched what I did and listened to what I said, but he mostly took few real notes and did not participate, brushing me aside with "Yes I know all that" when clearly he didn't. I was determined to complete the analysis of almost all the samples I had collected, plot the results and complete my reports before I left. That I did. Then, and under instructions, I left him to it. He had all the samples I had collected on the last field trip and would reanalyze them himself.

In those days we did a simple organic extraction of the sediments, using isoamyl alcohol, chloroform, carbon tetrachloride and other similarly volatile and unpleasant smelling chemical solvents. It was not realized at the time just how toxic and carcinogenic they were. Nonetheless, these extractions were normally done in the very large fume cupboard that covered most of the far wall of the laboratory. This was essentially a regular work bench lined with lead, with glass ends and glass sliding doors along the front. The top fans extracted the unpleasant fumes. In our analysis we were looking for tiny amounts of copper, zinc, selenium, and other trace nutrients that were complexed with appropriate reagents such that the product was coloured and extracted into the organic layer. The depth of the colour indicated the amount of the trace nutrient present. For other work, we prepared the extract and then sprayed the solution into the atomic absorption spectrophotometer flame, and using the appropriate element tubes, could measure the amount of colour in the flame and correlate this to the amount of the element we were testing for.

The amounts of these elements were tiny. We were looking for levels of parts per million, or, in the case of water samples, parts per billion. Once the test was done, the test tube contents were emptied into the sink. Because of the preliminary extraction process there was essentially none of the minerals left in the solution. Nonetheless, we rinsed the tubes thoroughly with distilled water. Any further testing of the pure water in the tubes invariably and correctly came up with blanks, showing that there was no contaminate or residue in the tubes.

This is where the trouble really started. Our new man decided that this procedure was not good enough; the test tubes had to be washed in hydrochloric acid (quite unnecessary), that it had to be concentrated hydrochloric acid (not only unnecessary but dangerous), and furthermore they had to be 'cooked' in boiling hydrochloric acid, not just washed out with it (possibly counterproductive). I could see a terrible accident happening here and I warned my two Fijian lab assistants who were looking predictably frightened and wanting me to intervene. I announced that the procedure was entirely unsafe. The Director then came along the outside corridor from which he could see in, and told me to let my planned replacement get on with it, and that he wanted to talk with me. We retired to my office next door without a sight-line to what was happening in the laboratory.

Soon after, there was uproar. "Marama, Marama, come quick, there has been a terrible accident." Loosely translated and in that context this meant, "boss lady, boss lady, come quick…" I did just that, and the Director, a confirmed civil servant (coward?), stood well back. The new chemist had decided to fill a metal saucepan with as many test tubes as he could pack in, fill them and the rest of the saucepan with concentrated (fuming) hydrochloric acid, and set the whole thing on a metal tripod with a lit Bunsen burner flame under it; all of this sitting on the lead base to the fume cupboard.

Any school student of even elementary chemistry will be able to predict the disaster. The hot and concentrated acid ate through the metal saucepan and then partly through the metal tripod. This then collapsed and the contents of broken glass from the tubes, and the hot and fuming hydrochloric acid, were tipped onto the lead floor of the fume cupboard, which started to dissolve in its turn. Acid, broken glass, and bits of melting metal went everywhere, and the entire laboratory was filled with toxic and corrosive acid fumes. I got the two girls out of the place, away from the fumes and into my air-conditioned office, thankful that I had it, even though its prime purpose was to protect my electronic equipment. I left the chemist to clear up. The Director said it was not a problem, and the man would surely learn. I figured his learning had so far to go that there would be many more mishaps to come. But it was clearly not my place to interfere. The Director was set on his choice of staff and I would be leaving shortly.

Eventually the time came for me to pack up and return to London. I thought about the car I had bought when I arrived and was wondering how to go about selling it. I was reminded that the sales people had confirmed they would buy it back when I came to leave the islands. With so many people coming to Fiji on one-year or two-year contracts, this was apparently a normal procedure. All I had left to do was have a massive farewell party, great fun as always, pass round all the possessions, food, and drink, that I would be leaving behind, and pack up my two or three trunks.

I went first to the docks, headed for Nadi and then for the airport and my plane home. When I had returned from New Zealand to London a couple of years earlier, I had planned my route most carefully, spending time in Fiji, though only one night and only in Nadi, then time in Hawaii and various cities across America, finishing up in New York. This time I planned to return to England by a different route. I flew from Fiji to Tonga, then Samoa both East and West, then Tahiti, Acapulco in Mexico, Jamaica, and Bermuda. That was quite a trip and added a number of places to my previous list of Pacific islands and the countries I had visited. At the time of writing, this total stands at sixty-four countries. This included my childhood visit to Pitcairn Island and my more recent visit to Hawaii. Now that I had been living within this greater island group, I was in the ideal setting to learn more about it, all of it – the various migrations from west to east, and more, and the very different influences that had come to bear. I had, in the previous years, read a great deal about all the places in which I was interested, and I was now keen to see these places for real.

Tonga was something of a disappointment. All the Polynesian character seemed to be missing. The English Church was paramount. I stayed for a few nights with a couple of school teachers. Nothing but religion was allowed on a Sunday – no running, no laughing, no ball throwing, or similar play. Nor could you be seen to be doing any housework or hanging clothes out to dry.

I flew from Tonga to Samoa and was surprised to find I was the only passenger on the plane – a large commercial one, though I don't recall what type. I was reminded that Queen Salote of Tonga had just died and that her extensive family members and friends, now dispersed around the globe, had been flown back to Tonga for the funeral and related events. They had chartered this plane. The plane had delivered the people to Nuku'alofa, Tonga's capital, and was now flying back, empty, to its base. As such it was an unscheduled flight and had not been offered to regular tourists, but since the date coincided with the specific date I had chosen, I had been given a seat on it.

I was moved up to first-class, of course. Would I like champagne? Of course. Would I like to visit the captain and sit in the cockpit? Of course, of course. It was a magical flight.

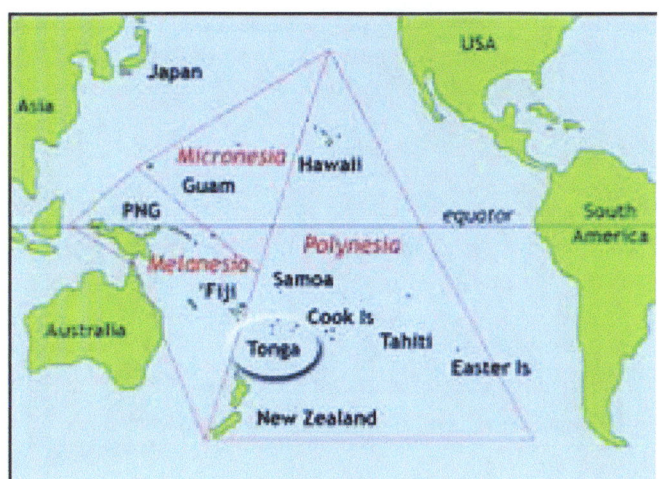

Samoa I loved. It had all the Polynesian magic I expected, the relaxed lifestyle, casual clothes, the warmth and friendliness. I loved the traditional Fale homes, circular structures with a conical roof. They had, no walls, but did have blinds round the sides that could be let down for protection from the weather, or perhaps for privacy. The reality of it blended perfectly with all the reading I had done.

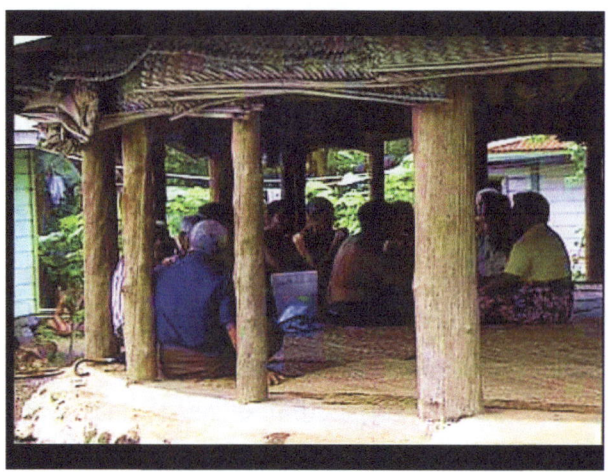

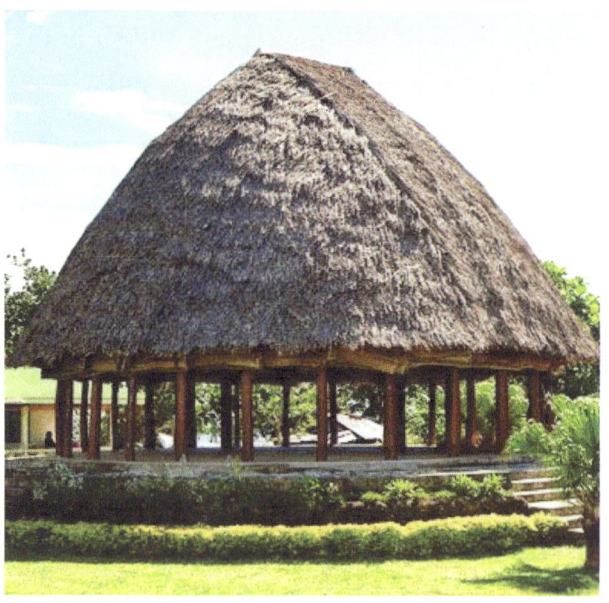

I made the short hop to American Samoa and back, but it was very different. I was interested in the contrast, but disappointed. In American Samoa the scenery was dominated by large hoardings advertising Coco Cola, and open-topped American cars – Studebakers, Cadillacs, being driven at crazy speeds along ridiculously short lengths of unnecessarily wide and tarmacked roads. It fell far short of the lovely Polynesian Samoa, largely left to itself.

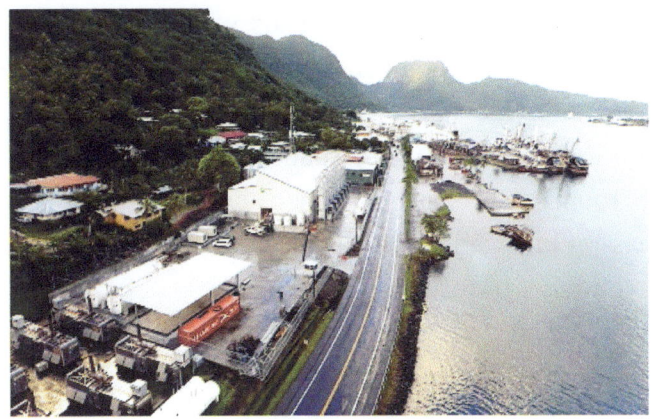

American Samoa

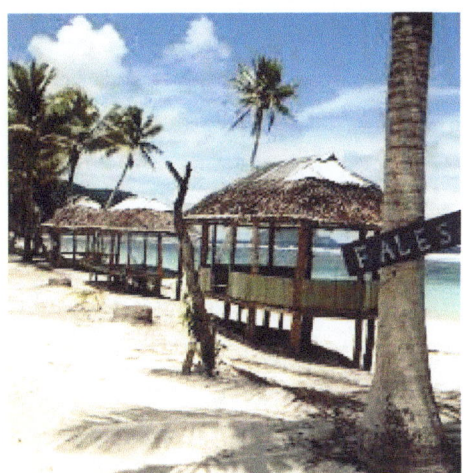

Polynesian Samoa

I was to find it was similar in other parts of Polynesia. The Americans in Hawaii had a very different impact when compared with the French in Tahiti. The Hawaiians had been absorbed into or seduced by relatively American ways of life. In Tahiti the Europeans had been relatively much more absorbed into the largely-unchanged Tahitian way of life.

Back in Apia, the main town in Western Samoa, I hired a scooter and explored the island.

Flying on to Tahiti I made friends with an English girl on the plane. She was travelling on her own as her friend had stayed behind in New Zealand. She was very apprehensive about this and was delighted to have company. I persuaded her to hire a scooter too and we drove round the Island together, exploring and enjoying the 'Frenchness' of this version of Polynesia.

Then I took off for Acapulco. I was keen to see the cliff diving. After a relaxed day on the beach, I was absorbed into a group of holiday makers and enjoyed a sociable evening, waking just in time the next day to catch my flight to Jamaica. Aunt had married her first husband before the Second World War and they had lived in Jamaica, so a couple of nights in Kingston were an essential part of my trip, as was collecting some real Jamaican Blue 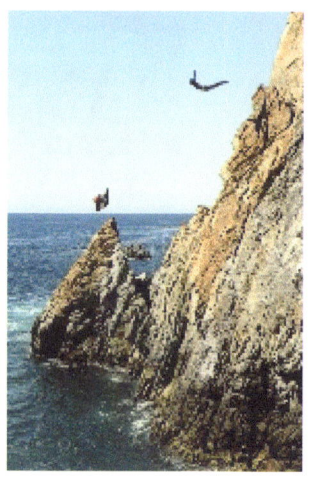 Mountain coffee beans that she loved. I enjoyed Jamaica, at least as it was then in 1966, but decided I could have skipped Nassau and Bermuda. Compared to the Pacific islands they left a lot to be desired. Then it was back to London, and Aunt.

Chapter 6

Imperial and Research

B ack in London I was not sure what I was going to do next, but my preference was for research. I was lucky in my searching for jobs. In those days only about three or four per cent of school leavers made it to university. A greater proportion went to technical colleges, teacher training colleges, apprenticeship training, or else straight into jobs that did not require higher education. Armed with a IIA degree from Imperial, I maintained a quiet confidence that I could get a job as, when, or where I wanted, though I think this 'quiet confidence' was based on events until this time, rather than arrogance. And so it turned out to be. It was rather as if something inside of me waited each time at these pivot points, to see what would turn up. Later, I was to liken this, and similar points in my life, to a case of waiting for my personal red carpet to roll out and show me where I was going to go next.

As a first stop, I went like a homing pigeon to stay with Aunt and her husband, rightly confident that she would be delighted to see me back. She had remained the one certainty in my peripatetic life, the relationship being enhanced and strengthened by the hour-long audio tapes we continued to send out to each other most weeks.

She found me a bed-sitting room and I moved in. In the style of the times, it was complete with single bed, one gas ring for single-saucepan cooking, one comfortable chair, and the use of a shared bathroom. All pretty normal in those days, and at least it was in Sloane Square. I needed no more until I knew what I would be doing.

Aunt had been living in Sloane Gardens when I was a student. I had come to live a couple of miles away, in South Kensington, when I was at Imperial. It is no surprise therefore that this edge of SW3 had become my favourite part of London. I had escaped there when I left home and Guildford. It was the place where I had first been happy or felt loved, liked, and welcomed. I had happy memories built around it – on top of which, of course it is a delightful part of London. In those days it was not so very much more expensive than other parts farther out, and definitely affordable to a student if you were willing to live in a cramped bed-sit, or share a small flat, as I was. It gave me a welcome and a sense of 'home'. By this time Aunt had moved south to a lovely house with half an acre of garden close to Reigate and Banstead.

When it came to looking for the next step in my career, inevitably my first stop was to the chemistry department at Imperial. Here I spoke with Professor West in the Analytical Chemistry department. I was fortunate, very fortunate. Within a couple of months I was given a research grant, a place in his laboratory, and a very small living grant. I was delighted, even though 'very' was the operative word in relation to 'small'. On account of the very reasonable income I had had in both New Zealand and Fiji, and on which I had lived comfortably, I did have a certain amount saved, although less than I might have had as I had travelled a lot. However, I had been trained well in the ways of living on a very tight budget by the exceedingly frugal arrangement that had been made for me from the start of my teens. Perhaps as a result of this, I have never made money a major consideration or driving force in my life. I saw no need to have more clothes than I could wear, and it never occurred to me that I could buy happiness by having more possessions. For the pure joy of being back at Imperial, with a place in a chemistry laboratory, I would definitely manage to live within my means.

My grant would be £11.00 a week. My rent was £7-10s. That left very little. I would make it work. I would have to. I badly wanted to take up this opportunity. A couple of years doing research into analytical chemistry at Imperial was too enticing to pass up. I managed, and found creative (and honest!) ways of managing. But it was going to be tight. In the meantime, I did some office work in the chemistry library until the academic year started and my grant kicked in.

I needed a car. That was not negotiable. Aunt lived in Chipstead by then. I would want to spend lots of time with her at weekends, and public transport was impractical. She worked with a friend, running Garden House School, off Sloane Square, and so for the next two years I would meet up with her for occasional lunches at Peter Jones. But I would definitely need a car to get to their house at the weekends. I bought the cheapest vehicle I could find, a Minivan, because in those days vans did not attract sales tax. Even so, that was another thirty shillings a week. That left only two pounds a week for eating and everything else.

Somehow, I managed. I gave dinner parties for six people on six ounces of lamb. This was all I could peel, flake by flake, out of the carved roast leg they had for Tuesday lunches at the school where Aunt taught and which she kindly gave me to take home after the lunchtime carving. I mixed this with onions and herbs and stuffed it into handmade ravioli; it provided a main course. The North End Road market closed at four-thirty on a Saturday. I was to be seen there at four-fifteen, racing round the vegetable stands and gathering up all the food they were virtually giving away, knowing it would not last until Monday.

On one occasion I saw avocado pears going for only pennies. Wow. How sophisticated, even elegant. I could serve up halves with a sauce. Back at home, I realized there was a problem. In all three avocadoes there was not a single half that did not contain a bad bit that had to be cut out. Quick change of plan. I scooped out all the good flesh, mashed that in with chicken stock (one cube), a few tablespoons of sherry and served it with a dollop of cream filched from the dish to be used for the dessert of fruit salad – the fruit also put together from the best of the fruit that I could retrieve from my nearly-old purchases. Faced with this green soup, the five guests, knowing or guessing something of my financial state, obviously thought "Ah well, pea soup is at least filling". Their delight after the first mouthful was wonderful! Sherry? An expense? Not really, it is in fact a lot cheaper than a bottle of wine, for the number of drinks it provides. I counted the pennies, walked rather than took public transport, got very fit, and had great fun. And, of course, I walked to Imperial, less than half a mile away from my flat, every day.

I settled back into life in the chemistry department. I was working on aspects of atomic absorption spectroscopy and trace mineral analysis, with a view to using this as a skill in future geochemical jobs, but in fact I didn't find it very interesting. I also found that while Imperial as an undergraduate had been enormous fun, being back there at twenty-six was very different. Most of my fellow research students were married, lived some distance away, and seemed rather duller. Or perhaps I was too used to mixing with people in so many different settings who were not focused on 'settling down'.

I was lucky in meeting up with the librarian in the Chemistry library, and through her I met some interesting people. As part of this, I was encouraged to sit the Mensa exam. I did this, thinking that there I might meet people who were really interesting. Sadly, this was to be a disappointment. Many of the people I met up with that way clearly did have a high IQ, but they had not necessarily found a comfortable niche for themselves. One was teaching maths at a boys' school and hated it. Another was a cleaner.

Then I heard about evening nutrition courses at Queen Elizabeth College and enrolled. They fascinated me. I learned a lot about nutrition, even though it was the very conventional nutrition of the dietetic way of thinking. Nonetheless, it was to stand me in good stead. It was the start of my thinking along lines of more sensible sustenance and the maintenance and restoration of homeostasis and good health. In fact, it was the start of opening my mind to naturopathic ideas.

This was the time of concern about the food and diet available to what were then thought of as 'Third World Countries'. I joined a study group. The particular concern was to provide poorer countries with a more protein-rich diet. Our project concerned making simple hand-turned equipment to extract the protein from various plants, one of which involved cauliflower stems. Other ideas were suggested, but the problem remained one of how to encourage villagers in far-flung countries to include these new and exotic foods into their traditional fare. The major emphasis at the time was on finding markets for the surplus milk powder of many western countries. Further investigations have since suggested that in fact the real problem at the time was a lack of the actual *amount* of food available, not just a lack of protein.

I was not familiar with vegetarian diets. They were not a concept I knew much about, with one exception. At a Girl Guide camp I had taken part in, a visiting Guider was a vegetarian and her choice was simply to replace the meat on our plates with some white bread, butter, and jam. That definitely had no appeal to me and I had not tried it. However, I did realize that vegetable-rich protein foods were a lot cheaper than meat and fish, and this definitely interested me. This focus on foods set me to exploring the essential amino acids and ways of combining vegetable proteins (cheap) to replace animal proteins (expensive) for incorporation into my limited food budget.

One of the text books I acquired at that time remains in my library to this day.[i] *Food Nutrition and Diet Therapy* by Marie Krause enabled me to work out the cheapest way of adding a proper amino acid balance to my diet. Another one,[ii] *Proteins: Their chemistry and Politics* by Aaron M Altschul also fascinated me. This project provided interesting biochemistry and was also useful in relation to my very tight budget. At home I became a near vegetarian, although when eating out I included fish and poultry. I have never much liked red meat and that dislike has remained. Some years later[iii], 1971, I read *'Diet for a Small Planet'* by Francis Moore Lappé and learnt more about amino acid balancing. My interest in nutrition aroused, I started to explore the offerings (very few) of the local health food shop (very small). B-complex supplements were mostly brewer's yeast, for instance, and the vitamin shelf was only a few feet long. Nevertheless, I found it interesting and continued to study.

In an effort to increase the scope of my chemical research I looked for further available applications of the trace element analysis I was working on. I did some work with the Agriculture Department, also in the Royal College of Science building, and under the professorship of the apply named Professor Cornfield. However, this did not come to much.

I came to recognize that I was not keen on 'pure chemistry'. What I really enjoyed was applied chemistry: geochemistry and its application to rocks, soil, mining opportunities, and more; food, amino acids, and how to supply the most nutritious needs at viable prices; ways of increasing the nutrient content of foods. I gave health little thought in those days, being young and having always had robust health myself. But it was already clear to me that truly improving good health would not be accomplished by the use of a variety of drug medicines with health warnings and toxic side-effects listed on the packages. I automatically and instinctively took the view of an applied chemist and figured that restoring normal chemistry would have a better chance of restoring optimal health.

From a family and emotional perspective, this two-year period was a wonderful time. During that time Aunt and I cemented our friendship and she became my whole family. Male parent was a distant memory and in New Zealand. Female parent was to be avoided as far as possible, unless I had to deal with her periods of incarceration. Brother came to Imperial two years after me and did Engineering. I loved him dearly, but he was a cool customer and impossible to get close to emotionally. It had been the same during our childhood – I took on the problem of a manic-depressive parent and he withdrew from it, as he could, being younger. Our time at Imperial had overlapped by one year, but inevitably we moved in different circles. Then I was in New Zealand, or Fiji. By the time I came back to London he and five friends had graduated and were driving across Europe and Asia, camping or living cheap as they went – you could do that then. He completed that trip in Asia, sailed to Darwin and worked there.

Thus, this two-year period in London was hugely enriched by the time I spent with Aunt, mostly at weekends but often with lunches or the occasional evening in town. She had a large garden, almost an acre, and I was in for a surprise. I had only ever known her for any length of time when she was living in a London flat. No garden. She had grown cacti on the kitchen window sill, but even that had not warned me. Now that she had a garden, she spent all the time she could out there.

Without giving it much thought, I had automatically assumed that when I went down for the day we would be spending the time indoors, talking, or whatever. After all it was autumn and cold outdoors. Not a bit of it. Each time I arrived she was in the garden preparing ground, weeding, digging, planting, and so on. I would stand around for a while chatting and hoping she would finish soon and come indoors. But no. She kept going. I kept getting colder and colder. Seeing me shiver she encouraged me to go back indoors. Hmm. Clearly the only way to be sharing time with her, unless it was pouring with rain, or dark, would be if I offered to help in the garden, an activity that was totally foreign to me. It wasn't much fun, but being with her was, so I did it.

Aunt took my involvement for interest and enjoyment, and suggested that I have a plot of my own. There was plenty of space at the bottom of the garden which I could use. Oh no! She marked it off, about fifteen feet by twenty. It seemed huge. It was huge. It was also covered with grass and occasional other vegetation that I could not identify – weeds. What was I to do with it? Growing vegetables had immediate appeal as that would ease my food budget. And so it became a pattern – she told me what to do and I did it. I didn't much enjoy the actual gardening, but I did enjoy sharing a project with her. Gradually I dug the ground over, cleared the weeds, raked and levelled the area and neatened the edges. Aunt gave me seeds, told me about composting, and added advice and information with each succeeding weekend. Fortunately, in time, I did become an enthusiast.

Eventually I wanted to spend more time gardening than one day a week or weekend. Together she and I considered the terrace outside my flat in London. It was probably about fifteen feet at the widest point, adjacent to the house, going down to a narrow end of about six feet, twenty feet away. Concrete. Walled on all sides. I had no money to spare so buying expensive pots was not an option. What I did have was my Minivan. What they had was a collection of flat wooden boxes. Each had been made to take either long mirrors or family portraits from their London flat down to their house in the country, in safety. They were now standing empty in Aunt's garage. Uncle suggested I could have them. We started slowly. Each time I was there we loaded the van with these boxes, destined to become large flat growing or planter beds, and then added sacks of earth plundered from the bottom of their garden. To this we added sacks of their home-grown compost. Each time we loaded up the van it seemed like a huge amount. Each time I unloaded the van and maneuvered this onto my terrace garden it seemed puny. Eventually, however, through that winter, I had enough compost and enough boxes to line both sides of the terrace with them, and across the far end. Luckily this space faced south and so had as much sun as England could offer. Against each side of the French doors I put smaller boxes or individual tubs, the sort she had bought plants in from the garden centres.

Aunt was very generous. Somehow, she always managed to have several seedlings left at the end of the day, and would say "oh, you take these, dear, there are more than I have room for". And so I would return to my flat and terrace with clusters of seedlings, various types of lettuce, tomatoes, leeks, spring onions, various herbs, and more – but not the large ones, broccoli, cabbage, and cauliflowers. These I continued to grow in my plot in her garden. Carrots, onions, shallots, and more I also sowed or planted in London. Peas and beans went in along the terrace walls and grew over them. Herbs grew in any vacant space and were available for harvesting close to the kitchen. Aunt had offered to water my plot on her land when I wasn't there, and in London I carried buckets of water through my studio room, to the terrace, doing my best not to walk mud through. Somehow it all worked and in time I thoroughly enjoyed it.

My research grant was for two years and at the start of the second spring I began to consider my next move. I still felt certain of getting a job, or even of having a choice of job offers, and I was lucky. Aunt and I regularly did the cryptic crossword in her copy of the Daily Telegraph. A newspaper was an extravagance I could not afford, but she generally encouraged me to take the Saturday paper back to London with me, insisting that in a few hours' time she would be deluged with the Sunday papers.

On one occasion I noticed a job being advertised in the West Australian Geological Survey. It was for a senior geochemist at a salary three times that of a new graduate. This was major, and of course I was pretty sure they would want someone a lot more senior and experienced than I was, at only twenty-seven. However, I watched the space, and when the advertisement was still there a few weeks later, I decided to apply. In no time I was offered the position, no interview required! Would I please arrange to be in Perth at my earliest convenience. The necessary government paperwork and authorizations would follow shortly.

I spoke with my professor and we wrapped up my current research. I wrote a dissertation, hoping for and subsequently being awarded a DIC (Diploma of Imperial college). A DIC was, at least at that time, somewhat akin to an MSc, but I already had that from my time in New Zealand. In addition, Professor West and I wrote and published three joint research papers.

This was still the time when most travelling was done by ship, so I booked my passage. Again, as when I was recruited to Otago University in Dunedin, they were in a hurry, wanting me there as soon as possible. Not having thought much about geology for two years I decided that, as it would take me three weeks to reach Perth, that would be the ideal time to read up on it again, and so I packed all my geology and geochemical books and papers ready for access in my cabin. I wanted a cabin to myself so that I had space and peace to study. I also wanted one with an outside porthole, for the view, so that is what I booked. Only sometime later was I informed that my pay level entitled me to something slightly less comfortable, but by then the less expensive cabins were fully booked, and as the WA Geological Survey wanted me in Perth asap, my booking was allowed to stand. I was lucky, and had a great trip.

Aunt, of course, was sad to see me go, but being who she was, and entirely unselfish, she hardly let me know this, congratulated me on this next opportunity, and saw me off with only a slightly rictus smile. As before, she preferred to say her farewells from her home base. It was back to tape recorder messages. We knew by then that we would be sending each other on average one tape each week, so with an hour of idle chatter every few days, it was amazing how closely we were able to keep in touch, follow each other's lives and share our thoughts.

This time I had my van, also another boyfriend. He and I had decided to drive out together, to Genoa, where I would pick up the boat. We would camp along the way, having allowed sufficient time for sightseeing, after which he would return to London and the van and I would embark. I watched it being swung onto the boat with some trepidation, but all was well. Time to say goodbye.

Boyfriends. I was lucky, I almost always had one, of some significant level of pleasure, seriousness, and relatively extended duration. However, the moment they got too serious, or started talking of marriage, I drew back. I remained deeply afraid of belonging to someone, of having someone else have any say over me, of a return to the manipulations and horrors of my childhood where somebody had 'rights' over my life, and who used them against me. My biggest concern was to avoid getting pregnant, and to remain free. This, thankfully, I managed.

An equally strong factor was that I loved my career, my professional life, and I certainly didn't want anything to take me away from this. I was barely conscious of this most of the time, I simply remained work-focused, but I did give it some thought during the trip out to Perth, when there was time for such reflections. My inner childhood refrain that 'I should never let anything matter to me' so that whatever happened I would be 'alright' and not get hurt, was greatly subdued by this time, but it was still there in the shadows. It made it easy for me to follow the work that I loved and could rely on, rather than risk anything like a total emotional commitment.

Again, I enjoyed the boat trip. Life on board was luxurious, comfortable, fun, and relaxing There were no new close friends this time on board, but there was plenty of interesting company, lots of time to play bridge in the early evenings, dance during the late evenings, and plenty of time for studying during the day. Certainly, I swam and played a variety of deck sports occasionally, but I felt duty bound, and keen, to study and earn the right to my upgraded cabin. I was, in any case, keen to brush up on my geology and prepare for life in Perth. I was travelling first-class, and most of the other passengers were a generation or two older than me, so there were no new boyfriends on this trip.

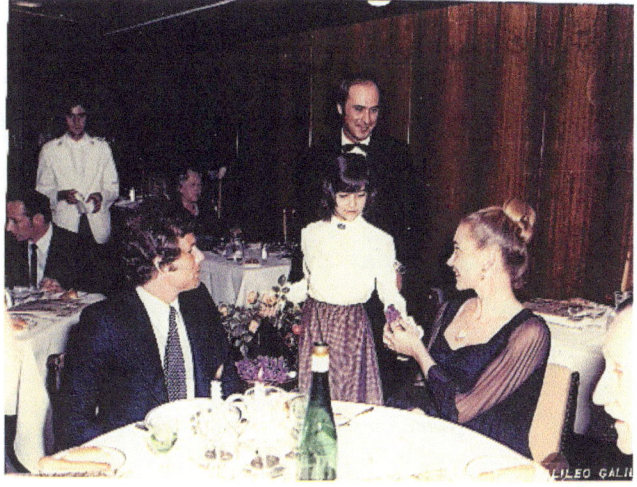

There might also have been almost no dancing, an activity that I loved. But I was lucky. There were two Swiss men on board, twins, looking so alike that they played the game of impersonating each other until they had all the passengers confused. They were wonderful dancers and loved it. Very few of the other passengers could be persuaded to do more than the occasional shuffle round the edge of the floor, so the after-dinner evenings were made up of the three of us, the twins taking it in turns, flying round the floor. Viennese waltzes were a specialty of theirs and any loss of balance I showed was surely due to rotating dizziness and not the occasional drink. Neither of them would tell anyone what they did for a living, only that they lived in Melbourne, worked nine months of the year, then spent the next three months going by sea to Vienna to visit their aged mother, and then back again by sea. Only on the last day, when I was about to disembark, did they tell me, under a vow of secrecy, that they were taxi drivers. They had one car and worked alternate twelve-hour periods. Thus they worked their car twenty-four hours a day, and saved up sufficient money each year for this luxury annual cruise.

On board we had televisions in each cabin, an innovation in those days, with regular items from the ship's communication centre and an evening news bulletin. As we were travelling first-class, we had one of the ship's officers at each of the dinner tables each night, and thus we were known to the officers. It was an Italian ship, but the second most common language among the passengers was English. To my surprise I was asked if I would read the English version of the news following each item that was given in Italian. Great fun. Thus, I recall the events of 1968 in Czechoslovakia almost first-hand.

My twenty-eighth birthday party was the penultimate night on board, and as many of us were disembarking, the celebrations, birthday cake, and farewells contributed to an exuberant evening.

---

[i] Marie Krause, *Food Nutrition and Diet Therapy,* 1952

[ii] Aron M Altschul. *Proteins:Their chemistry and Politics*, Chapman and Hall, 1965

[iii] Francis Moore Lappé, *Diet for a Small Planet,*1971

Chapter 7

WA Geological Survey

I imagine I was met at the docks as we disembarked, but I don't recall the details. A flat had been rented for me in Cottesloe, an attractive coastal suburb on the eastern edge of Perth, and a few hundred yards from the amazing golden sands that stretch along most of the Australian coast. I contacted the one person whose details I had been given by a friend in London, and arranged to meet up. I shopped for the necessary foods to start my kitchen off and stocked the food cupboards. I unpacked my two trunks, set up my books, and was ready for the next stage. The next morning I fronted up at the Geological Survey offices in central Perth, ready to make yet another, and I hoped, interesting beginning.

The WA Geological Survey was made up of four major departments: regional mapping; economic geology; oil geology; and palaeontology. Each was headed up by a senior geologist. Above these departments were four specialists: a palaeontologist; a mineralogist; a geophysicist; and, yes, me as the geochemist. Then there were the Director and the Assistant Director. The other three 'specialists' were a lot older than me by two or three decades. I didn't give this much thought. Many months later, the geophysicist told me how my appointment had been made.

It transpired that the Survey had advertised for a qualified geochemist with experience of both geology and field work, as well as chemistry and analytical laboratory work. They had had applicants from geologists and chemists. The geologists were tired of field work and the long stretches of time they had to spend away from home and family. The chemists were tired of being stuck in the city and wanted the freedom of being out in the country. The geologists tried to claim that they did, *really,* they did, have some chemical training (they didn't), and the chemists had tried to claim that they did have some geological training (they didn't), or so I was told. Then they came to my application. With 'W' as my surname initial, I was on the bottom of the pile. My application was read out. 'Three degrees with chemical and geological components, Imperial and Otago universities; two jobs with extensive field work in a variety of rough terrains and cultures; the setting up of laboratories and mobile and laboratory analytical work; and two years of chemical and analytical research at Imperial plus development in the two Geological Surveys.' Smiles all round. Until the Director, reading out my application, said "Oh my god, it's a woman". The fact that I was then only twenty-seven was probably also discussed, though I was not told of that. This was still an age when men did men's work and women did lesser jobs. Nonetheless, to my great pleasure, they had decided to make the most of it, and hired me. I settled in.

On one of my first weekends, and before I knew anyone, I had been pleased to find there was an 'Agricultural show' on the Saturday. I knew little of farming, but nothing daunted I went to explore. There was lots of farm machinery of course, about which I knew little, but then I spotted a wine-tasting tent. That's for me, I thought. The wines were handed out in small plastic 'cups'. OK, well, not too bad. After trying the first one I looked around for the spittoon as I endeavoured to make sensible notes on my tasting. There wasn't one. I resorted to spitting the wine out on the grass. There were several wines to drink and I did not want to get drunk, especially in that midday heat. I earned a few strange looks. The cost for the tasting was $1. I then learnt that no one really cared about the individual 'tasting'. The idea, pure and simple, was to get, drink, and enjoy as much wine as you could for your Australian dollar.

In the meantime, in the city, I needed somewhere more permanent to live. I was, by then an enthusiastic gardener and was determined that it would have an extensive garden where I could develop my newfound hobby, organic gardening, and particularly organic vegetable growing. This meant buying a house (the least important consideration) and some land (of prime importance), but of course I had no money. Nothing daunted, I set out to explore the possible areas. By far the cheapest place to buy was along the foot of the scarp that ran north-south, parallel to the coast line and east of the city centre. It was a good half hour's drive or more east of the city and generally considered a long way out with no accompanying benefits. It was not near the sea, considered to be worth a half-hour drive to the west of the city centre. By going about the same distance east, it lost any seaside amenities. Nor was it further east along the top of the scarp, which would have been further out but with wonderful views and cooling breezes.

I searched this economical strip to see what I could get for my limited funds. I was not a beach bum, nor were good views high on my list of requirements. Essentially, I wanted sufficient land on which to do some generous gardening, and the cheapest possible house. Finally, I found a couple of houses in the cheaper area that appealed. Neither of the properties had much going for them to look at, being made of 'clapboard' sheeting with corrugated iron roofs, but the land swung it. Given that this was my first property purchase, I seem to have been fairly relaxed about it. Ever the optimist. With the helpful advice of a couple of the geologists and their wives, I chose the one with over an acre of land, an odd-sized plot, placed as it was amongst a number of five-acre plots.

The house was an unadorned oblong divided into six rooms that simply led off each other, two by three. The two eastern rooms were bedrooms. The largest, to the front, I made mine, and the smaller back one was a spare room, of which more later. The two central rooms consisted of the living room, large, to the front, and a narrower back room with a concrete floor that I eventually made into my storeroom and gardening room, housing spades, rakes, hoes and the like there. Of the western two rooms the front, larger one was the kitchen. The back was divided into a small back entry way, a bathroom, and further space with a sink that might have been called a utility room – had it had any utility. I regularly took my laundry to the laundrette since equipment at the house was primitive. The hot water was heated by a small vertical cone with place for a fire at the bottom that heated the water flowing around the upper structure. In time I was to learn that by dint of standing ready within the bath and putting a match to the paper and twigs below the cone I could make this into an instant-hot-water system for a quick shower. It was primitive, but it worked. I had, after all, chosen the house for the land, and I had no money to spare. I thought myself very lucky to have found this place, and I loved it.

It was time to see the local bank manager and try for a mortgage. I was warned that this was an impossible task. Firstly, at that time single people could simply not get mortgages. Secondly, women did not count financially and were considered to be a totally unacceptable risk. I did not understand the concept of impossible, and so, undaunted, I applied. I pointed out that the house would cost $A10,000 and my annual salary was $A10,000. That was the amazing figure that had almost stopped me in my tracks when I had thought of applying for the job while back in London. I had references from my employers (a government department no less, how stable and secure can you be?) and others, and I offered these up, along with papers that showed an expected tenure at my job. I was told to wait, and they would inform me in due time. Luckily the house sellers waited too. Somehow it never occurred to me that I would *not* get the mortgage, although apparently the geologists had taken bets on this and all were sure I would fail.

A few weeks later I returned to the bank, where I was met by a temporary manager, the permanent one having gone on holiday. He told me that, somewhat to his surprise, the bank had granted my mortgage. At that time a new graduate earned about $A3,000, lived on it and even supported a family, if with some difficulty and careful budgeting. It was clear that I could pay off the full mortgage in little more than a year, which is what I did. When the permanent bank manager came back from holiday, he was aghast, saying he would never have supported my application. I guess I was just lucky that he took his holiday when he did.

After two years on a slim scholarship and counting every penny in London, I had no financial reserves. But I did have a handsome pay cheque coming in. I had no furniture, but luckily some came with the house. It was definitely nothing to write home about, but usable. I moved in, bought what else I needed, mostly the small items, and settled down, turning my immediate attention to the land, which was wildly overgrown with a few shrubs and a thick thatch of deeply rooted kikuyu grass.

At work I had a lot to do. West Australia was 'my' territory, my fieldwork area, and it is a large place, 2.65 million square kilometres. In European terms it would cover the area of UK, Spain, France, Germany, Austria, Switzerland, Italy and Poland all added together. A large field area for sure.

My first job was to design and equip a small caravan, about six feet long. Anything longer would not have ridden the rough terrain that I expected we would be driving over. It was equipped with a careful shock-absorbing base for the atomic absorption equipment. The days of solvent extractions and test tube comparisons on a small colourimeter were passed. I would be putting the skills I had learnt in Atomic Absorption Spectroscopy at IC in the past two years into full-time practice.

Unlike in Fiji, this time I could order what was needed 'locally', from the 'Eastern States'. However, this was all relative as Australia is a huge country, and the eastern coast with the majority of the population, industry, commerce, and retail business, was still a mind-bending 4,000 km away. "We'll have to order it from the Eastern States" was going to become a frustrating mantra. The WA market was small. The population of the entire state was only about half a million, thus there were few customers in Perth for anything but the most popular basics in the shops. Almost anything even slightly out of the ordinary that I wanted was subject to that proviso and delay. Buying over this distance also meant you couldn't access, touch, or try things out, and once bought, they were yours, no exchange. There was no internet shopping in 1968.

Going into the field (geological term), bush (Australian term) or countryside (UK term), was a serious business. We did not go for a day's field work, for a week or even for a month. During the winter months (the coolest time), the geologists, who would generally be heading north from Perth, went for three spells of two months each separated by one week back in Perth. Then they had five months in the city doing the associated desk work.

By the time I was settled it was mid-summer, Christmas, and I was set to do several relatively small field projects at about the same latitude as Perth, it being considered too hot to go further north at that point. I also had the Perth laboratory to set up and work to do on samples brought in by the geologists the previous winter. Consequently, I spent the next few weeks in town.

London friends had encouraged me to contact friends of theirs in Perth when I arrived. This I did. They lived on a spread of several acres, extending into open countryside up on the scarp. They were a delightful couple and became great friends. My first evening there was memorable. Before dinner ('tea' as they called it) we went out to milk her eleven goats. By day they roamed free. In the evening, with the promise of oats, they all came when she called, appearing out of different clumps of the surrounding bush. They were then tethered by long chains to their respective and individual small goat-sized sheds. I was delighted to meet them and was even given the chance to milk one of them myself, though it was a somewhat tortuous affair.

Over 'tea' (the evening meal) she encouraged me to do more than just grow vegetables, saying that with my acre or more I should endeavour to be even more self-sufficient, and how better to do that than to have a milking goat. The next thing I knew I was driving home with Chocolate Drop, an indifferent but lovely Toggenburg, in the back of my Minivan, the van that had come out with me from London. I had been given a halter and chain and instructed by my hostess in the art of tethering her. What about my absentee spells of field work? I asked. I was assured that I could take Chocolate Drop back to her for these times. So in spite of my concerns I was easily persuaded, another sign of my inclination for 'doing things naturally'.

Perth's summer is hot and dry, very dry. I was assured that I would not need housing for Chocolate Drop in the summer. In any case, I had a large, corrugated iron, mainly open-sided shed, about twenty feet square with walls on about two and a half sides. The plan, hastily concocted over that first evening meal, was that I would build a fenced 'run' extension of this at the back in which Chocolate Drop would, once it was erected, be able to sleep, and that I would tether her out during the day.

All this eventually came about, with the help of some of the geology bachelors who rapidly developed the habit of calling in on me during the weekends. These various 'geology bachelors' were not only single but relatively homeless. About eight or so of them worked in 'the field', hundreds if not one or two thousand miles away, for six months of the year and had only minimal accommodation, possibly only a single room, in Perth for the five months of the summer. So, my house (large) and garden (rambling), became a mecca for most of them during various parts of each of the summer weekends. In return for food (me), drink (them) and entertainment (Chocolate Drop), they were more than happy to help out, and we soon had the pen ready for Chocolate Drop, and in such a way that it included the back part of the very large shed-come-carport. But back to Chocolate Drop.

I woke the next morning in my usual happy state until I realised that, good heavens, I had a goat I must milk before I could go to work. The challenge was daunting. I can't even say the first attempt was a great success. I suspect it hurt Chocolate Drop more than it did me. But eventually I had a pint or so of milk in a bucket (she was no great milker but she was great fun). I stored the milk in the fridge, tethered the goat out, set a bucket of water close by her, and set off for work. I simply had to hope for the best, and that the tether would hold, as there was certainly no fence around my land. It generally held.

Some weeks later, after milking Chocolate Drop late one afternoon and having served three of the bachelors with coffee, I went out to do the milking. I came back with the usual pint and stored it in the fridge. One of the geologists asked me what I did with it. "You've been drinking it" I said, pointing to his cup of coffee, and a bit surprised at his question. "Is that *goat's* milk?" he asked, pointing to his cup. "Ugh". And he pushed it away. That was the last time he had milk or cheese in my house, refusing all my efforts to reassure him that it was safe to drink.

While focused during the weekdays on my work in the Geological Survey, both the laboratory and at my desk, the focus on the weekends was to turn at least part of my acre of overgrown wilderness into a productive garden. In the initial forays I was delighted to find there were two huge mulberry trees, a fig tree, a lemon tree, an olive tree, and an apricot tree in one segment of the garden, hence an area designated 'orchard'. I had already picked out another area that could most readily be cleared and turned into the vegetable patch. It was large, in full sunlight and dauntingly thick with weeds. Used to English weeds and ever the optimist, I assumed they could soon be dug up. It was probably just as well I did not know the challenge that faced me.

In the Survey offices, during tea breaks and similar, I had jauntily been talking of "digging the land over and planting my vegetable patch", unsure about the smirks this evoked. After all, although I was not an experienced gardener, I had spent many months under Aunt's tutelage in England. As a result, I had assumed, wrongly, that the same efforts would be sufficient here. What I had not experienced was the kikuyu grass with its lengthy, strong and deep roots that could extend many feet into the ground. Any tiny piece of root, broken off and left behind, had a near total capacity to start up new growths, developing rapidly downward, horizontally, and upward. Nor had I experienced the almost total lack of loam or organic matter in my sandstone soil, and the searing heat and lack of rain that lasted for most of the six months of the summer. It was, eventually, quite a relief to leave this behind after a few weeks and head for one of my small field areas, suitable for working in the relative cool of the late summer.

My first field area was to be close to Perth, a mere 550 km east, just beyond Coolgardie (itself beyond Kalgoorlie). It was to be a trip of short duration, about three weeks. Perhaps this was chosen to see if I could handle it. I did, of course, and thoroughly enjoyed it. It was a far cry from New Zealand with its compact short distances and huge variations of climate and vegetation and mild to warm temperatures. It was also totally different to Fiji's near-tropical islands and dense mangrove and coconut palm vegetation and generous rainfall. I collected my assigned Land Rover, hitched up the caravan laboratory, loaded up the tents and cooking and sleeping equipment, collected the two field assistants, who had been assigned their own Land Rover, and set off. We camped on the edge of one the salt lakes and the low level 'salt bushes' with leaves that did indeed taste of salt. The 'lakes' had once been aptly named, but with nowhere for the water to flow (inland West Australia is very flat, and somewhat like a saucer in shape, so little or no drainage out) and the hot sun beating down relentlessly, they were now more like salt pans.

We set up camp (tents) and set to, sampling on a grid pattern across the selected structures. Each Saturday, for the month we were there, I drove into Kalgoorlie for supplies, a rare luxury. One Saturday (shops all being closed on Sundays) I was standing in a hardware store – though they called it something entirely different – 'produce store' I think. To my surprise I heard one of the men ahead of me in the queue asking first for sunflower seeds, then molasses. Good gracious. I was used to buying these items in London from the local and much more elegant health food store. Surely there wasn't such a store here in Outback Australia? It was time to find out. I ordered a kilogram of the sunflower seeds and a tin of molasses, considered at that time to be a good source of minerals (true) and with less concern than today about the sugar level. Back at camp I opened them up with appropriate anticipatory enthusiasm, only to have it dashed. I should have known. The sunflower seeds were in their cortex or shell, obviously designed for very strong-beaked parakeets, and the molasses was the very bitter blackstrap form to be given to horses in their mash. Ah well.

The scenery was eye-opening. Salt. Almost nothing but salt planes and the aptly named salt-bush. I set out the grid lines and directed the field crew, who spent the days collecting the samples. I spent most of my time when not organising them, analysing the samples in my caravan laboratory. All in all, I was delighted with this job I had landed.

Back in Perth I was introduced to the Beethoven and Burgundy group that met on Saturday evenings when in town, through the summer. It seemed that several of the geology bachelors, plus Ian (the one married geologist in that group) and his wife Ann, enjoyed classical music. They also had a somewhat erratic social life as they were out of town for more than half the year and tended to fall out of more continuous social groups. So the group met on Saturday evenings when in town, through the summer. The plan was that each person brought an LP record (nothing digital in those days) hence the 'Beethoven' of their name, a bottle of wine, hence the 'Burgundy', and cheese. We tried to be original, but it was a struggle. Back in the late 1960s Western Australians drank beer, so finding any sort of wine other than red or white 'plonk' was a challenge. My earlier wine-tasting at the agricultural show should have warned me. Cheese was no easier. You had to be clever to find anything other than mild, medium, or tasty cheddar. We all endeavoured to be clever. The evenings were great fun and made up for the slim pickings for entertainment elsewhere.

One Saturday, Ian and Ann announced they were taking me to meet a couple of their friends the next morning, Mr and Mrs K. They said nothing more than that they were very keen vegetable and fruit gardeners and could help me get my garden started. Little did I know that this was to be my first introduction to the philosophy of anthroposophy and its application in the form of biodynamic agriculture.

I turned up as instructed at eleven o'clock and was made welcome with herbal teas, home-grown and home-made bread and cakes. Then the chat started. At least, I thought it was chat. But after a while, and certainly in retrospect, I realised that it felt more like being interviewed: I was. It all had to do with Rudolf Steiner, of whom I knew absolutely nothing, and the Anthroposophical philosophy and society, of which I also knew absolutely nothing. At this time, I thought of myself as a pure physics and chemical scientist, even if I was showing certain tendencies into a vegetarian diet (financial), protein nutrition (to add interest to my DIC), and gardening (to be able to spend time with Aunt). Ian's father, in Sydney, was head of the Australian branch of the Anthroposophical Society. Ian and Ann were very interested in the subject, and Mr and Mrs K were deeply involved in it and in biodynamic gardening. Somehow, with all my talk of gardening organically, they had developed the idea that Mr K might teach me both the gardening and the anthroposophy, though I knew nothing of the latter at the start.

By the end of that morning it was agreed. Mr K would come to my house each Saturday morning and help me with my garden. I was almost overwhelmed at this generosity but very grateful for his help. And so it started. He was a wonderful help and a dedicated worker. No slacking. Saturday after Saturday he cycled the ten miles to my house and we worked on clearing the ground. He found an old wire six-foot bedframe that could act as a sieve. That was propped at forty-five degrees to the ground, and foot by foot, moved along the first row of the plot while we threw the dug-up earth and weeds against it. The weeds, the largest proportion, were then barrowed to the spot he had designated fit to be the first compost heap. The soil that fell through our crude 'sieve' formed the basis of the soil in which we would eventually sow and plant. It was back-breaking work. The sun was high, the sweat dripping. He steadfastly insisted that we drink only warm water – why? I was gasping for an iced drink.

In this way the weeks went by. Most weeks I was invited to spend one evening with them, exploring their garden while he explained to me all that he had been doing. His home was close to the coast and his garden had been pure sand. Over the years he had nurtured it, composted, sown, and harvested. It was unbelievably dense with rich growth of fruit trees, vines, rows of produce, and neat compost heaps.

Then came the time that he announced we could think of sowing some seeds.

"Put the carrot seeds in on Wednesday, the area is ready."

"Why Wednesday? Why not now?" I was impatient, keen to get started.

"The moon is not right."

What did he mean, 'the moon wasn't right'? What had the moon got to do with it? I was a pure scientist. This didn't make sense. But then I thought of how good he had been to me, how much he had done for me, so much help, so much talking, so much teaching, so much I had learnt. The least I could do was sow the carrot seeds on the day he had requested. But I wasn't going to leave it at that.

On the Sunday I cleared another square metre of land, way off, across my acre and behind some shrubs, out of sight. I sowed carrot seeds there, in parallel rows, every Wednesday. In time it became obvious that the seeds sown on the fifth week, when I assumed that the moon was again right, produced seedlings that caught up with those sown two or three weeks earlier. I was a scientist, wasn't I? I had done a test and found that the plan worked. I might not know how or why, but I could not ignore the fact. And from then on, I endeavoured to do things on the days of the lunar cycle as he advised.

Mr K gave me books to read, including *Occult Science*. I thought that any man who could put those two words together and make some sense had, at the very least, an interesting mind. Other books were *Knowledge of Higher Worlds*, and *Theosophy*. They were all by Rudolf Steiner. Again, by way of thanks for his help, I started to read them (heavy going) and discuss some of the ideas with him on subsequent Saturdays (mind-bending). At that time I didn't realise what a significant part of my life anthroposophy was going to become.

Mr K also taught me about the various anthroposophical preparations used in what I now learnt was the biodynamic farming method.

The first geological field trip had gone well, and it was soon winter and time for a full-scale field trip in the north of the state where the temperature had reduced to a comfortable level. Chocolate Drop was duly sent back to her first home, and with only minor adjustments to the laboratory stock we were soon off again, this time for a full-length trip. This one involved working to a grid and sampling soils and outcrops of rocks located on Twin Peaks, a sheep station (farm) a mere 850 kilometres away. I had six field assistants, and we were accompanied at the start by a geologist who would be working further on, but calling in to our camp occasionally.

We set off in three heavily laden Land Rovers. As usual, mine was towing the six-foot, air-conditioned caravan laboratory. Also as usual this was not for my comfort, perish the thought, but for the temperature-protection of the atomic absorption spectrophotometer. It was small, of course, to cope with the rough roads, tracks, or sand, and had to be driven carefully. The load also included what we hoped would be sufficient food and drink for the two months of our stay. It had a small fridge, allegedly for the chemicals, mostly organic solvents, but the field crew soon made inroads on the space in it for their cans of beer.

We set up camp, with a central area for the cooking fire and then various food and equipment stores, plus three two-man tents beyond, on the far side. My tent was on the opposite side with my ablutions tent a hundred yards farther back among the few scrubby trees that existed in the very dry environment. Walking the path to and fro at night, I enjoyed the dark sky, unaffected by any city lights or reflections, and could observe the progression of the moon cycles. Orion was familiar, although upside-down to my England-trained eyes. I soon found the

Southern Cross, but of course, most of the constellations with which I was familiar were hidden on the other side of the planet.

We were camped on a sheep station of sufficient size that it took the owner twenty minutes or more to drive to us. When he came by one evening, after the first four or five weeks, he brought with him a few precious cans of beer, and, for me, an invitation to fly in to Geraldton the next day, Saturday, and buy any supplies we might need. I loved my life in the bush, but the chance to shop, mostly for fresh food plus supplies the guys wanted, and to have a shower in the hotel where we would have lunch, was not to be turned down. I drove down to the homestead the next morning and met up with the station owner. The two of us took off in his two-seater Cessna, landing at Geraldton, some 300 km southwest, soon after 10.00. We arranged to meet up at 1.00 for the promised lunch before we returned. Back then, Geraldton was not a very big place, and I could easily have covered every shop in just one of the three hours until lunchtime, but I set off to enjoy myself.

After a morning of shopping (a bit) and exploring (mostly), a hot shower (in the hotel), clean clothes (my own), and feeling unfamiliarly well dressed, I was introduced to my host's friend, and the three of us went in to lunch. Sitting in a chair, eating at a table, in a room with walls, all were a treat after over a month of camping out, and the lunch was delicious. I was offered wine, cold, crisp, and white, perfect for the winter. Even the winters in that part of the world are sweating hot during the day, though nippy cold at night. The wine was a treat, but I was a little concerned to see what my two male companions drank, given that one was my pilot back to camp. Chat, coffee (black, I was glad to see), and the two of us walked off to the airfield, climbed into the Cessna, and took off. All was normal until we got to a few thousand feet up. We had just cleared Geraldton air space (I assumed), when the pilot (station owner and owner of the plane) cut off the radio, slumped down in his seat, leant back, said "shoo tay kover" and closed his eyes. No nervous prodding on my part could rouse him, he just snored, so after a while I focused instead on what I had to do.

That part of West Australia is essentially flat for several hundred miles in any direction. The homestead name, Twin Peaks, was an essential clue. Looking due east, I could see two small humps on the far horizon (inland). That seemed to be the place to head for. I failed entirely to get the radio to work. We had a full fuel load, so I figured I would head for the two peaks, keep an eye on the fuel gauge, fly round the peaks once I got there and keep hoping that he would wake up. If he didn't, I decided I would rather crash near the Geraldton airfield and hospital (if they had one) than out in the bush. Given that decision, I would head back west and hope to arrive with a minimum of fuel that could catch fire. Wild thoughts. I hoped it wouldn't come to that.

I had been a passenger several times, on various other field trips, but never, of course the pilot, although I had held the 'stick' occasionally. I experimented. I moved the 'stick' to the right, and yes, we turned right, but we also headed down to earth. Not a good idea. I leaned back, somewhat automatically, and wonder of wonders, the plane levelled off. I took us back up to 10,000 feet. That seemed pretty safe to me at the time, though I'm not sure why I thought that. In any case, there was no other aeroplane to be seen, and I didn't anticipate any. Back on track and once again heading for the hills, I pulled the stick back and up we went. I was beginning to enjoy myself – just as long as I didn't consider the long-term picture.

On we went, me digging him in the ribs from time to time, but to no avail. Over the Twin Peaks homestead I took a circular path. I could see his wife down below waving at me, but there was little I could do to explain the situation to her. I waved, but I doubt she saw that. Finally, and just as, with a wary eye on the fuel gauge, I was considering heading back west, my digging and prodding had the desired effect. Bleary eyes opened, a grunt, vertical movement on the seat and he got his feet on the controls and said "ah, es, shoo you got us here. I'll tay kover now". Of course he would, there was no way he was getting out of that. I don't recall if, once we landed, I crawled or dropped out of the plane, my legs were so shaky.

I was to learn later that he and his friend had spent the entire morning drinking whiskies in the pub and had had a great deal to drink even before the lunchtime wine. It was apparently his normal week-end routine. I was also to learn that he drank a bottle of whisky at home most evenings. I guess I got off lightly.

Back in Perth and my house a month or two later, I woke one morning feeling dreadful. Exhausted. No energy. And by 'no energy' I do not mean just 'tired'. It took me many, many minutes to drag myself onto the floor, and then crawl across the room and finally to the phone to call for help. After a visit to a doctor, it was put down to nearly zero thyroid function and I was put on 175 mcg of thyroxin. It was attributed to the time at Hammersmith Hospital when I was a student on a summer job and had walked along corridors littered with radioactive iodine for around five hours. I found that as long as I took the thyroxine I was fine. If I forgot, or stopped, just to experiment, I was lost.

My garden flourished, in spite of my erratic departures. I learnt to make cheese with Chocolate Drop's milk, but wished I had a greater quantity. At one time I thought this wish had been granted. Inspired by Chocolate Drop, my neighbours, a few hundred yards away and with more land, also bought a goat, though I felt rather sorry for it. They had built a shed for it with walls that stopped a foot above the ground and a foot below the roof, so there was moderate air circulation. They only let her out for a few hours each day, tethered close to good green feed, but I felt she was a bit restricted. Chocolate Drop, on the other hand, had an open pen about thirty feet square, with my open-sided car port along one edge, and could run around that during the nights. Each morning I would milk her, a process at which I soon became a dab hand, and take her for a walk before going to work. The process would be repeated when I got home in the evening. She made the most of those times, eating all before her. During the day I left her with an extensive tether, close to generous vegetation and with a secure bucket of water within reach.

Then came the day the neighbours were going on holiday. "Would I milk their goat for them?" Of course I would. She would be all right left in her shed all day, I was told, and they provided plenty of dry feed for her. Two weeks of generous milking – she gave about four times as much as Chocolate Drop – I focused on all the cheese-making I would be able to do. But it was not to be. After the first morning of milking, I was only halfway back across the land between our two separate acres, when the smell got to me. I turned swiftly to my left and tipped the milk onto my compost heap. I had just learnt what people meant when they called goat's milk smelly. Thinking about it, I came to the conclusion that it was not so much the goats, but the way they were kept, maintained, and fed, that adversely affected the taste. Chocolate Drop was definitely an outdoor goat. No smell. This lovely white Saanen goat was kept almost indoors almost all of the time, and fed on concentrates. The smell was terrible. I milked her for the rest of their holiday, but made no effort to turn the milk into cheese.

The timing worked well. By the time Chocolate Drop's milk output was falling off I was ready for my six months of field work. Chocolate Drop went back to her first home, completed her pregnancy, dropped the kid and was in full milk production by the time I was back in town for the summer.

During the several long periods that I spent living in tents and hundreds of kilometres from even the smallest township, I did have time for reading. I read some of the books that Mr K had given me, based on Rudolf Steiner, and thought about that in conjunction with Buddhism and other Eastern religions. It was all very interesting, and food for thought, but definitely, at this stage, a side interest.

Another field area involved surveying an outcrop of carbonatites. It was hoped that this would be a significant find, similar to some of the deposits in other parts of Western Australia. My job was to plan a sample grid and then analyse the samples for relevant indicator trace elements, carbonatite rocks being a significant source of valuable rare earth elements. As well as this, I worked in several other field areas during each of the winters of my two years in Western Australia and thoroughly enjoyed them. Social life in the city was relaxed, the geochemistry was fascinating, and I loved the camping and exploration of the Australian way of life 'out back'.

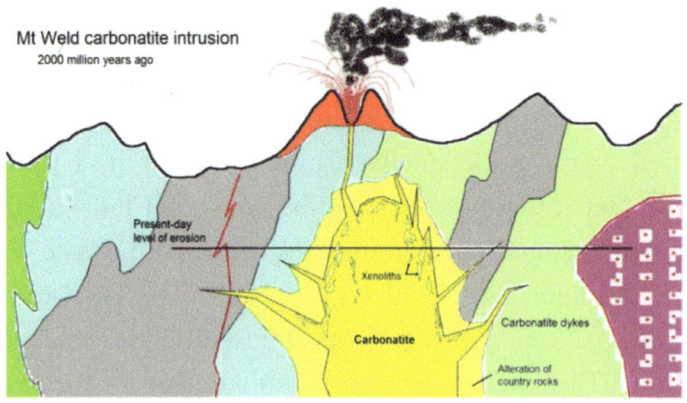

During these lengthy camping trips out of town I generally worked all day on the practical aspects of the job, planning and inspecting the sampling grids, checking and sorting the samples, getting them back to my caravan lab, and setting up the analytical tests. Come dusk – rarely later than seven – we would have 'tea'. The guys would then retire to their tent, drink beer and play two-up. It was cold at night during these winter field trips, so inevitably I retired to my caravan to work on samples and results, or to my tent to read. I read a lot, and to be sure that I could, before each trip I would choose and stock up on a stack of books on a particular topic. Once it was on comparative religions, another time it was on various civilisations from the Early Egyptians through the Greco-Roman period to the middle Europeans. Another time I followed all the history of the royal families of the UK. Sometimes I took books on philosophies. I read such books as Toynbee's *A Study of History*, and Churchill's *A History of the English-Speaking Peoples*. All of these are subjects outside my professional interests, the latter having been built around chemistry, and I have often thought that if I hadn't studied chemistry, it might have been history. But then I come to the question of what would I have done in the way of making a working career of it, never mind one as interesting as this one, and that is when I reverse rapidly back to my fascination with chemistry.

During my next period in Perth I woke one morning, around four o'clock, to the sound of the sliding door between my bedroom and the spare bedroom closing. That was odd. Certainly it was not closed when I went to bed and equally certainly I never closed it. Could the wind, a strong one sweeping down off the scarp, have moved it? No, not a sliding door. Then I heard footsteps moving around in the back of the house. An intruder? I remained still, clutching the sheet to my neck and feeling stupid for doing so in such a conventional hold, but wondering what else to do. More footsteps, then bed sounds, and a muttered "You beut!". Silence. Had the intruder really gone to bed in my spare room? Should I stay quiet and hope he slept? For a short while that seemed like a plan, then I figured I should try for escape. To get out of bed and go through my bedroom door into the sitting room meant getting a lot closer to the door to the spare room. I eyed the dress I had been wearing the day before, slid out of bed, grabbed the dress and rushed through and out the front door. In the relative safety of the open veranda I stopped to dress, then with a sudden burst of fresh adrenalin raced the few hundred yards to the neighbour's house.

This was summer and by this time it was heading for daylight. I knocked on the neighbour's bedroom window, called out to them at the same time so as not to frighten them, and explained the situation. The police were called. The husband went across to greet them when we saw their car arrive. His wife and I watched from the safety of their house. Husband came back. Had I seen the intruder's trousers anywhere? They were later found in my van – a vehicle that, being so small, must have been a thoroughly uncomfortable option for him if he was trying to sleep there. No wonder he had opted for breaking into my house in search of a more comfortable place to sleep. Husband came back again. Had I seen a Mercedes anywhere? It was found a hundred yards down the road. And finally: would I go and identify the man they had found? Was it perhaps someone I knew? Oh no, was my thought, don't say it's one of the mad geologist bachelors dropping in, I'd feel a right idiot. But I needn't have worried. Even from a distance, as they brought him out, he was clearly a complete stranger. They took him away. Apparently, he had been on his way home, clearly very drunk, got confused and, he claimed, mistaken my house for his (though he had had to break in via the window next to my back door). I wondered, slightly hysterically, if that was how he normally got into his own house when he arrived home drunk.

I might not have learnt anything more about the incident, and certainly the police didn't tell me, had not a friend seen a tiny notice in the local paper sometime later: 'Man breaks into house claiming he thought it was his own home. Judge tells him to get a homing device and charges him ten dollars'. Ten dollars? That was definitely insulting. I had to do battle with my nerves every night to remain living in that house on my own. But I was determined not to give up my way of life. It was quite a relief when it was time to go off on my next field trip.

I'd been in Perth for over two years at this time, and the mining boom had really taken off. Small start-up companies with big dreams and insecure starts were all looking to find the next great bonanza. The larger mining companies were also looking for staff to fill the developing gaps. People with geological expertise were in high demand. I was all packed and ready to leave on my next field trip when the phone rang. I answered it, all unsuspecting. Had the call come an hour or two later I would have been on my way to my next field area trailing my caravan. Had I missed that call, my life could have been very different. The caller was from a geological consulting firm with head offices in Brisbane and Perth. I was being head-hunted. They wanted a geochemist. Would I be interested in working for them?

He explained the job, and that they were about to set up a Sydney office with one senior geologist and a secretary. It was too expensive to house the field crews there and they would operate out of Perth and Brisbane where the company already had directors. They really wanted me in Brisbane, but I could live in Sydney and commute as appropriate if I preferred (I did). The casual way they talked of flying a thousand or two miles nearly took my breath away, used as I was to tight government budgets, but I was soon to get used to it.

What areas would my work cover, I asked. Good gracious, this was to be my largest field area yet, extending from New Zealand and the Pacific islands across Australia to Southern Africa, depending on the needs of their clients. However, most of their work, they anticipated, would be in Australia, but this time the whole of Australia, not just the West, so fully the size of mainland USA.

I certainly liked the idea. The job was professionally challenging and interesting, and I loved the thought of the travel that could be involved. After some discussion, a plan was formed. I went off on the immediate field trip as already planned and thought over their offer. Fortunately, the trip was expected to be a short one. I decided to accept the job. Once the decision was made, I managed to get into a township not too far from our camp and phone to let my future employer know of my acceptance, and the date by which I could complete my current projects.

Back in Perth a few weeks later I packed up and enjoyed a hilarious leaving party built mostly around my recently homemade wine. It was really far too young to be drunk, but I was hardly going to take it with me, and as ever, geology bachelors and friends were not too fussy! I gave away all I didn't want to take with me and let the house. I was very attached to it, as I have been to almost everywhere I've lived, and was reluctant to sell. I had great memories of all I had done and achieved there. However, a few months after arriving in Sydney I was contacted by the tenants. They loved it there, it was exactly what they wanted. Could they please, please, please buy the place and all the furniture such as it was? They could. Of course they could. It made sense.

Working as a confidential consultant did not lend itself to publishing research data, so for a while at least, my publications stopped here.

Bibliograpy

- *Preparation, purification and analysis of Iron 52,* Internal report, Hammersmith Hospital research group, 1960
- *Applications of Analytical Chemistry to Geochemical Prospecting*, A.R.C.S. Dissertation, Imperial College, 1961
- *Applications of Analytical Chemistry to Geochemistry*, M.Sc. thesis, Otago University, New Zealand 1964
- *Geochemical Prospecting for copper, nickel and zinc in the Longwood Range, Southland, New Zealand*, New Zealand Journal of Geology and Geophysics, vol.10, No.3, pp.742-758, 1967
- *Chemical Variations in Stream Waters and Sediments in the Moke Creek area, West Otago.* New Zealand Journal of Geology and Geophysics, vol.10, No.3, pp.759-770, 1967
- *Statistics in the interpretation of Geochemical Data*, New Zealand Journal of Geology and Geophysics, vol.10, No.3, pp.771-797, 1967
- *Atomic-fluorescence spectroscopy of magnesium with a high-intensity hollow cathode lamp as line source*, Analytical Chimica Acta, vol.42, pp.29-37, 1968, With T.S.West
- *Atomic absorption and fluorescence spectroscopy with a carbon filament atom reservoir,* Analytica Chimica Acta, vol.45, pp.27-41, 1969, with T.S. West
- *Investigations in Atomic Absorption Spectroscopy and Atomic Fluorescence Spectroscopy*, D.I.C. Thesis, Imperial College, 1968
- *Investigation of Ministerial Reserve 453H, Lake Yindarlgooda, Bulong District, West Australia*, J.Safoulis, X.K.Williams and D.L.Rowston, G.S.W.A. Record No.1968/17

- *The Geology and Geochemistry of a Cupriferous area at Twin Peaks, Yalgoo Goldfield, West Australia.* J.Safoulis and X.K.Williams, G.S.W.A. Record No 1970/2
- *Selenium as a guide to Mineral Exploration,* G.S.W.A. Record No.1970/3
- *Geochemical Prospecting for copper, lead and zinc in Northampton Mineral Field, West Australia,* G.S.W.A. Record No.1970/4
- *The Geology and Geochemistry of some Carbonate Intrusion in the Mount Fraser Area, Peak Hill Gold Field, West Australia.* J.D. Lewis and X.K.Williams, G.S.W.A. Record No.1970/

Chapter 8
Sydney – Layton and Associates

My original idea was to drive over to Sydney – only 4,000 km after all! But when a friend who had been interested in coming with me, changed plans, I decided to fly to Sydney rather than drive all that way alone.

I booked into a hotel in Sydney for the night, visited the office the next morning, met the senior geologist and found an estate agent. I was, remarkably, going to be on an even slightly higher salary than in Perth, and so I was looking for a pleasant place. It could not be too big as even a one-bedroomed unit (flat) in the centre of Sydney would cost a lot more than my rambling acre on the outskirts of Perth. I told the agent exactly what I wanted: one bedroom, new unit, balcony, on the north shore of the harbour facing the sun, and close to the ferry across the harbour for work. I informed him that I would be away (I was to go straight on up to Brisbane to meet the boss) for a few days and would look at the properties he had chosen for me on my return. I admonished him to keep my strict criteria very much in mind.

I left for Brisbane and spent four days there, meeting fellow employees and potential clients. I liked what I saw, enjoyed the people, and realised I had moved into a different world. Gone was the laid-back government department mode. I had spent ten years since I graduated in a succession of university chemistry departments and government-run geological surveys. The focus had been chemistry with a geological application. It had been somewhat academic research with a strong applied background, all run at the rather stately pace of applied academia.

Working as technical consultant in mining and mineral (occasionally oil) exploration, the focus had changed. I was thrust into the high-speed world of consultancy and making every minute something that could be charged out to a client. No waiting for buses. Grab a taxi, move fast from here to there – several meetings, projects to be explored, plans to be made. It was all very exciting. So was the wining and dining, which was a new experience for me. I had until this time lived a generally economical lifestyle, even down to student-poor. As a result, I had paid off the mortgage on one house and was about to buy a unit that cost nearly twice as much. I knew nothing of real estate investments, or any other financial strategy, but it seems I had inadvertently made some wise decisions. It remained to be seen how much I would like this change. For the moment it excited me. I saw it as a chance to apply many of the ideas I had developed during my applied research over the past ten years.

Four days later I was back in Sydney and looking at the units that had been chosen for my selection. I looked down the agent's list, picked out the one that was closest to my list of requirements and asked to start there. It was perfect – brand new, single bedroom, top floor, balcony, wonderful view, near the ferry. "I'll buy it." However, the agent was having none of it. Apparently, it was simply not done to buy the first place you saw. I was dragged round to three more on his prepared list. None of them suited – not new, not facing the sun, not near the harbour, two bedrooms and too expensive. As soon as he started to droop, I said "Right, now can we go back and can I buy the first one I saw?" Defeated, the poor man gave up and started on the paperwork. I think I wanted brand-new as an antidote to the bucolic house and setting of the previous two years. I loved this Sydney unit and never for one moment doubted my choice. In between fieldwork and consultancy trips I spent the next few weeks furnishing it and getting established.

There were three directors in the company and, almost in turn, they asked me to advise on different clients. One request came in from an exploration company in Cape York Peninsular, in the far north east.

The client company had a lease close to an area where antimony had been found. They could even see the stibnite (antimony-sulphide mineral) on the ground in parts of their own land. But when they had analysed soil samples to look for further evidence of it nearby and under the soil, they couldn't find it.

"Which soil horizon have you sampled?" was the obvious question I asked. I knew by this time that geologists were far more interested in the solid rock samples they studied than in the broken-down rock that constituted the soil samples. I was right. The bemused expression on the director's face told me that the concept of soil horizons was foreign to them and I assumed this was a dead end. I was so used to the great reluctance of government departments to authorise expensive field trips, that I asked the next question with little hope of getting a positive answer. It was, after all, 2,500 km away.

"Would you like me to go up there and have a look?"

"Oh, yes please, could you do that?"

I could and did. I was delighted.

With no other project yet 'live' on my schedule, the next morning saw us both flying up to Cairns. There we were joined by the client's local director of exploration.

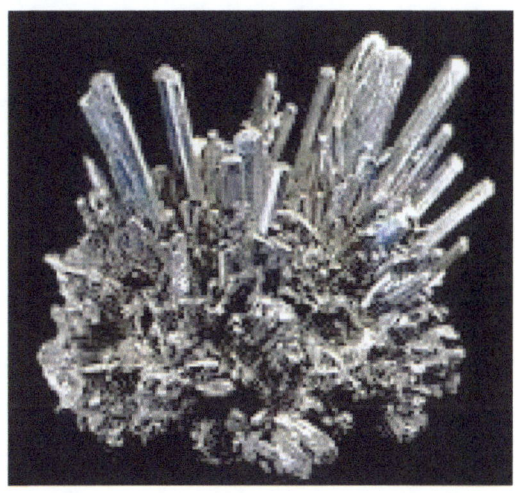

A sample of Stibnite

The three of us piled into a four-seater plane and took off to fly even further north. Landing was more difficult, as would be taking off the next day when we were ready to leave. We flew in over the 'strip' they had carved out of the 'bush' – trees and scrub. We flew the length of the runway twice with the aim of scaring off the kangaroos and other wildlife, and then came in to a successful, if somewhat bumpy landing. It was only a short walk for the three of us through the scrub to the exploration site. There was an extensive field crew there of between ten and twenty men. The head man, as we arrived, was on his knees on the ground, engrossed in some equipment he was trying to repair. He clearly heard us coming, but he didn't look up.

"Just a minute," he said, keeping his eyes fixed firmly on what he was doing. As we got close, he looked up slowly, seeing three pairs of legs encased in jeans. Only when his eye climbed above our waist level did he realise that one pair of legs belonged to a woman. Clearly, he had not been warned, but he took it well, as did the whole field crew. As usual, even in the sub-tropical heat I wore a T-shirt style top with a polo neck and long sleeves, and jeans rather than shorts. It precluded possible complications.

I was shown the site that evening, so was able to have a more detailed look at the soil horizons and the nature of the area in general the next morning. Although they could see small lumps of stibnite on the ground, when it came to sampling, they had clearly been sampling the wrong soil horizon as I had anticipated. I explored this, explained the soil chemistry in some detail, and advised as to how they should plan their future sampling program. And that was it.

Then it was time for the three of us to leave. But there was a problem. The strip was too short to take off with four of us (including the pilot). So he took two of us, flew us to a nearby cattle station with a much longer strip, returned for the remaining man, came back and picked up the two of us, and we headed back to Brisbane taking off from the longer strip. I was thrilled. This was clearly going to be an exciting and interesting job. I enjoyed the work itself, and that was obviously an essential pre-requisite. I also loved the travelling, including to places I would never otherwise have visited. I loved the huge range and variety of interesting people I met, and, as always, I also revelled in sharing information and knowledge.

Other advisory requests came in, some requiring field trips in various parts of the country. Others involved desk work, looking at geological maps, studying drill cores and geochemical profiles.

One trip had added fun. The local Sydney director of one client company asked me to go with him to an area north of the Borosso Valley in South Australia. The work was interesting and straight-forward and finished early one Sunday morning. He and I then drove back down to Adelaide. However, there was to be a detour. On the way, he asked if I would mind if we stopped at a local aerodrome where they had gliders and a gliding club. He explained that he had a licence and club access, and he was keen to 'glide' over the valley. Would I mind? Not at all, after all, his company was paying for my time, and would do so until I got back to Sydney. Layton Consultants (my employer) would gain, of course – not me personally – but a relaxing hour or two was no trouble. When he came back to the car, possibly feeling slightly guilty, he asked if I would like to fly in a glider. Yes of course I would. Fantastic. He explained that as it was not his club he could not take me up himself, but that he had arranged for the local instructor to do so. Wow.

I was to sit in the front, the instructor behind me. I wasn't sure exactly what to expect, but I was excited by the prospect. In fact, it was nothing at all like the small, single-engine, two-seater planes I had become used to on field trips. The strip of metal flooring was less than twelve inches wide, the rest of the floor, walls, and roof were clear plastic, as was *everything* in front of me. Talk about a bird's eye view. Full spherical view. And the silence – no throbbing motor and no rotating propeller to spoil the view. The take-off, being dragged up behind a small plane, was noisy and a bit bumpy, but once we were set loose it was unbelievable. Swooping, turning, rising, falling, we soared over the Barossa Valley in breath-taking style. Then I was asked if I would like to take the controls. Of course I would. He explained how to 'find' the thermals and then more or less left me to it, presumably confident that he could take over if I goofed it. Happily, that did not seem necessary. I could have stayed up for ever, but of course, and far too soon, the time came for us to land. Oddly I had absolutely no fear. This is generally an inevitable if minor part of flying a single-engine plane, as you know you are entirely dependent on the engine continuing to function. In the glider there was absolute confidence, perhaps wrongly placed, that because there was no engine to go wrong, you could, when required, glide gently down and land wherever you wanted to, and that was what happened. We landed back on the strip we had left. I returned to my client and his car and we resumed the much more prosaic drive to Adelaide airport and the flight back to Sydney.

Another technically interesting field trip occurred when I was consulted by Noranda mines. They were looking for assistance in their search for further uranium deposits in their site in the Northern Territory, over 3,000 km from Sydney. Several strategies were relevant. These included the analysis and correlation of certain plants to the levels of associated trace elements in the surrounding soils.

That was followed by another consultation in the north, this time in northwest Queensland. I flew in to Mount Isa where I was met by that company's geologist. We drove in a southerly direction for several hours along dusty dirt tracks through near desert, keeping a keen eye out for any free-roaming cattle or kangaroos that might leap out across the road and into our Land Rover. Eventually, our way led across adjoining cattle stations, their boundaries marked by timber gates through the dividing fences.

Finally, we arrived at an extraordinary house. It was a timber-built thirty-foot square of three rooms, built on a platform four feet above dry and dusty earth (for fear of snakes). The inside was divided by walls as tall as the external walls, but not reaching the pitched roof, so privacy was impossible. One half was the living space and the other half was divided into two to form bedrooms. The one I was offered had a bed, a low cupboard, and hooks along one wall with a variety of clothes hanging from them. It had been the couple's son's bedroom. The walls were upright planks of timber. The 'windows' were also made of planks of timber. These were hinged at the top and could be pushed open from the bottom if you wanted daylight and held open by yet another piece of timber. There was no glass. It rarely rained there, so the main problem would be a sand storm. The company geologist who was with me was quite content to sleep outside. The oblong living room half of the 'house' contained a table with space for four chairs around it along one wall. Along the opposite wall was a vast 'radio' for communication with the rest of the world. For the few days that I was working there, the four of us (Mr, Mrs, the geologist and myself), sat around the table in the evenings with a single kerosene lamp, the only illumination available, in the middle, and our four books encircling it so we each of us could just about see to read. At the end of the evening we went separately and in darkness to our bedroom or, in the case of the geologist, his bunk on the outside veranda.

The kitchen was a lean-to at the back, down at ground level and on the earth floor, with a stove and beside it a table. On the floor under the table were the cooking pots and plates, and on the table top, the tins and packets of food. Preparation was done on trays on the floor and the washing up in a bowl of water, also on the floor.

In place of a bathroom, I was directed either to a small shack with a trench some fifty yards from the house itself, or to a large corrugated iron tank, further away and in a slightly different direction, that housed the precious water supply. For a shower I went as directed to the far side of the tank, away from the house, stood on a sheet of corrugated iron, and grabbed a length of hose. I threw one end of this into the tank and sucked on the other end sufficiently to draw enough water through the pipe to set the syphon going. By holding it over me with one hand I was able to wash with the other. No hot or cold tap here, in fact, no taps at all. It hardly mattered as the temperature was generally in the thirties. A cold winter's day was in the upper twenties. All of this was eyed in silence by a gathering of the station's cattle. Their son was away at University in Townsville. I could only wonder what he thought of the contrast in lifestyles.

It was rough living, but very interesting, and I revelled in the countryside, miles and miles of flat near-desert with amazingly stunted scrub trees. It was quiet. The work, the surveying and sampling, was relatively straightforward, and we left with a large stack of samples. I have wondered since if the clients ever found anything approaching another Mount Isa, but somehow, I doubt it.

Back in Sydney there was more desk work to do, and more clients to meet with and to search for. I was in my early thirties. Up until this time I had only eaten out in restaurants when invited out by and, of course, paid for by boyfriends. Anything else would not have been considered correct back then. I had not even done anything so wildly extravagant as to hail a taxi. In fact, when I first flew to Brisbane from Perth I had sat in the airport for a while waiting for the (non-existent) airport bus into town until I plucked up the courage to get into one of the taxis, wondering if the company would pay for it – they did, but of course, the government would not have done!

However, while in Sydney I soon got used to the high life, the business lunches in smart hotels and restaurants, the frequent dining out with friends, or clients, and the company car. Ah, yes, the company car. By then I was running the Sydney office, the initial director there having chosen to return to West Australia. It was a small office, just myself, a middle-aged geologist mainly there for gravitas and the marketing of our services, and a secretary, but it was a good shop window for the company. What car would I like? I knew exactly what I wanted. My beloved Minivan, that I had had since in London, was immediately sold. I would like, please, an MGB. Good gracious, what would the clients think when I had to drive them around in that as a company car? There must have been quite some discussion among the directors. However, it seemed that they decided, that as they were unconventional enough to have a woman, and a young one at that, running one of their three geological offices, she could also be humoured with her choice of car. The clients seemed to enjoy it – so did I.

With the erratic nature of my work-related travel plans it was lucky that my current boyfriend was also in the mining industry, as a company geologist. We shared a lot of work interests (though of course my client information had to be kept confidential) and he understood the unpredictable nature of my diary. We also had a lot of other interests in common and shared many geology friends.

In the middle of this period, it occurred to me that I was busy working for, and making money for, another company. I was writing million-dollar contracts between my consulting firm and many large mining companies. I began to wonder if I could run a business of my own. Having thought that far, it occurred to me that I could use my 'hobby', the studies of foods and nutrition, and open a health food shop. When in town I could work in it at the weekends and some evenings and advise people on what I had been learning in those study courses while in London, and with all my general reading since. It was a crazy idea, but enticing. A woman I knew thought this sounded like an exciting project and so we drew up a plan. I would finance two-thirds of it and she would put in one third. I would advise on it and work there when I could. She would run it for the regular shop-opening hours. So far so good.

Having seen a district of Sydney near to where I lived and where there was no competition, I bought out a cake shop that was for sale. I took the holidays that were due to me by then and took great pleasure in turning what I thought of as a nutrient-negative, unhealthy cake shop into a nutrient-positive, healthy health-food shop. We designed and built the shelving, ordered and unpacked the stock, and set too. It was great fun, at least for me. Once it was established and my holiday leave had run its course, I returned to my mining and geochemical consulting. She ran it full time, although I spent all the spare time I had there.

It worked – at least for a while. After a time she found she was bored and didn't like being tied to the shop for regular hours. She wanted out. That created a potential problem for me, particularly as I *didn't* want out; I was enjoying myself and finding it interesting. I was fortunate and found Frieda, an excellent assistant and keen to run the shop. She had always wanted to run her own health food store but had no money to invest. In those days in Sydney most health food shops were run by the owner with an occasional after-school helper, so she couldn't get a paid full-time job in one. Until she met me. I needed a full-time assistant to take over from my one-time partner. That was the start of an excellent and prolonged relationship.

Initially, the shop ran as a conventional health food store. However, there were two additional rooms at the back and so in time I extended these. To begin with, I added an extensive book shop, my aim being not just to sell products but to teach people about nutrition as well. The second became a take-away snack bar, and eventually a herbal and homoeopathic dispensary.

I worked in the shop on the Saturdays when I was in town and on Thursday late-shopping nights, advising people on nutrition as much as possible. This was in the early 1970s, when nutrition knowledge and classical naturopathy were little known, although the key elements did have an extended history, followed by a few. I enjoyed it all and it became an increasingly absorbing hobby, functioning behind my 'day job'.

My day job continued to be as absorbing and demanding as ever, with lots of interesting field work. I used to joke that I knew more about the great Australian bush than about any of the towns around the coastal periphery where the vast majority of people lived and worked. I didn't, during this time, have my own geochemical laboratory. My caravan laboratory would have been impractical as I could be travelling a thousand or more miles a week, supervising sampling teams and advising clients on the possibilities of their various mining claims. Instead, samples were sent off to one of two specialised analytical laboratories.

As usual, most of the searching was for economic mineral deposits, mainly nickel, copper, and zinc. Uranium was of interest in the Northern Territory. Uranium does not travel far through the surrounding rocks and soil, and is difficult to detect at the low, but economical concentrations that might be present in the underlying rock, or overburden, or surface rock. However, selenium is often associated with uranium deposits in geological structures. Selenium does travel and it can be more readily detected. It is also concentrated

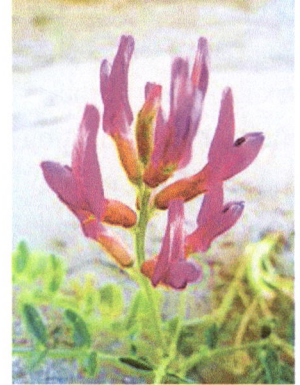

in certain plant species. One project involved looking for and mapping the beautiful mauve plant Astragalus (A). In some instances, the mere presence of these plants in unusual abundance could be a positive indication of underlying uranium. We also subjected samples of *A. pattersoni, A. preussi, and A. thompsonae* to analysis for selenium. Another plant, whose name I have forgotten, responded to unusually high levels of uranium in the soil by changing its growth pattern, from vertical stems to stems that lay flat along the ground.

If this sounds easy, it wasn't, though I thoroughly enjoyed it. Almost all the field work involved covering vast areas, often on foot or over rough ground, in Land Rovers and similar vehicles, in generally dry but sweltering heat, dripping sweat and endeavouring to avoid sunburn. Heavy boots were essential almost all the time, as was a heavy back-pack for sampling and other equipment. I was always working with men. At no time did I meet or work with another female professional geologist, and no other geochemist at all. In my entire time in the mining industry I was a rare bird. I always dressed circumspectly, well covered up, never flirted, and never had any of the problems one might have expected. As part of that I insisted on carrying my own share of the samples and equipment and doing nothing that indicated I was different to the rest of 'the guys'.

One unusual project involved the idea of searching for indications of underground oil by sampling the soil hydrocarbons. We thought this to be impossible in areas where there had been much activity with the use of vehicles causing industrial pollution of any sort. It could also be difficult in areas of active and varied geology where gases would readily escape. But the idea we looked at was the possibility that, in Australia, where the vast central land mass was not only flat and stable, had a fairly uniform geology and was essentially devoid of vehicles and so of exhaust gases, the idea might have merit. I was keen to explore this further. After all, geochemical prospecting, which would involve the collection of soil samples with indications of hydrocarbons only a metre or two deep, would be vastly less costly than the very expensive deep hole geophysical drilling. The idea was not taken further, at least while I was there, although it was considered a few years later when a fellow geophysicist and I were asked about the possibility of its application in Greece.

I was absorbed in my work and thought little of the future. Then, early in 1970, Poseidon shares crashed. Other shares slumped like dominos. It was the end of the mining boom. The smaller companies that had floated on a wing and a prayer, often based more on and hope and hype and very small soil anomalies, than sense, also went broke. Mostly they had spent their start-up funds but generally found little or nothing in the way of an income source. The larger companies reduced their exploration budget or began to train their own geochemist and brought the work in-house. The writing was clearly on the wall. I was sent out on more and more marketing efforts looking for clients. I have never liked marketing. Staff were gradually being laid off. I had to sack the final Sydney senior geologist. The company's third, though very minor partner, left the different company he had been working for and came with the expectation of taking over the Layton office in Sydney. It was plainly time for me to look for something new.

There was now going to be little money for the type of large-scale consulting firm I had been working with. I had in the past few years, both in Sydney and while being a commercial consultant rather than a government employee, had the wool pulled from my slightly naïve eyes. In the various geological surveys in which I had worked, I had been largely free to follow my research bents, free from the commercial pressures of financially viable finds, and able to avoid political manoeuvring. In the last years with Laytons I had begun to see below the surface. I had started to dislike what I saw. In the last couple of years I had become aware of slight pressure to 'rejig' the results for clients, to write a more optimistic report, to make the maps look as if the area of 'interesting anomaly' was larger than it actually was, so as to please the shareholders. I did not like this. I remained focused on 'finding the truth, whatever that was', just as I had imagined I would when contemplating a career as a forensic chemist. Commercial reality was coming face to face with my focus on 'truth'.

I considered my options for the future. I could apply for a lecturing post in one of the universities, but that did not seem exciting, especially after the glories and freedoms of the past twelve years. I had been a geochemist throughout this time. My career had been perfectly balanced on the lead up to and the duration of the mining boom of the late sixties and early seventies. I had spent three years in New Zealand, and two or three each variously in Fiji, in London at Imperial, and then in West Australia, and the remaining time in Sydney. I had loved the work and the travelling all over such a huge proportion of the southern hemisphere. But this did seem to be coming to an end. I had been lucky. I had been in the right place at the right time with just the right amount of training behind me, and as such I had risen up rapidly in an empty and growing niche. Now, at the top, I had to rethink.

I was clear that I was not interested in pure research, in knowing more and more about less and less. Thus, as I thought about it, the idea of university life quickly lost its appeal. So that idea was out. On top of that, with a large number of geologists losing their jobs in exploration companies, there would be few vacancies. I was very interested in applied research, such as I had been doing for the past decade or more, taking an idea and applying it to see whether or not it proved valid and useful, or what more could be learnt from it and applied later. However, there was clearly little financial appetite for this, at least for the foreseeable future.

Furthermore, I was interested in the chemistry aspect of geochemistry, much more than in the geology aspect of it. I had spent the past decade analysing river and stream water samples, river sediment samples, soil samples, vegetation samples, and more. I loved trying to understand what the results meant in relation to the current project or search and the underlying geology. I thought back to my earlier career plans, back in my student days at Imperial in London. Then I had planned to be an analytical forensic chemist. That had appealed, many years ago. But how I could enter that profession at this later stage if I really wanted to, was unclear. The next possibility I considered would involve learning even more about my current secondary interest – food, food chemistry, and health, and build on the nutrition studies I had done both on my own and at Queen Elizabeth College in London. Perhaps it was time to think about that?

The day came when Layton and I decided to part company. They had reduced income to pay me as a consultant. Neither did they have clients that needed or could any longer pay for my skills. In all conscience I could not stay. We decided this in the morning of a day of high summer. I left the office and went for a long walk through the nearby Sydney botanical gardens and thought things over. I realised clearly that I had never had any specific career plan. Until now it had all seemed to roll out organically. I looked back on three undergraduate years, and later two research years at Imperial. I thought of the ten years or more in the mining industry, largely in mineral exploration and mapping. I'd loved it. Most of that time I had been associated with or employed by the Geological Survey departments of a variety of countries – New Zealand, Fiji, and West Australia. In these I had had the luxury of being able to research and explore ideas without undue commercial pressure. These last two or more years I'd been employed by Layton and Associate Consultants based in Sydney, and available for their clients all over Australasia and even beyond. There had been this fantastic and heady mining boom. I had been fortunate in having several large companies as clients, Noranda Mines, Anglo American, and others. These companies were still active, and occasionally in need of help, but they were well over-supplied with applicants, at least with geologists. It was time to clear my desk in Layton's city office and consider my future.

Chapter 9

End of an Era

It was the end of an era. Not a geological era, exactly, but perhaps a geologically associated era, for me at least But what was I to do next? What did I want to do?

I had my home on Sydney's lower North Shore. I had my business, the health food shop I called the Natural Gourmet, about a mile away. I had a reasonable amount of money saved and set aside, so had no desperate or immediate need of a new income. I adored Aunt – she was an integral part of my life, and she was in London, but I could not build a life around her, and England had little other pull for me. In all the time I had been living outside England, she and I had kept in touch via our audio cassettes. That would certainly continue. Amazingly, she had always been there for me, a backstop of support and approval. I was very lucky to have her. It didn't occur to me, until decades later, that she might have felt just as lucky to have me, the daughter she could not have.

I recalled the time in London when I was doing research for my Diploma of Imperial College (DIC) and had nearly no money. I had realised then that I could stretch the food budget by moving towards a vegetarian diet. Vegetarianism was almost unheard of in those days and I had been unsure of the wisdom of this diet. So I had studied it with a focus on protein chemistry and the balancing of amino acids. I had given rein to the part of my brain that had considered doing biochemistry instead of analytical chemistry for my final Honours year as an undergraduate at Imperial. I had enrolled in studies in Nutrition at Queen Elizabeth College and found it fascinating. One of the great benefits of having chemistry as a starting degree is that it can be the basis of studying all types of spheres of activity and interests. I had had only a tiny research grant for those two years but I had made good use of it and the time I spent getting my DIC. The more I had thought along these lines during these years, the more it had seemed obvious to me that you could not look for improved health by consuming toxic drugs, even if they carried the adjective 'medical'. The chemist in me veered instinctively to putting right what was wrong, what we now call 'restoring homoeostasis', by improving nutrition, rather than battering the problem with foreign substances (drugs). It had not, at the time, occurred to me to make a profession of this.

Perhaps now it was time to consider this option. I thought about taking on the shop as my full-time occupation, but swiftly decided that that was not enough, either intellectually or financially. So would I travel, look overseas for a future opportunity? Somehow I felt inclined to remain in Sydney and I did not want to disrupt Frieda from the job she loved. I continued to put in many hours at or above the shop while I thought about this. Above the shop itself was a generous four-room apartment. I set up the main room as my office. I expanded the book section of the shop downstairs and read the majority of the books I bought as stock. At that time 'alternative health care' was not even an accepted term. No one spoke of 'naturopaths' or 'alternative nutritionists'. There were, however, many books on nutrition, and I read them with growing enthusiasm. I also spent a more extensive amount of time chatting with and advising the customers, or clients, in the shop downstairs, though without charging them.

I had another interest too. As a kid I recall having to go to church every Sunday. This memory goes back to my childhood year in New Zealand where I recall walking back from the church with Father and Brother (the latter aged about seven), having just been given our Sunday treats of copies of 'Dandy' and 'Beano'. In the various boarding schools that I had been to in the subsequent years of my early childhood, I had been fed the standard English version of 'scripture'. I hadn't questioned it. During my first year at Tormead (aged eleven), while I was a day girl, Mother and Maternal Grandmother, on the rare days they weren't fighting each other, took us to church on Sunday mornings. As a border at Tormead we went to church every Sunday morning, walking crocodile style. At school we had a scripture lesson every week, based totally on Church of England protestant beliefs. The Bible was a given, as were all the stories in it. It was presented as a history, and the only true one at that, rather than as any sort of a philosophy. There was no debate.

I clearly lacked any sort of religious conviction, and it didn't occur to me to go to church once I left home for university, and peace. However, in my last year at Imperial, the Church of the Latter-Day Saints (a Mormon church) in Exhibition Road, South Kensington, was opening and, for the first six weeks visitors were allowed inside. DZ and I had gone in. Inevitably I had asked a lot of questions, to which the answers were invariably along the lines of "that is what the bible says, we follow it strictly". Then we came to the baptismal pool. This was about four feet square and ten inches deep. I was told that people were baptised as they walked through it. My logical brain had protested at this. "But you just said you followed the bible exactly. The bible talks of total body immersion". The answer "We have to be practical, and there isn't the space here" set me thinking. The more I thought about it, the more I realised that there were many inconsistencies in Christian writing, thinking, and stories. I was to come across many more in the years ahead. I had always wondered at the different stories of the gospels, the different versions of Christ's birth – stable or luxury, shepherds or wise men, and so forth.

London in the 1950s and early 60s was largely Protestant, at least the part I knew. I had had little exposure to other religions or belief systems, and little interest in exploring them. I was, after all, a scientist. Soon after I had arrived in Dunedin, aged twenty-one, the flat I first moved into overlooked a church. As I watched the congregations arriving and leaving, it occurred to me that I saw no point in religion. There were clearly many of them. Christianity was not the only one.

They disagreed: "My god is better than your god". Countless wars had been fought over religious beliefs, both between the major religions and between sects within a religion. None of it made sense. I had decided then, that as a chemist and a scientist, I would be more comfortable focusing on chemistry and the physical evolution of ourselves and our world and leaving religion alone. How our world and our individual lives both started and ended was of little interest to me at twenty-one.

I thought back to my time in Perth when I had bought my house and land with the aim of building an extensive garden. I thought of all I had learnt from Mr and Mrs K who had become good friends and opened my mind to Rudolf Steiner and Anthroposophy. From time to time Mr K would lend me more books in addition to *Knowledge of the Higher Worlds*[i], *Theosophy*[ii], and *Occult Science*[iii]. All of them were by Rudolf Steiner. I had felt no particular inclination to read them, but had felt that I owed it to Mr K to do so and had struggled through them. The curious thing was that they gradually made more and more sense to me. I was particularly intrigued by Steiner's *Occult Science*. How could those two words belong even in one sentence, never mind in the two-word title of a book?

The time had come, while I was living in Perth, when I was introduced to the BD (Biodynamic) preparations. An ounce or so of each preparation was mixed with water and stirred, then stored until used. The preparation called '500' was to be sprayed on the earth, another, called '501' on the leaves, and five others into the compost heaps, one at each corner and one along a central hollow at the top. All this seemed very strange. After all, I was only given an ounce or so of each to use. How could they work? Mr K chided me for my impatience and lack of imagination. Worse was to come. I was to put each of the first two preparations into large tubs of pure water and stir them in. But no, not just any stirring. I was to create a vortex in one direction and then, as soon as that formed, to stop and reverse the rotation until the alternative vortex was formed. And to increase the challenge this was to continue for a full hour. I went in search of the radio. No, this was not allowed. I was to focus and 'meditate' (me, a pure material scientist, meditate?). I was not even allowed to read one of Mr K's books while I stirred. Then, once these preparations were complete, I was to walk all over my acre of land with a very large brush, dip it in the gallon of treated water and flip it over the leaves, and another at ground level. That, I thought, I would not be doing in daytime, in the sight of my neighbours, I'd look a right idiot. I did do it however, but during the late evening hours. I was keen to test the outcome.

For the rest of my time in Perth I had continued to work with, and be helped by, Mr K. But I learnt little more of the great scope of anthroposophy. During the extended field trips in WA, I had read up on many of the world religions; interesting, but none had fully appealed.

When I had first arrived in Sydney, my time had been fully taken up with mineral exploration and my career within the mining industry. But now that the demands of work had been so radically reduced, I decided to explore Anthroposophy further. I was not encouraged in this by a desire for any spiritual or religious development, but I had become intrigued, during my two years in Perth by *Occult Science*. As I picked up my copies of the books, I was again struck and intrigued by the juxtaposition of the two words. Rudolf Steiner (1861-1925) had also intrigued me. In all the reading I had done in Perth, and on field trips in discussions with the Mr and Mrs K and IW, it was clear that Steiner was not a religious leader, nor the head of a cult or similar. I was not asked to follow him, obey him, or believe in him. I was asked to explore his ideas for myself.

As I saw it, he seemed to be a man who could perceive non-physical forces and events in a way that most of us could not, certainly back then. I likened it to someone who could see, in a community of blind people. They lived in the same world, but the one who could 'see', in this case Steiner (perhaps better to say 'could perceive') could say things like "over there, about ten yards away, is a beautiful tree".

Everyone else, those without eyes (or organs of perception) failed to understand what he was doing or saying, but when they went over to it and felt it, they found it to be as the sighted one had described.

Steiner, in his lectures and writings, seemed to be describing a spiritual or non-physical world that he could 'see', or perceive, and describe to other people. There was no suggestion that anyone else should 'believe' anything he said. Instead, he encouraged people to study and explore for themselves. He encouraged would-be biodynamic farmers and gardeners to experiment with his ideas for the use of compost accelerators and more. He encouraged doctors to experiment with his ideas for a different approach to health care for people in a wide variety of walks of life. I had done just that when I ran the carrot seed test as described in chapter seven, which required the moon to be 'right'.

Even after I had arrived in Sydney I hadn't immediately followed up on this interest. I was too busy. I was away from Sydney on field work and consulting visits too often to do anything on a regular basis when in Sydney. But once I resigned from geochemistry I decided to follow up on this interest. With the aim of learning more I met up with BW and was welcomed into several of the study groups. I enjoyed them all. On Tuesday evenings there was a group led by MS, young, dedicated and inspiring, as well as being an excellent teacher. He worked in one of the residential Anthroposophical homes for children in need of special care. Under his guidance, this group explored the ideas that Steiner had laid out in his book *Theosophy*, though it had nothing to do with the Theosophical Society. Steiner had joined the Theosophical Society near the start of the twentieth century, finding it a place where other people had some of the same perceptions as himself. Theosophy, the wisdom of god. That was a high ideal and level of knowledge to aim for, but Steiner soon grew frustrated with it, and with the Theosophical Society and some of its politics. He then established the Anthroposophical Society, based on exploring an understanding of 'the wisdom of man'. This better reflected Steiner's striving to become more aware of the true nature and depth of individual humans, and perhaps from that to move on to an understanding of higher things.

On Thursday evenings the senior Sydney group met for general discussion. This was largely made up of Germanic Europeans who had come out to Australia round the time of, or because of, the Second World War. It was interesting, but in truth a bit dull, at least to my exploring mind. On Friday evenings there was a group led by a very interesting couple who focused more on the science behind Anthroposophy and projective geometry. They were very stimulating, and excellent at teaching what they had learnt. During several weekends throughout the year there were also various events and discussions. The Tuesday and Thursday evening group members were roughly around my age and I started to go to all of those meetings. Thursday evenings were a fallback option, but I attended most of them. Increasingly I was drawn to learn more and try to make sense of it all. It was a positive banquet of new ideas, new ways of viewing the world, new ways of thinking, and meeting up with the most delightful and interesting people. I loved all of it and lapped it up with boundless enthusiasm. Thus, I gradually shed my geological friends, in the way one does when one's daily life and interests no longer coincide. Instead, I had found a wonderful group of friends all interested in and excited by the ideas we were exploring.

I learnt just how highly practical were the applications of Anthroposophy. I learnt much more of its testable concepts. I found the whole topic an intriguing and satisfying blend of spirit and science. I soon learnt that Steiner's ideas covered not only biodynamic gardening and farming, but nutrition, health care, medicine (he gave many lectures to doctors), education (the Waldorf schools), the needs of people who needed special care, the arts as in eurhythmy (expressive movement), and more, very much more. I was also amazed at the way all the various topics blended and melded with each other. Everything 'made sense', like the pieces of a complex jigsaw, coming together and explaining the great tapestry of life.

I learnt of a type of chemical analysis that Steiner and some of his colleagues or co-workers had developed that showed up the specific and subtle aspects or energies of many substances. The term they used was 'chromas', but this had little to do with the conventional chromatography of science laboratories that I knew. As a one-time analytical chemist, I was intrigued by it, and had already done a few experiments with it. I now had the time to set up a small laboratory above the shop. Here I analysed and compared the different ways of making juices, and then the different 'chromas' made from these juices by different methods. I studied juices made by hand-squeezing, and by machines with ever stronger (rougher) physical methods. I compared the chromas of juices made from biodynamically grown, then organically, and then commercially grown fruits and vegetables. I studied the chromas of foods cooked in containers made of different materials: glass, pottery, aluminium (as was common in those days), steel etc. The results were fascinating, and can be found written up in books available from Rudolf Steiner Press.

BW, IW's father, ran the Biodynamic section in Sydney, but another man, AP, ran it in Melbourne, nine hundred kilometres away. I was intrigued to find that there were differences. There was a very large number of biodynamic farms throughout Victoria, and many of the farmers were not even remotely interested in anthroposophy. They simply farmed that way because it was more economical, more successful, and healthier for the land, for plants, for the animals and for humans, than the produce grown commercially and with chemical sprays. Better still, the produce was tastier. Surely that was proof of some of the concepts.

So there I was, living happily in my lovely unit and working part-time in the Natural Gourmet 'playing shop'. It was great fun. I started a snack bar in the space behind the shop and I was experimenting in my laboratory. I had built up the book stock and was reading avidly all the books I could find on nutrition, then helping to answer the questions of some of my customers who were in search of better health. And finally, I was enjoying my evening and weekend studies and friendships. It was all very pleasant, interesting, and satisfying. It was also a great contrast to my career in the mining industry. But I knew it was not a long-term option.

And that was when GWA walked into my life.

---

[i] Rudolf Steiner, *Knowledge of the Higher Worlds. How is it achieved?* Rudolf Steiner Press, London, 1969

[ii] Rudolph Steiner, *Theosophy: An Introduction to the Supersensible Knowledge of the World and the Destination of Man*, Rudolph Steiner Press, London, 1922

[iii] Rudolf Steiner, *Occult Science, An Outline*, Rudolf Steiner Press, London, 1963

Chapter 10

South Africa

Fortunately I was in the shop on the day that GWA walked in. I soon learnt that BW had sent him, convinced that the two of us should meet up during GWA's visit to Australia and compare our shared interests. GWA was a dedicated anthroposophist, living in Johannesburg and involved almost single-handedly in running an amazing number of anthroposophical activities and organisations. 'Pharma Natura' was his head office and factory. From there he supplied and masterminded five health food stores, one each in Capetown, Durban and Pretoria and two in Johannesburg. He had a large importing company that brought a whole range of health foods into the country and supplied many other health food shops and chemists, as well as his own. He was instrumental in establishing Rudolf Steiner's Waldorf schools. He employed a Swiss anthroposophist who was well trained in manufacturing the Wala medical remedies, and was also a strong and efficient business and accounts manager. His wife, from whom he was separated, ran the Weleda (anthroposophical) pharmacy and their biodynamic farm outside Johannesburg. Other than that, he was on his own with largely unskilled workers under him, none of whom shared his deeper interests and enthusiasms. He was dynamic and driven, choleric in temperament and with a passion for all things anthroposophical. Thus, he was full of ideas, but short of other people to lead and run them and share and work with him. We had a lengthy chat about our shared activities and interests and arranged to meet up later for dinner.

Dinner was quite relaxed, but it rapidly became clear that he saw me as exactly what he had been dreaming of for his business empire, the one person who was precisely what he was looking for, who had commercial and business sense, practical knowledge and experience and with an anthroposophical commitment. Would I move to South Africa and join him in his business empire?

As he saw it, I could take over the supervision of his five health food shops and start up the restaurant(s) he wanted. I could write useful nutritional articles for their regular health magazine. I could set up the laboratory he wanted so they could run the chromas (me being a chemist), and contribute to the Weleda pharmacy and the biodynamic farm if I felt like helping his very independent wife. He was convinced I could train up on the anthroposophical approach to medicine,[i,ii,iii] [vi]and lecture to the doctors who were starting to apply the Wala remedies his company was making. I thought this could take some time. However, by our next dinner during the second day of his Sydney visit, he had it all planned out. I would be the fourth director in his business, with him, the Wala medicine manufacturer, and the business manager. His wife seemed to be running the Weleda pharmacy on her own with a different personal partner.

I did recognise how I must seem to him to be an amazing 'fit'. Not only did I have the skills and experience that he wanted, or the makings of them, but I enjoyed and was interested in all he was doing. I was also keen to explore the practical application of anthroposophical concepts.

However, I would have to consider leaving Australia and moving to South Africa. At that time, I had rarely lived in one place for much more than two or three years, so I was used to that, and it did not seem to be a major complication, but I hung back. I was just developing an interesting life for myself. I had created a niche in Sydney that I was enjoying and I had made many good friends. Yet I was also tempted. The opportunity offered much more of a challenge than what I was doing in Sydney. I was tempted practically, commercially, and intellectually, and I loved a challenge! I thought about apartheid, but I had lived comfortably in Fiji with two other races so assumed, wrongly as it turned out, that that would not be a major problem. I would also be closer to Aunt and might even manage a few visits, costing, I hoped, rather less than the cost from Sydney, which at this time was prohibitive.

Nonetheless, I still continued to hang back. In fact, that evening I said no, I would probably not accept his offer. Then I thought about it that night, knowing he was leaving Sydney the following afternoon. Even so, at our farewell lunch the following day, I again declined his offer. His disappointment was obvious. I said that there were too many uncertainties; it was all very sudden and unexpected and I would be giving up a lot here in Sydney. That was when he applied the heavy persuasion. He would fly me over to Johannesburg (Jo'burg) for a three-week visit to give it a try. I could even fly back, via Ireland, and visit my beloved Aunt. It amused him to be able to tell me that although that meant I would be flying many more miles (two sides of a triangle), it would actually save him seven rand on the fare. It didn't seem fair as it was a win-win situation for me on many fronts, whereas he ran the risk that I might visit and still not want to leave Sydney. He was adamant that he thought the risk was worth it to him and he was confident that I would decide in favour of South Africa.

Finally, and at the very last minute, just as he was leaving that afternoon, I agreed to consider the three-week trial visit. He was a very strong and persuasive choleric! As the idea began to take root, my mind focused as usual on all the positives, all the opportunities this offered. Also as usual, I focused on the near future, trusting that, should I finally accept his offer, the long-term future would somehow take care of itself.

The decision made, I made arrangements for my affairs to run in my absence, and a few weeks later I took off for Jo'burg. It was an eventful month. I was met off the plane, introduced to the two senior staff and shown around his various establishments – the office, factory, and health food shops. We drove to Pretoria and visited his organisation there, followed by a drive down to Durban to his south-coast shop, stopping off along the way and talking with a number of the doctors who were already getting interested in anthroposophical medicine. The scenery was amazing, as was the route along the coast to Cape Town to his other health food shop, and more anthroposophical doctors. Then back up to Jo'burg. It was a lengthy drive, but the roads were good and fairly empty, and we had plenty to talk about. GWA was certainly keen for me to see the best of the country and to meet as many interesting people as he could arrange. In this he was successful. There were still pros and cons in my mind, but in the end I decided on the move to South Africa. My first priority, though, was the quick trip to Ireland to spend a week with Aunt, who was understandably delighted with this aspect of my proposed move. It was a few years since I had seen her and had the funds and opportunity to travel. It was very much more expensive in those days.

I returned to Sydney, sold the Natural Gourmet, at that time a successful and thriving business, and let my unit (apartment)fully furnished. That left me with a minimum of luggage which I sent over by sea, while I headed for Jo'burg by plane again.

It started well. I had a loosely defined area of responsibility, mostly retail and medical. Clearly, he was headstrong, but he had a right to be and it was undoubtedly this that had led him to achieving so much. He was also determined as to what *he* wanted to do, but generally our ideas meshed. I observed for a few weeks and then made a variety of suggestions, following up on all the ideas he and I had discussed. He had taken on the lease of an Italian restaurant in the centre of Jo'burg and so this I had to fit out and get started. Déjà vu, really, but in previous jobs it had been fitting out a geochemical laboratory. I greatly enjoyed the company of HA, the Swiss manufacturer of the Wala remedies, and had great discussions with him. I spent some weekends camping out at the company's biodynamic farm and encountered my first snakes. Ironically, I had seen none in Australia. The sales manager was not interested in Steiner's ideas and was refreshingly practical and logical. GWA, on the other hand, showed progressively more and more of his irascible side. Clearly his strong determination had got things done – getting the remedies into the country, the Steiner schools started, and more, much more, but he was not an easy person to work with. Nonetheless, there was much to enjoy and I learnt a lot.

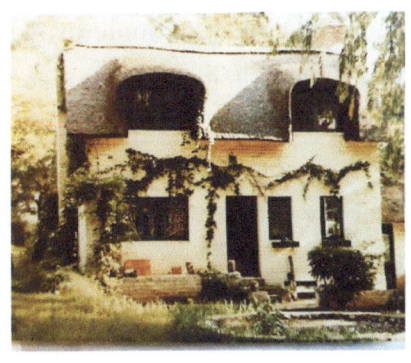

Initially I lived in a lovely Dutch cottage owned by the company, on two acres of land near, actually too near for safety, to the Soweto township. There was to have been a chap staying in the other half of the cottage as it was deemed to be unsafe for me to live there on my own. Unfortunately, his work took him away some nights, and even with a friend there for company on those nights and a Doberman for protection, it was difficult to relax. Several nights a week I would wake up with the dog growling and moving around inside the house, me following, nervously clutching my geological hammer for protection. As a result, I soon moved into a large and neatly furnished flat in Hillbrow. I'm told it is now an unacceptable area, but at that time the flats were efficient and attractive. The house girls lived in accommodation on the roof and came in to clean each day. There were locks on all the cupboards, even in the bathroom, and on the fridge door, all with keys provided. I found it difficult to get used to having to lock the doors on all the cupboards every time I went out, and managed to lose one or two precious items when I forgot and left them lying on an open shelf.

My first job involved establishing the restaurant, fitting it out and defining the menu. Based on my middle name, I suggested we called it Kate's Kitchen, which seemed to amuse the kitchen staff. I was determined it should not be totally vegetarian but that it should have a generous selection of meat and fish as well as vegetable dishes. I knew from personal experience that if I was in a group of diners, the meat-eaters would generally insist on a non-vegetarian restaurant, maintaining that "there would always be something there you could eat". As a result, a purely vegetarian restaurant could struggle for customers (this was of course fifty or more years ago and a lot has changed since). Therefore our fixed menu included a couple of meat dishes, chicken and fish, but our variable menu, changed daily, always comprised several totally vegetarian dishes. Desserts were no problem, nor were the coffees as we had dandelion, chicory, and others, but teas were different. We offered the three herb teas that were available in those days, chamomile, peppermint, and rosehip, and of course China tea. But what about our 'ordinary' tea? You could hardly call it that on the menu, never mind that we aimed to be 'interesting', not 'ordinary'. I opted for calling it 'Indian' tea. A surprising number of people ordered it but then complained that it was indeed 'ordinary'. Explanations were required.

Initially it was a challenge to find all the foods, the ingredients, and the quality that I wanted, but in time we managed. I had one Australian manager in the restaurant and the rest of the staff were African. I enjoyed them all and as we grew together a positive camaraderie grew. I spent the lunch hour of each day supervising the restaurant and its running. A few times I forgot to count all the knives, forks, and spoons at the end of the day in the restaurant. It was the staff that often had to remind me, for their own safety and to avoid being blamed if some were lost. I was troubled by this, but conformed. When a member of staff failed to show up for work one morning, this was brushed aside with "They're probably in jail", or "They may have lost their permit". This was the one they needed so they could have free movement round the city, beyond their own townships. The casual way this was said disturbed me as much as the event itself.

I then focused on the health food shops, looking at and learning the products they carried and researching others that I had been familiar with in Australia. They had several products that we had not had in Sydney, all, I suspected, due to the initiatives of GWA. Weekends were holidays then, no 'shopping till we dropped'. Perhaps we worked part of Saturdays, my memory is unclear.

At that time there were no such things as 'health bars'. In Sydney we had had 'sesame snaps' and a couple of others, but not much else. I had developed several while at the Natural Gourmet: flapjacks, walnut slice, date slice, coconut squares. This was easily done there in the space that I had. It should have been easy in South Africa and I envisaged sending them out to all our shops, not just Kate's Kitchen. However, there was a problem. Without a bakery licence we could not use flour. I could use nuts and seeds – oil-rich seeds, though, not starch-rich seeds such as wheat and other grains. Without flour all my attempts had a strong tendency to fall apart. But I persisted. It was then a question of what to do with all the broken bits that broke into crumbs. In this way was born by far our favourite dessert, Kate's Delight. This was a layer of cooked brown rice, a layer of fresh fruits, and a layer of the nuts and seed crumbs from the broken health bars, all topped with plain yoghurt.

We employed several people in the restaurant and shops, almost all African, and I noticed them becoming very nervous on the day, each month, that they were paid, in cash. They explained that "the township trains are dangerous". Men knowing about the pay day were in the habit of attacking the women and stealing their wages on their way home. They each wrapped their pay in stockings and tied these around their waist, hidden by layers of clothing. I offered to give them their pay weekly, or in some other way, instead of a month at a time, but they didn't seem too happy about that either.

I was still taking thyroxine for the after-effects of the accident at Hammersmith Hospital with radioactive iodine, but I did not like doing this. When I spoke to one of the anthroposophical doctors, he told me about a Wala remedy called Thyroidea Thymus that would improve and restore my thyroid function. He advised me to take this for three months and then gradually reduce the thyroxine intake until I felt I no longer needed it. This I did, at least for a while.

I focused a lot of my studies on the anthroposophical medicines and the chromas.

A friend I made worked as a tour guide and he included me in a trip through the Kruger National Park, a magical experience. But I made surprisingly few friends. There was no congenial professional focus such as the university, into which I could slot, and I missed the anthroposophical study groups of Sydney, so my brain began to feel addled. But there was worse. Increasingly I struggled with the laws and cruelties of apartheid. I had foolishly thought that having lived in and visited other multi-racial settings, this could not be so very much worse. There had been relatively few Māoris in the South Island of New Zealand where I had spent most of my time when living there, so New Zealand hardly counted, but I thought that Fiji, where I had lived and been happy, and Samoa, Tonga, Tahiti, and other islands that I had visited, had given me a fair bit of experience. But the unfairness of the apartheid system, and the inbuilt mistrust, I found abhorrent.

My time was routinely dispersed over several of our Jo'burg locations – the shop, the restaurant, the two city centre shops and others. I would occasionally get back to the head office late in the afternoon and on two occasions I had thoughtlessly allowed myself to be the very last one to leave my office in the main building where we had the factory and administration offices. On each occasion I was approached by Africans wielding knives. My speed at reaching my car, getting in and slamming and locking the door should have earned me a place on the Olympic team. On the second occasion the knife left a serious scratch along the driver's window. I gradually learned to think defensively, but all in all, I was beginning to wonder about my stay in this country. I certainly did not feel at home, not in the way I had instantly done in the past, each time I relocated.

I enjoyed the work, but it became clear to me that I could not envisage a long-term future here. Yet I felt I owed it to GWA to stay on for a while longer as I remained impressed with his dedication and ideals and the amount he had accomplished. I stayed for longer than I might have wished, but in the end, after some careful planning both in South Africa for the company, and back in Australia where I had to make plans, I left.

I returned by boat, and it was only as I went on board in Cape Town that I realised I had packed my backup stock of thyroxine in my trunk and that it was now inaccessibly buried in the hold and could not be reached for over two weeks. It was a Sunday, no pharmacy was open, and I had no prescription with me and no chance of seeing or getting one from a doctor. I had four thyroxine tablets left and was supposed to be taking three a day. Fortunately, I did have my Thyroidea Thymus. Faced with this situation I decided the best thing was to break each thyroxine tablet into four pieces, making a total of sixteen, take one of those each morning and, if necessary, double up on the frequency with which I took the Thyroidea Thymus. In this way I managed to reach Australia and my trunk without running totally out of energy.

I then considered the matter. I had always been reluctant to take any medical drug at all, and certainly not on an ongoing basis. I decided to see if I could continue on the present regime, but take only the Thyroidea Thymus. I had been told it would help normalise the thyroid function. I waited to see how quickly and how well it would accomplish this. With only minor energy slumps, I found that it worked. There was no anthroposophical doctor in Australia so when I got back there, I ordered more of the product from Germany and hoped for the best. It continued to work. Over the next four or five years I carried on taking it. Gradually I found I could take it less and less frequently and not run out of energy. Eventually I felt emboldened enough to give it up altogether. That was fifty years ago and I have had a well-functioning thyroid gland ever since, even though, some years later I was to learn that the original accident had apparently caused a lot more harm to several people than I had realised.

On my way back to Australia I gave considerable thought to my next move. I was used to uprooting and moving on to the next country and the next opportunity, but hitherto I had known what I was moving to. This time I had certain ideas, but all vague, without a definite plan, and no backup or material support, either practical, conceptional, or financial, However, what I was sure of was that I wanted to be involved in some way with health and nutrition, and with anthroposophical philosophy, concepts, and activities, particularly biodynamic gardening or farming and the anthroposophical medicines. My exploration of these concepts had started with all the anthroposophists I had met and talked with, but I also built on such books as [iv,v] Rudolf Hauschka, *The Nature of Substance*, and Rudolf Hauschka, *Nutrition*. I had been communicating for some time with AS, a distinguished anthroposophist in Melbourne, and was particularly eager to spend some time working and studying with him. I was keen to research chemistry within the anthroposophical concept and with the chromas. With this in mind I had arranged, on my return, to discuss a working relationship with him.

As a result, I was considering settling in Melbourne instead of Sydney. I had thought of funding this move by setting up a wholesale structure to market the biodynamic-grown produce that already existed. DW, son of BW, had a large wheat farm in New South Wales but could only sell his BD wheat to the wheat board, which immediately milled it to white flour and so lost the benefit of all his dedicated growing. There were many farmers in Victoria who were farming biodynamically, simply because it was more efficient and productive than standard chemical farming, and they too were looking for specialised outlets rather than just the occasional weekend market stalls. To top this off I was even considering long term, a chain of health food shops and outlets for the anthroposophical medicines that I was considering importing. I believe in thinking big!

Since the fare was the same, I had booked passage on to Sydney, rather than stopping off at Melbourne. In Sydney I planned to spend a week or two catching up with friends before selling the Natural Gourmet, gathering up the possessions I had left stored there, and then heading back south to Melbourne for the next phase.

---

[i] Rudolf Steiner, *Rudolf Steiner and Medicine*, Rudolf Steiner Pub. Co, London, 1948

[ii] Rudolf Steiner and Ita Wegman, *Fundamentals of Therapy*, Rudolf Steiner Press, 1925

[iii] Victor Bott, *Anthroposophical Medicine: An Extension of the Art of Healing*, Rudolf Steiner Press, 1978

[iv] Rudolf Hauschka, *The Nature of Substance*, London, Stuart and Watkins, 1966, Substanzieermann Frankfurt Am Mainehre Copyright 1950 cy Vittorio Klostermann Frankfurt am Main. This translation first published in 1966, 45 Lower Belgrave Street, London SW1

[v] Rudolf Hauschka, *Nutrition*, Loeilehrndon, Stuart and Watkins, 1967, Ernahrungslehre © 1951 Vittorio Klostermann Frankfurt Am Maine

Chapter 11

Formal Training as a Naturopath

So there I was, somewhat over three years after leaving the mining industry, returning from the South African experience. I could not say that it had been entirely successful. But I had learnt a lot, had experiences I would not have had in Sydney, seen anthroposophy on a world stage and, I hoped, contributed a lot. Back in Sydney I caught up with friends, went to some of the anthroposophy meetings, canvassed ideas, and planned my future in Melbourne.

Yet again, fate intervened, this time in the form of EB. EB was an artistic but practical Hungarian who, with his wife AB had taken the dangerous walk through communist-controlled territory, to cross the line and escape from Hungary to the west. I could only imagine what some of their memories must be like. In Sydney, he had developed his own photography business and artistic studio, but he was also seriously keen, as I was, to make biodynamic produce more widely available. This was particularly important as, at that time you could buy almost no produce that had been even organically grown, and we certainly considered biodynamic-grown produce to be of much better quality than the organically grown and the organic forms commercially produced.

Yet again, I rethought the present situation and turned things over in my mind. DW, son of BW, secretary of the Australian Anthroposophical Society, ran a successful biodynamic farm in inland New South Wales. EB was just starting an experimental bakery to use the biodynamic wheat. This was wheat grown with the best possible biodynamic procedures, but since there were no specific outlets for it, DW had to sell it to the wheat board where it was milled, stripped of most of its nutrients, chemically treated, and sold on as regular white flour. Little had been gained in the food market. Beautifully grown as it was, it benefited the soil, but not the consumer.

EB's idea was to use the flour to bake bread, and then expand from this into cakes and other wheat-based products. Could I help? Well, in theory yes. I had developed a line of cookies while running the Natural Gourmet, and done more since, in Jo'burg, but did I want to? EB was funding the project and had two men who were baking the bread, but at this stage the rest of the help was casual, voluntary, and erratic, so deliveries were unreliable, and without a steady supply the customers were losing interest. Exactly as GWA had, a year or two earlier, EB and his wonderful wife saw me as just the person they needed to help them develop and fulfil their dreams.

In the end, friendship with EB and AB, in combination with the wealth of anthroposophical activities and friends I had built up in Sydney over the years, and the offer EB made to me, were too good to refuse. I joined EB, we formalised the Demeter bakery, and later incorporated Helios Enterprises. In addition to the bakery, this was to include the importation and sales of the Dr Hauschka skin care products and homoeopathic remedies. I was glad of all I had learnt in Johannesburg about Dr Hauschka and the products he had masterminded, all based on the ideas of Rudolf Steiner.

As my unit apartment was still let on a long-term basis, I needed a place to stay. A couple I knew were going overseas for three months and would be delighted if I would house-sit for them while I looked for one of my own. It was a convenient, though somewhat depressing building, facing south (so cold) and damp, but a useful stepping stone.

I sold my own unit (costly and no garden) and looked for my next home. My main aim, as in Perth, was to have a large garden, one that I could use to continue my fast-growing gardening hobby. I was less fussy as to the state of the house. This was fortunate as I could not afford the best of both. The first house I looked at was set at the distant end of a long slim half-acre garden. It had even more land behind it that belonged to the local bowls club. The part of their land closest to my boundary was too rough and wet for their use, so I was also assured of a 'green' view at the back.

This house was an hour out of Sydney centre but slightly closer to EB and the bakery that he was using on a time-share basis. As in Perth, when buying my home, my main concern was for a good-sized garden where I could explore the possibility of a very mini smallholding and garden and cultivate them biodynamically. I bought it, moved in, and immediately found I had my half acre of land plus the addition of a friendly and helpful if taciturn neighbour. What I did not have was furniture as it had all been sold along with the unit. By this time I also had very little money, and I had agreed to work for a minimum wage while EB and I developed the Demeter bakery and Helios. It was time to tour the local second-hand furniture shops. I can't say that anything was very beautiful, but it was all functional and my main goal was to fund my activities.

I spent about a year working with EB and the bakery, Jill-of-all-trades, until such time as the business was large enough, and sufficiently well established that he could hire the individuals that were needed to take it over: two bakers, two delivery people, and one office worker, plus me trying to hold the whole thing together. We were all very part-time. I had achieved a small goal, but did not see this developing further for me.

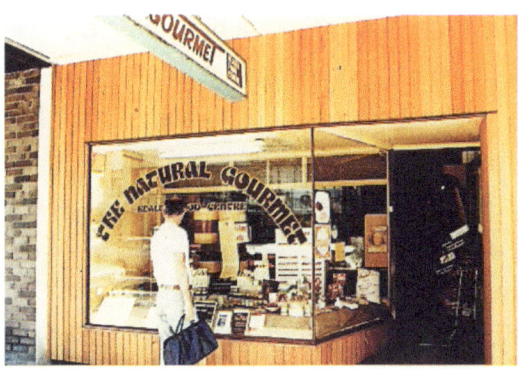

Fate again. The Natural Gourmet came on the market and the owner, to whom I had sold it when in South Africa, asked if I would like to take it back. I would. It would fit in well with everything else I was doing and planning. In a way I had perhaps taken a sidestep by going to South Africa, and was now resuming where I had left off. Yet there had also been many benefits to this detour, some interesting contacts, a few friends, several new skills and an immense amount of learning.

So there I was, reading and studying, advising on nutrition, albeit in a general way, running the shop, helping with the bakery, and at weekends gardening my half acre. I enjoyed all of it, but I was also looking for something more.

Fate intervened once again. A well-meaning but ill-informed friend, who was studying at the Sydney Chiropractic College, assumed that as I was some sort of chemist and had a health food shop and an interest in nutrition. He assumed that I must be a biochemist. He spoke to the head of the Sydney College of Chiropractic and told them he had found the biochemistry lecturer they were looking for. When he told me this, I tried to correct him:

"No, CL, you don't understand. I am a geochemist not a biochemist".

But he was not to be deterred. "That's alright, Garry will phone you next week."

Garry did, somewhat prematurely welcoming me onto his staff.

I had to dispel his illusion. "No, Garry, I'm sorry, you do not understand. I am a geochemist, not a biochemist."

That's alright," was his response. "I'll send you the text book."

I tried again. "No, Garry, you don't understand. I am a *geo*chemist, not a biochemist, and I am fully employed at the moment."

Garry was still not to be deterred. "That's alright, classes don't start until 6.30 in the evening."

And he put the phone down.

The textbook duly arrived. *Introduction to Biochemistry* by Routh, a slim book of 160 pages, published three years earlier in 1971. I opened it with some trepidation, and as I expected, I was not familiar with any of the material. Equally though, as I read it, I could understand it all. It was possibly the subject matter I would have been studying had I indeed chosen organic and biochemistry for my honour's degree at Imperial, instead of analytical chemistry. The difference this time was that I would have to learn it on my own and then teach it. Instead of deterring me, I found the idea challenging and exciting, so I agreed.

This was the infancy of natural therapies in Australia. Teaching was via part-time evening classes and was not extensive. The amount of basic biochemistry known to natural therapists at the time was virtually zero. The amount that was generally available and appropriate for the study of metabolic nutrition was also virtually zero, and certainly not overwhelmingly great compared to the present day.

My tasks for the next year would be to study, prepare lecture notes, and teach this new material once a week. I had the summer during which to make a head start and then the job of staying six weeks ahead of the chiropractic students. I gave two hours of lectures on Thursday evenings. It was a challenge that terrified me initially but that I ultimately came to love ad enjoy. As I accomplished this, I also learnt a number of deflecting strategies in relation to the students' questions.

"What is this FAD you talk about?"

"We'll find out about that next week," I told them. *You and I both,* I thought.

"Where are these red blood cells that you talk about, formed?"

"Ask your physiology lecturer, we don't have time to go through that" covered the fact that I hadn't a clue. But I did make a mental note to find out about each item before my next lecture. I loved it, and soon started reading more and more biochemistry, amplifying the lecture notes and making them increasingly relevant to chiropractic.

There was good reason for my fear As a postgraduate student, from Otago days onwards, I had had, from time to time, to give talks to the various geologists with whom I was working, or at conferences. This meant that I had generally been lecturing about geochemistry to geologists, while knowing a lot less than them about their own subject. They were disinclined to learn about the chemistry that I could have discussed with them in detail, and I was perpetually afraid of and on the defensive about falling down that crack. Now I would have to get used to giving a two-hour lecture every week. I took a solid slug of tranquilising herbs before each lecture. This was in the form of Nervnnahrung, an enriched form of honey laden with the appropriate herbs. I knew little about them then, but the product, in the form of a large spoonful before each lecture, certainly did the trick. I also wrote out my lecture notes almost verbatim to still my quaking nerves. I still have these notes! Obviously, I tried very hard to make it look as if I was *not* reading them, and gradually I came to relax more and eventually love the activity of lecturing and sharing knowledge with interested students.

With that accomplished I was delighted by a further challenge. The chiropractic college told me they were hoping I would take on the task of teaching nutrition. They may have heard of my relatively brief nutrition studies at QEC in London, and perhaps thought it more than it was, but who was I to disabuse them? Besides, there was really no one else. There were a number of traditional 'natural hygienists' at the time, who were practising in the 'hygienic' system, based largely on fasting and massage, but there was no one with a biochemical background and a scientific approach to nutrition. That still needed plenty of study and growth. This was, after all, only the mid-1970s.

Back home, the friendly neighbour, JO, was an interesting character – a retired bachelor, grey haired but very fit. I had no idea of his age. In the six or seven years that I lived there I didn't see him once have any visitors. He had no family except his mother who lived an hour's drive away and never visited him, though he drove there from time to time. She died during the time I knew him. His garden paralleled mine, but continued for a further few yards and then backed onto the same waste land.

JO quickly learned that I was out all week but usually home at the weekends. As in Perth, I had bought a garden that was wildly overgrown. He would walk through the gap in the fence between our two gardens and gaze disapprovingly at a segment of my patch. He would then mutter that this tree should come down, or that patch should be cleared, and he would then get stuck in and do just that. He said little, did a lot, and was rarely cheerful, but he seemed to like the company.

My vegetable garden began to flourish, but he would not accept its produce, preferring to stick to his supermarket frozen vegetables.

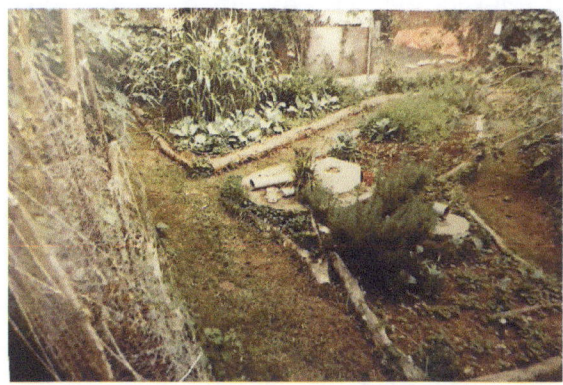

I bought some hens early on and we built a coop for them. He learnt that I wished I had enough room for a goat or two and seemed intrigued at the idea. He suggested that he could build a pen for them at the bottom of his garden and they could be tethered out during the day over the wasteland beyond his back fence. It then seemed a good idea to put the hens down there too.

Each morning I would walk through the gap and down through his garden to milk the two goats, feed the hens, and gather up the eggs. Each Saturday or Sunday, my neighbour would appear and comment on what he thought I should be doing next on my land, and proceed to make a start. People of melancholic temperament range from sensitive carers to down-hearted pessimists, and are often introverted. That was JO, temperamentally an unsociable melancholic. The glass was always half empty, not half full.

He always expected the worst. On rainy days he worried about the mud on his car, or a possible leak in his kitchen roof. On hot sunny days he worried about the paint on his house blistering. Initially I commiserated with him and tried to cheer him up, but this was not the best approach. Instead, I tried an alternative approach as I greeted him. On a wet day I would commiserate that he could not put his washing out to dry, and the mud would damage his shoes, and on the days of hot sun I expressed my concern that he didn't get sunburnt. Once he realised that I fully understood the problems he faced, he almost always became more relaxed and less concerned – not happy, though, that would have been too much for him. I never once saw inside his house, although we had innumerable chats on his back step. He accepted milk, cheese, and eggs, and threw himself into our joint activities.

After I started teaching biochemistry to the chiropractors, I realised that my interests lay firmly with nutrition and the chemistry of the body, not with chiropractic and the physics of the body. I still wanted to study and learn more. I considered enrolling for a PhD in nutritional biochemistry. After much questioning, it seemed that none of the three city universities in Sydney could offer anything suitable.

I turned to the Hawkesbury Agriculture College, a half hour drive from my house and further out of town. They did have an indication of nutrition on their syllabuses, so I went out there to explore. The discussions got off to a good start. They approved of my previous education, my three degrees in chemistry and particularly the two from Imperial. Then they asked about the topic I would like for my research. They wanted something specific and detailed. General topics were frowned on at this time, at least for a PhD thesis. This was the reason I had made little effort to do a research degree in the past few years. That reason still applied, but now I had a stronger desire to study more and develop further into new academic circles. I wanted applied research and had a general idea of the topics I wanted to explore.

They continued to ask about a topic. I hadn't been able to get a clear idea of the interests of any of their lecturers, except that they involved mainly animal foodstuff. This was not a good start. But they did have a food technology department and I asked about that. To my horror I found that it was focused on the best way to manufacture and process foods for longer shelf life, good appearance, and sales appeal. I was hoping for something I could develop along the lines of biodynamically grown foods and the use of the chromas to indicate quality. I decided to explore this slowly and gently and suggested something along the lines of human nutritional benefit.

"Such as what?"

"Possibly vitamins or minerals?" I was struggling here.

"Which?"

"Vitamins." I figured that these offered the wider range of options.

"Which ones?"

I thought for a bit. "Vitamin B6 perhaps."

"Which enzyme system?"

This was not looking good. This was in the days when a PhD generally took three years of solid practical research work. I would have to work long hours if I was to keep my existing life going and accomplish this research with chemistry within the anthroposophical concepts and with the chromas. I arranged to discuss a working relationship with them. It was doable, but it seemed that it would be three years spent learning more and more about less and less and with no room at all for considerations of biodynamic agriculture. This did not appeal, and I wasn't sure where it could lead, A future in general human nutrition and health with a biochemical basis was clearly not on offer.

It was time for fate to take a hand again, or give me a pointer as to where I might go. I already knew of an evening-class college that had been teaching short 'soft' courses in nutrition, herbs, and related 'general interest' subjects. I believe there were other similar short teaching courses at that time. I had looked at them briefly, but coming from an academic training background of university-level teaching and rigor, it had not occurred to me to get involved with them. The chiropractic college had been different. It was, if I recall correctly, a five-year intensive course. You could not do something like chiropractic half-heartedly, and so their training had been meticulous and thorough.

I then heard that this evening-class college was to be taken over by new owners, and that they were starting a three-year full-time

Naturopathic course with high standards. They knew of my work at the chiropractic college and wondered if I would I be prepared to head up, organise, and teach in their biochemistry and nutrition department. It was time for me to explore this option.

The course was to last three years, soon to be three and a half years, full-time, and consist of three eight-hour days of lectures each week, plus additional clinic time, mostly at weekends. In the course they planned, I would be teaching two hours of chemistry and two hours of nutrition each week to their first-year full-time students. In the second year, when we got to it, I would be teaching two hours of nutrition and two hours of biochemistry a week. In their last year and a half, it would become four hours of nutrition a week. The same course would be followed for the evening students and span five or six years.

Right at the start they were also very keen for me to do the full naturopathic course myself. Was I interested? I most certainly was, just so long as it was rigorous enough. However, that would mean twenty hours a week as a student on top of my lecturing. Could I cope with this? I thought I could. It meant hiring a full-time assistant to run the Natural Gourmet, but that was not a problem. I would then oversee it and focus on college life. I would also continue to do the office work for EB at Helios-Demeter.

Working on the truism that "In the eyes of the blind the one-eyed can see," I accepted this challenge and started a further program of self-study. At this time there were no fully qualified naturopaths or nutritionists and few text books. There was no internet. There were many general and popular-level books. Authors such as Adelle Davis[i], Pavo Airola[ii], Francis Moore Lappé,[iii] and Roger Williams[iv] come to mind and are still on my library shelves, others giving way for lack of space to the numerous other books I have bought since.

My delight in lecturing developed and gradually increased, and I relaxed into it. Lecturing to the very interested and enthusiastic naturopathic students was even more exciting than lecturing to chiropractic students who were far more interested in the physics of the body than in its chemistry. I was in my element. I had found my niche. I was earning a lot less than as a geochemist, a job I had enjoyed, but I was now of the frame of mind that I could pursue a hobby I loved and was still getting paid at least a sufficient amount to live on.

By pure chance the Natural Gourmet shop was still perfect, and large enough for my needs. Over the next few years I rearranged the rooms slightly, both on the ground floor and on the floor above. Upstairs I had a bathroom and four rooms. I could have actually lived there, as was the normal pattern along the street, but I had my own house plus, more importantly, the large half-acre garden.

I again commandeered the large room for my office. From here I ran the business, prepared my lectures, pursued my own studies, and occasionally advised clients on nutritional matters. One room I converted into a laboratory to explore the chromas[v, vi, vii,] and do other tests I would have done with AS in Melbourne had I gone there.

The far-seeing organisers of the college were also setting up the Australian Natural Therapists Association (ANTA) with one college in each state doing a similar course to the one in Sydney. This meant that the graduates of each of the colleges could join ANTA, which became the standard for naturopathy in Australia.

The study of naturopathy, and the chemistry of the body, had instant appeal. Even though I had spent my first decade, post-graduation, firmly entrenched in the applied sciences, or perhaps because of this, as before, it continued to make no sense to me to aim for improved health using toxic chemicals instead of restoring normal function. Although we didn't call it such then, we now refer to this as restoring homoeostasis.

It was 1977 and I enrolled in the first full-time course the college ran. Fortunately, by then the Demeter bakery was fully up and running and I was no longer needed. The Naturopathy schedule covered three days a week of four lectures a day, each of two hours, so three eight-hour days each week for two eighteen-week semesters. By the time I graduated, the three-and-a-half-year course had run for 3024 hours.

There was, apparently, something to be proud of in having a course of more than 3,000 hours' teaching time. Then there were the clinics and, of course, the exams. Fortunately, I had some exemptions, including the chemistry and biochemistry, and nutrition, which I taught.

The college ran an evening part-time course as well as the day course, so suddenly I was teaching for something approaching twenty hours a week, studying for my own Naturopathic Diploma, and running my business, though with Frieda's full-time committed help. Fortunately, as a student and as a time-saving study aid, I had got into the habit of 'talking' my lecture notes from the other lecturers, onto cassette tapes that I could play in the car on my hour-long daily commute each way. My enthusiasm was such that I listened to these at all hours of the day and wherever I happened to be. A large bag of files and folders became a necessity.

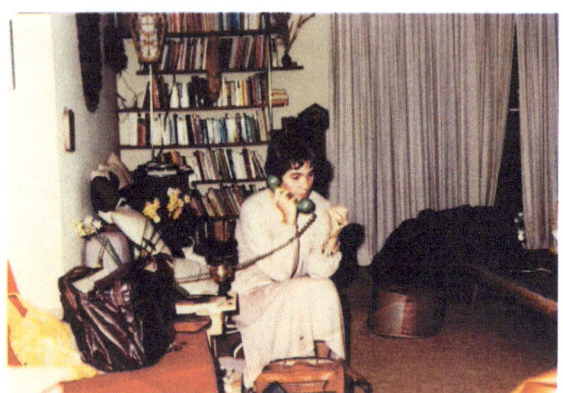

As a lecturer, the holidays were usually taken up with writing and marking the exams for all the classes I taught – a task that I did not enjoy and the dark spot of each year. We were very lucky with these other lecturers. Since at that time there was no established body of fully degree-level naturopaths or nutritional therapists, all the medical subjects were taught by doctors. They provided a rigorous training, each in their own specialty. We also had good lecturers or teachers in the CAM (Complementary and Metabolic) modalities with a particularly excellent lecturer in botanic (herbal) medicine, and another in homoeopathy.

In spite of all the pressures, I loved the chance to study again. As a geochemist I had, of course, kept up with the research literature. Then I had become immersed in anthroposophical studies. Now this was again serious, demanding, challenging, and enormously exciting.

It was at this time that I met TM. Like me he had lived, studied, and worked in several countries. He had returned to Australia and enrolled in a PhD course in Ecology at Macquarie University. He was living in one of the University bachelor apartments, part-way between my home and the Sydney North Shore where I had the Natural Gourmet, and the city where I taught. We shared an enthusiasm for gardening, and what with our lengthy work hours plus our respective gardening hobbies at the weekend, we found it difficult to see much of each other. The obvious answer was for us to live together, and the obvious place for us to do that was in my home.

He was a wonderful thoughtful and kind man and we shared many interests. We made a point of dining out on the one evening a week when I wasn't lecturing and would talk for hours on countless different subjects. We didn't argue, we didn't try to be right or wrong in any discussion, but open-mindedly explored each subject's pros and cons.

Living economically, it seemed stupid to have two cars, so we sold one. I could then drop him off at his university as I passed each morning and pick him up as I returned each evening. As that was often after 10.30 at night, it gave him plenty of time for his PhD work. At the weekends we gardened. An ecologist with deep environmental concerns, he was in favour of gardening organically rather than biodynamically, in which he was less interested. Additionally, as the biodynamic method demanded more time than organic gardening and at specific times in the day, or more particularly in the moon cycle, than we could give, and as he was less interested in BD gardening, we stuck to the organic method.

Two people can certainly do more than one, and I was able to expand my interests. Together, TM and I bought a variety of different types of hens, and several ducks, for which we built a pond. We also had guinea pigs, though I am not sure why. He was a wonderful cook, mostly Asian style, and loved to do it, so I was spared what to me was a chore. He was more gregarious than me and loved to entertain. Yet it was always up to me to meet and greet and get the party going while he immersed himself in the kitchen. Then, over the meal, he would relax, open up, and talk way into the night while I fell quietly asleep in a chair.

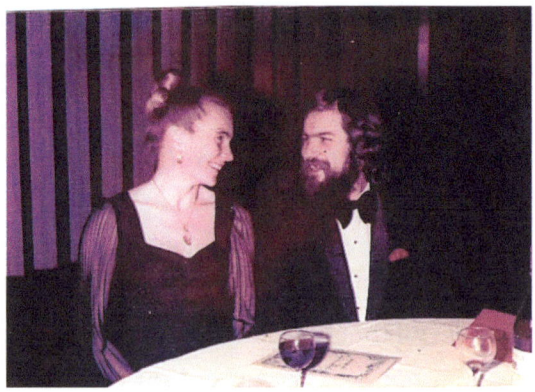

This had been an immensely busy time, with long hours of teaching, studying, and learning, interspersed with the energies I threw into gardening and, in a minor way, my smallholding. It was also a well-structured time with a steady routine built round academic schedules. But I have since thought of it as the lull before the storm, before the great explosion of activity and diversity that was about to follow.

The course had included many different topics, all bulging with information and opportunities. It was clearly time to consider which topics or modalities I would focus on. I loved chemistry and nutrition and this was obviously a front runner. I was fascinated by botanic medicine, even though, initially, it had seemed unlikely that such delicate plants as chamomile and others could actually pack a therapeutic punch. However, I soon came to respect their potential and was delighted when I was offered a supply of almost a hundred herbal tinctures and fluid extracts by a company that was closing down. This meant I was able to set up as a herbal dispensary within the back part of the shop premises, and not only prescribe but also dispense preparations of my own devising, for my own clients and for other practitioners.

There were two ranges of products, both of them consisting of toiletries and remedies, both herbal and homoeopathic, that were firmly based on and within anthroposophical standards and concepts. These were produced in Switzerland and Germany for Weleda and Dr Hauschka respectively. I had worked with them both in South Africa. The local Weleda distributor here in Sydney, who had been supplying the local society members, was keen to hand over to someone (me) who would take on the whole range, and supply on a larger scale. EB, with backup support from me, was already importing the Dr Hauschka range. With these, the herbal tinctures and extracts and a growing section selling books, more space was clearly needed.

After three years of a very full schedule, it was a welcome change to graduate, give up my own undergraduate classes and focus on building a practice instead.

---

[i] Adele Davis, 1966, *Let's Get Well*, George Allen and Unwin Ltd, London

[ii] Paavo Airola, *Dr Airola's Handbook of Natural Healing: How to Get Well*, 1974, Health Plus Publishers

[iii] Francis Moore Lappé, *Diet for a Small Planet: High Protein Meatless Cooking*. Friends of the Earth/Ballantine Books

[iv] Roger Williams, *Nutrition Against Disease: Environmental Prevention*, 1971 Bantam Books

[v] Ehrenfried Pfeiffer, *Sensitive Crystallization Processes: demonstration of formative forces in the blood*, 1936, 1975, Anthroposophical Press, NY

[vi] Agnes Fyfe, *Moon and Plant: Capillary Dynamic Studies*, 1967, Society for Cancer Research, Arlesheim, Switzerland.

[vii] Ehrenfried E Pfeiffer. Chromatography applied to Quality Testing. Biodynamic Farming and Gardening Inc

Chapter 12

1980s, My Early Years as a Practising Naturopath

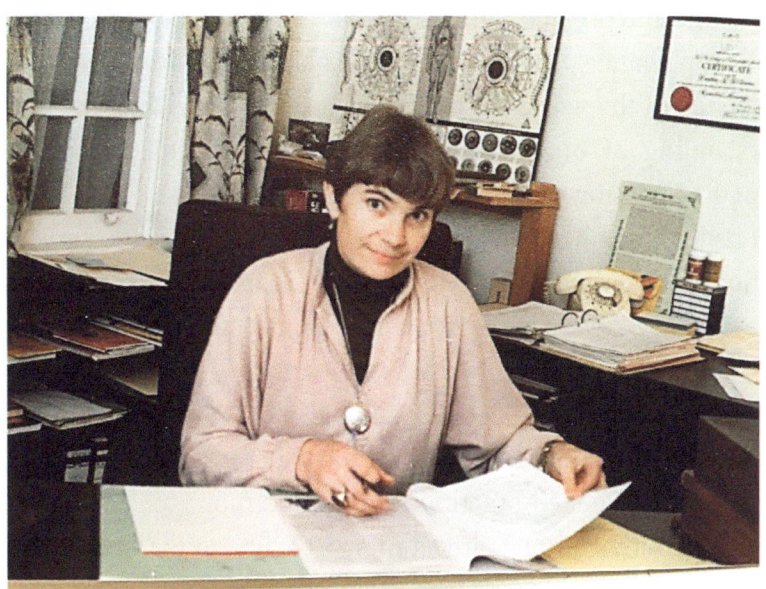

$\mathbf{F}$inally, in 1979, aged thirty-nine, I added to my nutritional training when I graduated with a full Naturopathic Diploma (ND), a Diploma of Botanic Medicine (DBM) and a thorough training in homoeopathy, though no separate diploma was given. This was all in addition to the nutrition that I had taught, and that was so taken for granted within 'naturopathy' that it wasn't given a separate title or certificate of its own.

I was part of the first group of well-trained graduates from the first full-time three-and-a-half years, 3,000 hours of training, to begin to set up in practice.

It had been an interesting exploration, learning and reorienting for years, travelling from being a geochemist working in mineral exploration to a fully qualified Naturopath working in the Health Care field. I had loved the process and now was glad to have arrived. However I also appreciated that this was in its own way a new starting point, one which drew together my many different interests: medical biochemistry, health restoration, nutrition and naturopathy, biodynamic and organic farming and gardening, Rudolf Steiner's ideas of philosophy and spiritual science, the balance between understanding this version of the world we live in, in combinations with the scientific understanding of our material world, and lecturing as a means of sharing and passing on this knowledge.

I had by then been teaching the same lectures in biochemistry and nutrition several times each year for more than the previous three years, so these subjects were well entrenched in my brain and could be called on at will. Teaching is the best way of learning. I felt fully able to start out in full time Naturopathic practice, as opposed to the nutritional support advice I had been giving for the past few years.

As a fully-fledged practitioner I needed more space. I moved my consulting room from the largest room upstairs, to the best of the three smaller rooms. The largest room was then subdivided and became Reception, waiting room, and (suitably partitioned off) the massage room. In time the other two rooms would be used by new graduates for massage or consulting, as they made their first tentative steps into seeing their own clients, prior to setting themselves up independently elsewhere. I kept my experimental laboratory. I employed a full-time receptionist and set about building my practice. I also converted a space as a phlebotomy room as I was soon to start taking blood samples from my clients for various tests, particularly cytotoxic food tests, more commonly but wrongly referred to as allergy tests.

Up to this point clients had mostly come of their own accord and with nutritional questions. Now I needed to think seriously about building the practice. I had more time, as I no longer had to deal with my own student's twenty-four hours of lectures each week plus clinic hours at weekends. I needed a proper secretary. There were stationery and cards to organise, and more. The routines that had been developing slowly over the recent years had to be fast-tracked into shape.

I arrived at the building before nine each morning, opened up The Natural Gourmet and dispensary (Pharma Natura) and let in the shop assistants who worked there. Upstairs, the receptionist and I organised the practice for the day. As a fully-fledged naturopath, with general nutritional experience behind me, I rapidly attracted more clients.

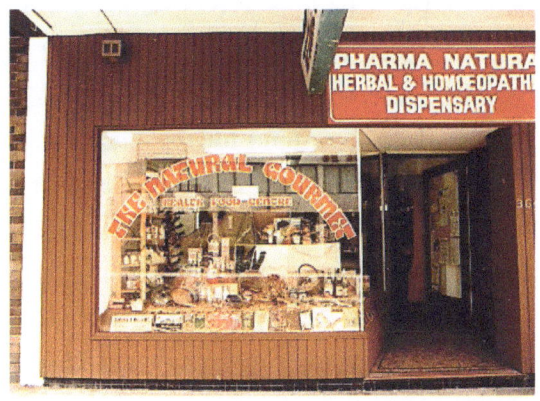

Having graduated from clients with nutritional queries to ones with general health problems amenable to naturopathy, I took on more interesting cases. Many of my clients came as referrals from the shop downstairs, when people who came in shopping asked for advice. I continued to teach at the colleges, of course, and so other clients came from referrals from the students. Others came from a variety of word-of-mouth referrals. At no time have I ever placed advertisements for clients.

Part of the Naturopathic Diploma course had included training in Swedish massage. I was not particularly drawn to doing massages, but clearly this could be a way of attracting people and building up my practice. On my first Monday morning after qualifying, I had a man booked in for a massage at 10.00 a.m. I was excited. He didn't arrive.

My enthusiasm and slight apprehension turned to disappointment. I heard nothing more until later in the day when someone phoned me to say that he had had a heart attack that morning and died. I was, of course, sad for a man I hadn't met or known, but also a bit shaken to realise that he might have died during the massage I could have been giving him.

In spite of this, and in very little time, I had a steadily growing practice. By then a College of Botanical Medicine had started up, and they too asked me to teach. In time I was sometimes lecturing for up to eighteen hours a week. Somehow, I was able to fit in all the other activities involved in my schedule. We closed at six o'clock each day and slightly earlier on Saturdays. But I also lectured for three or four hours for four evenings a week.

With no more lectures to attend for myself, I took on more active lecturing and scheduled it such that I was at the college on Tuesdays, where I did four hours each morning, another four each afternoon and finally, after a half hour break for dinner, yet another four hours each evening. Twelve hours of lecturing in a day. It could be considered a punishing schedule, but I loved doing it, and thrived on it. I loved the subjects themselves. I loved the teaching, the sharing of information, and the interaction with the students, and I loved formulating and expanding the responses to their questions. I drew energy from their feedback, rather than lost it.

At the colleges and in my various teaching roles I was keen to balance my relatively extensive science background and scientific approach on the one hand with, on the other, the concepts embedded within the philosophy and concepts of naturopathy and those of anthroposophical spiritual science and the developing understanding of the other energies. Throughout my career I have worked to interweave these two parallel streams.

Part of my involvement at the college, from the start, was as head of the biochemistry and nutrition department. With three degrees in chemistry and several years of university education behind me, I also had clear ideas as to how thorough and structured a suitable academic course should be, and I cared deeply about the way the profession should develop. Some may say I pushed the standards too hard. Certainly, a few of the students enjoyed the full depth of biochemistry that I gave or expected of them, but generally the majority found it somewhat overwhelming.

I was very conscious that at this time in Australia, early in the 1980s, Naturopathy, the colleges, and the association were twenty years or more ahead of the UK. We were fortunate in having a group of people leading the way who set very high standards that were uniform across the continent and in most of the states. Overarching this was just one association (ANTA, of which more later) to which you simply *had* to belong in order to qualify, so there was no chance, as there was here in the UK when I arrived in the late 1990s, of doing a cheaper and easier course and *then* joining the association.

I have been delighted in the years since by the positive feedback from several of these students as I have met up with them later in life. Many of these graduates have been grateful for the depth and extent of the training I gave. Conversely there was a large appetite for more and more nutritional information as we all worked at keeping up with the research and development going on in other countries. As such I was also able to play a role, though a smaller one, in shaping the whole course at the main college where I taught.

I enjoyed the work so much that I made little distinction between time spent working at home and time working in my office. During most of the three years of my training I had been living with TM, the very special partner who, thankfully, expressed no interest in marriage, and who has remained a very good friend, if not partner, ever since. We would do the necessary watering and feeding of our various plants and animals, goats, poultry and pets such as guinea pigs, early each morning, before heading off to work at eight o'clock, then work away on the garden on Saturday afternoons and all of Sundays. It was great fun and very rewarding. I had a hankering for a larger small-holding but wasn't prepared to give up any part of my day job to travel for the sake of having more land, so that was not possible.

I soon felt it was necessary to specialise. The entire offering on the naturopathic approach was too vast for one person to embrace it all to any great depth. I considered all the health problems and all the different modalities and wondered where to start. I was intrigued by homoeopathy but not fully comfortable with the underlying concepts. I suspected that classical homoeopathy with its various 'provings' had worked well during the nineteenth century when there were relatively few toxins around to interfere with the clinical pictures and 'provings'. I suspected that in this latter part of the twentieth century, the toxins would interfere.

I have so far maintained a lot of sympathy for homoeopathic processes and results, but I use them on a 'trial and see' basis. Ever the scientist. During these early years I explored various ranges of low potency multiplexes such as those of Dr Reckeweg, plus the Oligoplexes. In recent years this has extended to the Guna and Heel or Biopathica ranges and others.

Of the tissues salts I found their fundamental assessment, that there are twelve tissues salts in the remains of a physical body after combustion, to be unsatisfactory as a stand-alone modality. However, I have used some of them in my practice, along with more general nutrition.

I used herbal products extensively, valuing their composition and chemical components. I rarely gave Bach flower remedies or homoeopathic potencies above 6C, feeling that they impact on the emotions and the astral or soul forces of the individual. As a result, they could be assisting the person's spiritual development to an excessive extent, rather than leaving them to drive their own development. On the other hand, I have always kept a very open mind and explored all other suggestions that crop up from the research literature or in the professional journals or newsletters.

I feel our job is to support each individual as they proceed through life rather than do their work for them. If given the higher potencies to help their emotional state, they might have to come back again and develop those emotional skills for themselves next time. That was my position at this starting point. I thought it would be interesting to find out how this progressed.

In this way my way of working gradually settled. My first speciality was in nutrition, that was never in doubt. This was supported strongly by the use of herbals and, to a somewhat lesser extent, by low potency homoeopathic remedies.

I was never tempted to take on any form of the various physical therapies, from massage on to the more targeted strategies such as osteopathy or chiropractic. When our class had divided, halfway through the course, into Oriental health care (oriental massage, Chinese Herbal medicine, acupuncture and more) versus western health care, there was no question. I was going to follow the Western approach.

It was time to get started on my new role.

Hanging my Shingle

I was, I suppose, understandably slightly nervous at the very start of my time in practice as a full time Naturopath. It is, after all, one thing to learn the theory and to 'practise' in the college clinic with one of the lecturers, mostly doctors at that time, as a supervisor. It is another to be entirely on your own, and faced with a client who is relying on you.

Nonetheless, as a fully qualified Naturopath I put that shingle on my door with pride. I was delighted to find that people responded fairly quickly, coming in with a variety of health problems, not just questions on nutrition.

First Clients and Migraines

One of my first clients was a tall, slim, elegant and self-assured woman. This did nothing to help my own not-as-yet fully-established confidence! She explained that she has been suffering with migraines that would lay her low almost every week. Trying to reassure both of us, I explained that I would run a series of tests, check for toxins and for food intolerances and allergies, and for any nutrient deficiencies. I told her I also had a number of herbal products available that had proven to be helpful. I further explained that, if necessary, I could refer her on for chiropractic or osteopathic help.

"Oh, good heavens, I thought you could just give me a pill that would fix it," was her response. *So*, I thought, *that is what clients want!* I recommended feverfew tablets and she was on her way.

By coincidence, I had a second client later in that first week who also complained of frequent migraines. Feeling a bit more confident by now, I assured her that she needn't worry, I had the perfect herb for her that I was sure she would find helpful.

"Oh no," she said. "I don't think you understand. The pain starts at the base of my neck and works upwards. In the evenings, over dinner and when the boys are home making a noise, it is a sharp piercing pain. If the weather is thundery, it affects my right eye, and if I have been reading a lot, it hurts behind my nose." It was nearly a half hour before she had finished telling me about all the symptoms that attached to her various migraines. Clearly, she was not going to feel that I had provided the best assistance until I had fully understood every aspect of her symptoms and how they were affecting her life.

That set me thinking and wondering. How could two people have such different needs when seeking help for the same problem? It reminded me of a book I had read several years earlier on one of my field trips in Western Australia, and which I still had. The book[i] was *Understanding Our Fellow Men* by Knud Asbjorn Lund, an anthroposophist. In this book Lund describes the Four Temperaments based on the philosophy of the Ancient Greeks. Their belief was that our physical world was made up of four elements: fire, air, earth and water. They also believed that our health was a balance of four fluids, or humours: blood, phlegm, black bile and yellow bile, and that an excess or deficiency of any one of these fluids could directly influence both an individual's temperament and health. This view of the human body became the most widely held view by European physicians until the start of modern medical research in the eighteenth and nineteenth centuries.

These groupings were eventually discarded in the light of more modern knowledge and understanding. I was later to discover, however, that the theory of the Four Temperaments was, and still is, considered to be valid and is embedded in the very detailed and complex Myers-Brigg's personality test. Back in 1970 or so, I had devoured Lund's book with enthusiasm, and I recalled it that weekend as I reviewed my first week in full-time practice.

Through my own subsequent research, I have been able to find and expand on the use of four quick questions that help me to determine the temperament, attitudes, and personalities of my clients, or more accurately, to which of the sixteen sub-temperaments they belong. I have used this tool many times over the years, and it has helped me to respond in ways that are most helpful to them.

The Four Temperaments are traditionally named as Choleric, Melancholic, Sanguine and Phlegmatic. In the language of today I might better call them, respectively, Dynamic Leaders, Sensitive Carers, Fun-loving Butterflies, and Loyal Traditionalists.

The following is a brief summary of the questions I would ask a client, generally working them into our conversation, rather than formally.

1. *"In relation to how we work together, would you like to start with an overview and know where we are going?"*
   If the answer is 'yes', they are either choleric or melancholic, and so the second question is:
2. *"Do you want to focus on the facts, figures, and explanations?"*
   If so, they are part choleric (T). Or:
   "Do you prefer to be understood and emotionally supported?"
   If so, they are part melancholic (N).

If the answer to question 1 is 'no' and they prefer to get started by taking some immediate action, they are either Phlegmatic (J), or Sanguine (S).

If so, their next question should be:

3. "*Do you want your program to be pre-planned?*"

   If so, they are part Phlegmatic (P). Or:

   "*Would you prefer it to be open-ended and flexible and we will see how it develops?*"

   If so, they are part Sanguine. (S)

4. A final question I like to use is:

   "*To recharge your batteries, do you prefer to be alone?*"

   If so, they are introverts (I)

   ". . . *or do you prefer to be with people?*"

   If so, they are extroverts (E).

Once I have answers to these questions, I have four letters that help to define which of the possible sixteen sub-types best describes the individual, and I have good idea of the client's mentality and characteristics and how to relate to them and better understand their needs. This has proven to be an incredibly useful tool in developing rapport and understanding with my clients, and establishing successful therapeutic protocols and relationships.

Clearly my first client had been a woman with a strong choleric temperament, and the second one a strong melancholic.

For more detailed information, see my own book *Love Health and Happiness*, UK edition, or *The Four Temperaments* USA edition. Both are out of print as I write this, but copies can be obtained from xandria@xandriawilliams.co.uk. You may also find second-hand copies online, as we do, to keep our own stocks up.

Fasting

At this early stage before the development of naturopathy as a fully recognised profession in Australia, there was the group of people who called themselves Hygienists. They built their protocols round water fasting, juicing, and massage.

One morning I was called down to the shop to help a customer. He said he had been on a liquid-only fast for several days, and he felt terrible. He also looked terrible, and I could see that his hands were shaking. In those days it was normal, especially amongst the Hygienists, to assure people that it was quite normal to feel 'bad' when first going on a fast. They called it a 'healing crisis' and attributed it to the release and elimination of toxins as a result of the cleansing process. People were assured that their symptoms would improve after a few days. In the years since, we have learnt much more about fasting and how to avoid much of this 'crisis' without losing the 'healing'.

"I've been on a liquids-only program for ten days. It's not getting any better," the customer responded.

That, I thought, did not sound good. Fortunately, I asked him if he had been on a water fast or a juice fast, and if so, what juices he had been drinking. I was beginning to think he might have had an overload of sugar from juices he might have chosen. I was thinking of pineapple juice or grape juice. But worse was to come.

"Oh no, none of those," he said. "I have stuck to Coca-Cola and black coffee."

No wonder he was feeling terrible and jittery. On such a high caffein and sugar diet, combined with their diuretic effects and a lack of food, it was not surprising. Unfortunately, when I suggested he give up his two favourite drinks and go to diluted fresh vegetable juices or water, he was appalled. That was possibly his last venture into 'health foods', which he clearly derided. We didn't see him again.

Writing

In 1973, when the Chiropractic College had first contacted me and asked me to lecture, I had insisted that I simply couldn't lecture, I would be far too frightened as I had not done any significant lecturing before. What little I had done had generally been on chemistry, and because of my position between the two departments, chemistry and geology, had been presented to geologists. I had felt out of my depth when faced with their in-depth geology questions. However, I was persuaded, and soon found that I loved lecturing.

In the same year as I graduated, I was asked by a number of magazine editors to write articles. Again, I had demurred, insisting that lecturing was one thing, but writing articles was a skill beyond me. Yet again I was persuaded. Yet again I succumbed to pressure, and I soon found that I loved writing too, at least writing articles of 500 to 2,000 words.

In the first edition to which I contributed, a magazine called *Nature and Health*, I wrote four articles of varying lengths, the longest 2,000 words, the shortest 400. At this stage, writing was still done on a typewriter. I thought my ideas out, then wrote a first draft, and then cut and pasted the material until I had edited it into the shape I wanted, retyped it again, and sent it in. This was a time-consuming and tedious process and might have deterred me from any further writing. Up to this point, all my lecture notes had not even been typed but hand-written, yes, pen and paper, the old-fashioned way. I was now being encouraged to purchase what would be my first computer. The main driving force behind this purchase was my need or desire to be able to apply a homoeopathic program that made determining the homoeopathic similimum a lot less arduous and uncertain than if I had to rely on memory and mental analysis. I had as yet little idea of what a computer could do and no understanding of the concept of a word-processor. I was intrigued, however, by the idea, and particularly keen to see how it would facilitate homoeopathic prescribing.

The computer cost three thousand dollars and came in three distinct pieces: a large and very heavy box that housed the workings and the slots for two eight-inch floppy disks. The second item was a screen the size of a small television set, and the third was a keyboard that would completely dwarf any of today's laptops. It had what was then considered to be an amazing 64K of memory (that's true, not a typo) and we all thought it was wonderful! The instructions were clearly a literal translation from idiomatic Chinese and difficult to comprehend, especially as I had no understanding of what I was even trying to do. I read the instructions: 'First boot the computer', and wondered which part of it I was supposed to kick. Fortunately, TM could help. In time, it lived up to my expectations of its capacity to simplify homoeopathic prescribing, at least up to a point.

This first computer arrived before the next article was due, two months later, and by that time I had learnt the capabilities and creative freedom of word-processing. This totally transformed the process of writing, whether for articles, lecture notes, research data, or, later, books. It made all these forays into authorship much easier and more enjoyable than the old-fashioned pen and paper method.

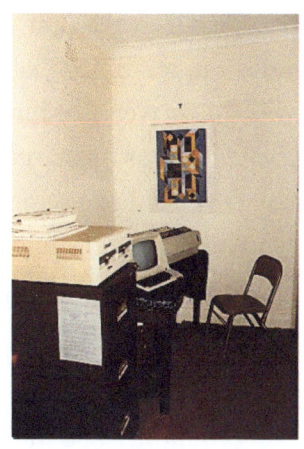

I was eventually to write over four hundred articles for several magazines, often on a monthly or quarterly basis. Invariably the various commissioning editors, not being naturopaths themselves, would eventually run out of ideas or topics, and so happy to leave that choice to me. This gave me the stimulus to explore and write about topics as I learnt about or became interested in them, and it gave me an 'audience' for what I wrote. This was wonderful. The various magazines I wrote for eventually included: *Nature and Health, Australian Wellbeing, Prevention Magazine, Discover Better Health, Inside Vitamins, Here's Health, Health News, Good Health*, and other smaller and more occasional titles.

A few years later, fate was to give me another prompt. The publishing house, Allen and Unwin, tried to persuade me to write books for them. Such was this rapid growth in and enthusiasm for naturopathy and the natural therapies in general during the 1980s, that they wanted six books to start with. Again, I demurred, insisting that writing short articles was one thing but writing whole books was quite another and I wasn't sure I could do that. However, a few years later I finally did start writing books, and, considerably helped by my developing computer skills, I soon found I greatly enjoyed it. This, I believe, could well be my twenty-second book.

Giving Interviews: Early Topics

Writing so many articles put my name somewhere in the public view, and I was soon asked to give interviews, either on radio or television, on topics that had hit the headlines. Two of the early topics I was given were: 'Aluminium, is it safe or dangerous?' And 'Which is better, butter or margarine, and why?' This was about the time that trans fatty acids were being recognised as dangerous, at least in some of the more thoughtful quarters.

Trans fatty acids, Butter and Margarine

One evening I was at a drinks party where the hostess knew that I had just published such an article. She took me over to meet a man, saying to him, "You must meet each other. Xandria has just published an article on the dangers of the trans-fatty acids in margarines, and as you work on butter and in the dairy industry you two will have plenty to talk about," after which she moved on to her other, presumably easier, hostess duties.

Such was my enthusiasm for what I was doing that I was happy to talk enthusiastically on the topic, elaborating on the dangers of margarines, trans-fatty acids, and the processed fats. We chatted for quite a while, both, I thought enjoying the interchange. However, at the end he finally said, "I have enjoyed our chat, however there's just one thing, she had it wrong, you know, I work for the margarine industry, not the butter industry." Whoops. I do not recall any continuation of that friendship. However, I do recall his parting comment which, for obvious reasons, has stayed with me: "Actually my company and I do know the dangers of trans fats. However, it is much easier and cheaper to make them from the various oils and fats than the healthy cis fatty acids (Cis fats are the typical form of unsaturated fat found in nature), so we have two research teams going in parallel. One is evolving ways to make the trans-fatty acid margarines for the current market even more easily, and another to making the cis fatty acid margarines (healthier, but more difficult and costlier to make). We do this so we can swap to the cis forms and have the methods available when the public realises the dangers of the trans forms. It was to be several decades before the public did begin to realise the dangers of trans-fatty acids and processed vegetable oils – in spite of my lectures.

Dr Alan McLeay and his Laboratory

Early on I meet up with Dr Alan McLeay. He ran an innovative pathology and nutritional testing laboratory. Among many of the tests his laboratory offered was nutritional analysis for both alternative practitioners and general doctors. He also provided the Bryant cytotoxic test for food sensitivities. This latter involved an assessment of the amount of white blood cell breakdown caused by individual foods to which a person might be sensitive. It was of immense help in determining which foods each individual client should avoid. Years later, in London, I was to find that while some of these were, presumably, specific food sensitivities or even allergies, unique to the individual, others were in fact the foods that the particular client should avoid because of their unique metabolic type or needs and the way that their individual bodies processed not only foods, but also vitamins, minerals, other nutrients, and more.

Both Alan and I were interested in nutrition and we applied this, when asked, to the athletes training at the Institute of Sports in Canberra. Alan also trained me in phlebotomy, and listed me as one of his outlying phlebotomy collection centres, hence my need for a room in my office for sample collecting. This meant that I was able to collect all my own clients' blood samples and have them collected each evening and taken to his laboratory. Thus, we did a lot of work with food sensitivities, and also with athletic performances.

Masked Food Allergies

We started from a basis of recognising that there are opiate receptor sites in the brain that respond to internally produced opiates, such as morphine or morphine-like substances. These form the basis of the internally produced, or endogenous, opiates (endorphins) that help us to reduce the experience of pain. After an accident, for instance, the immediate experience of pain is generally delayed, and that is thanks to our own endorphins. Most people will know of, or know someone who has, for instance, experienced the ability to break a bone in their foot but keep running in an emergency, or in an important game of football, only to feel the pain sometime later.

There are other compounds that have chemical structures similar to these internal opiates. They are known as exorphins, or externally produced (m)orphines. It is not that whole molecules of an exorphin are identical to an endorphin, just that a part of them, possibly a very small part of them, has just the right structure (like a key to a lock) to 'lock' on to the opiate receptor sites in the brain. This is the basis of many of the food sensitivities, wrongly called allergies, since they are not allergies in the true and original meaning of the word. True allergies generally produce an immediate and more obvious reaction. This might be the experience of coming out in hives after eating strawberries, or going into anaphylactic shock after eating peanuts.

A curious fact about food sensitivities is that they are often masked. They may produce no immediate reaction. In fact, the foods concerned may even make you feel wonderful, the opiate 'high'. I have tried to explain to many people who are 'sensitive' to soy, for instance, and who feel great after drinking soy milk and are sure that it must be good for them, that the contrary is often true. The 'high' or seeming good feeling that they are getting when they drink soy milk could be due to the harmful, and addictive, reaction of the compound, usually a small stretch of a protein (a peptide) that is reacting with their opiate receptors.

I recall Geraldine coming in to see me one morning, saying she had a drinking problem. She told me that every morning when she woke up, she said very firmly to herself "I will not have a drink to-day". She looked crestfallen as she spoke. "But I generally only last until about eleven o'clock, by which time I am desperate for a drink. I go to the fridge, promise myself that I will only have just this one small drink, and then no more."

"And?"

"Well, that lasts a few hours, but then in the afternoon it is just too much to resist, and I have another one. And then another one, and then another, with ever decreasing gaps between them, until by the time I go to bed I have drunk a couple of pints or more."

"Of what?" I had the sense to ask.

"Of milk. It's so ridiculous. It's not as if it's alcohol, but I feel like an alcoholic. If I don't drink milk, I have to eat cheese."

Both her addiction and her chosen food were upsetting her.

In the end I was able to help her avoid *all* dairy products for a few days and then assure her that for as long as she avoided *all* dairy products, she could probably prevent the return of the initial craving. This turned out to be true.

It was a similar problem with Charles. He and his wife came to my office together. His wife explained that recently Charles had become tense, irritable, and moody. This was making him very difficult to get on with. He also complained of indigestion and low energy. Following further questioning, I decided to run a test for food sensitivities. About a week later, both Charles and wife came in together to get the results. They looked expectant.

I anticipated a straightforward consultation, something along the lines of, "These are the foods you are sensitive to and you should avoid them if you want to feel better." I got as far as explaining that he should avoid wheat and dairy products. I was a bit surprised when his wife burst out laughing! She turned to her husband and said, "See, I told you that you drink too much milk!" She then turned to me and explained that her husband consumed several pints of milk each day, and also ate cheese like there was no tomorrow.

Out of the corner of my eye, I could see that Charles was nearly in tears. I quickly warned his wife not to laugh. It was possible that her husband was actually addicted to milk. He would most likely have a difficult time giving it up and would most certainly need her help and support. I explained that he would have to avoid all dairy products, either on their own or in combination with other foods. If he was able to do this one hundred per cent, perhaps even for just a few days, he might find that the addiction was broken, though it might be a struggle for a few more days. "So, he can then go back to having dairy products?" she asked. Charles looked hopeful. But I had to disabuse him. "No", I said. "At least certainly not for a long time. It could be all too easy for you to become sensitive to the foods again. However, once the addiction is broken it is unlikely that he will crave those foods. The real danger is, at least initially, that he will accidentally consume dairy food that is hidden in a recipe, which will then start the whole process all over again."

This turned out to be true. I didn't see them again, but I had frequent updates from his wife for the next year or more. If he completely avoided all dairy products, he was fine, maintained his relaxed, easy-going temperament, had no digestive problems and his general health improved. However, on the occasion that he did consume some dairy product, even inadvertently, he found himself heading straight for the fridge and a large glass of milk. For the most part, his wife was successful in monitoring his eating habits, and the last I heard he had overcome his dairy addiction.

Most people with food sensitivities soon learnt the benefit of avoiding them and chose to do so, but this was not always the case.

Sinus Congestion

When Denis walked into my office one winter afternoon and sat down, I could hardly make out what he was saying. It was as if he had been holding a clothes-peg totally over his nose, he was so muffled.

It all became clear when he said "I've 'ad dreadful sidus problems. I've 'ad them for a long time." As he talked and told me more, I came to suspect food sensitivities, possibly milk and wheat, and I organised the appropriate tests for him. The results showed he was clearly allergic to milk, wheat, peanuts and foods with moulds or yeasts in them. I explained that this meant he should give up all breads, milk and cheese, wines and beer and a few other things. His face fell at breakneck speed. "Bud I luf all dose foods, a glass of wine, bread ad cheese, a beer in th'evening. Oh dear. They are de basis of my social life." He looked doubtful but agreed to give my instructions a try.

A few days later I received a frantic phone call from him. He was almost in tears. "I don't know what has happened, what you have done, but it is something terrible, I have such pain in my face I can hardly bear it. It is sharp, cutting, excruciating." He was almost shouting, insisting that I had to DO SOMETHING. As a fairly new practitioner my first thought was a tendency to panic along the lines of "Oh golly, what can I have done!" My second was to tell myself "Do not worry, think professionally, stay calm and listen to what you can learn." And in the third split second I tried to reassure him and suggested he come into the office as soon as he could, which he was more than happy to do.

He arrived the next day and the first thing I noticed was the clarity of his speech. This was just as well since he was rubbing his hands over his face in an ineffectual effort to reduce his 'pain'.

"How has the sinus problem been?" I asked. "Have you managed to avoid all the foods I listed for you?" We had to start there, and I was determined to get to the root of the problem.

"Oh, it's fine, I can breathe freely now, talk more clearly and all the deep sinus congestion has gone."

We continued to talk around his problem for a while until I had a clearer picture and asked the obvious question.

"How long is it since you have been able to breathe through your nose, as you are doing now?

"Oh, years, ever since I was at school, and that was about thirty years ago."

"So, in fact, what you could be feeling is the cold air passing in and out down your nose for the first time in thirty years?"

"Ye-e-s," he said doubtfully.

"Look, this is the middle of August, it's winter (in Australia), the temperature is down to about 12C and the air is cold (very cold for Sydney). For the past thirty years the lining of your sinuses has been a warm and moist place, undisturbed, with no air flowing through them. I suspect that what you are experiencing now is simply the normal respiration that other people enjoy daily."

And that is what it turned out to be. He soon adjusted to this and phoned to say he had come to enjoy the new sensations. Imagine my surprise, then, about a year later, when I met him and heard the original voice of the totally congested sinuses.

"What happened? I thought we had solved your problem."

"Well, you 'ad, bud I couldn't live wid'out bread and beer, cheese and wine. My social life is centred round the 'barbie' wid loads of beer and wine, bread in all forms, and cheese to nibble on." He went on to explain that he could live with blocked sinuses, and it seemed that his friends could too, as long as I keep throwing the parties, laying on the wine and offering the typical Ozzy- barbie food."

As far as I know he continued to consume his allergies and put up with the sinus congestion.

Initially, few people were really aware of the leap that had recently been made in the development of the naturopathic profession with the current thorough training. Many clients continued to come with typical and traditional nutritional questions, such as what to do about fatigue, how to lose weight, or possibly what to do about skin problems, or even, more daringly, what to do about indigestion. But these questions soon led on to further discussions and questions as to how they could be helped with other or associated health problems.

Candidiasis

Candidiasis was a common, though frequently unrecognised problem in those days. *Candida albicans* is one of the many types of microorganisms in or on our bodies, or in the various crevices. It and other similar moulds are most commonly found within the digestive tract and the vagina, and take their name 'albicans', from the white colouration of the overgrowth that they produce. This can most easily be seen on the tongue and in the mouth cavity, as well as in a discharge from the vagina, often noticed on underpants. We knew at the time (1980s) that its overgrowth was encouraged by sugar and a high intake of refined carbohydrates in combination with a diet that had a lot of yeast-based foods.

Jennifer was one of the many people who came to see me early in my practice years, with problems that were easily recognisable as candidiasis. Her tongue showed the visible signs, and her description of her digestive problems and persistent vaginitis with a white discharge reinforced the diagnosis. I explained the necessary dietary changes that would help her to get rid of it. She looked somewhat dismayed but left my office saying she would give it a try. However, she met up with her friend in the waiting room. As they walked out, I heard her say, "This is impossible. I'm going to find another practitioner, one who doesn't make me give up all those foods that I love". She didn't return, at least not then. But many months later she was back. She still had the problem. It seemed that nothing had worked and she had decided, after all, to give my suggestions a try. Luckily they worked, and her problems became a thing of the past. There was also an additional benefit to this change. She had become moody and depressed. She put it down to marital problems, but with the change in her diet her mood improved – and so did her confidence in her marriage.

From clients like this I soon came to recognise the need to pay attention to emotional and psychological issues, and, in time embarked on a number of studies related to psychotherapy.

Multiple Sclerosis and Lead Toxicity

Some aspects of client care required unusual sleuthing. Geraldine had been diagnosed with multiple sclerosis (MS). She told me that she was allergic to vitamin C and she could not eat any food that contained it. If she did, her symptoms would rapidly worsen. These restrictions ruled out almost all fruits and vegetables and thus her diet was dreadfully inadequate in almost all respects. I found it hard to believe she was allergic to a natural vitamin when consumed in combination with its frequent co-factors such as many of the bioflavonoids, as in this example. I might have thought otherwise if she had been reacting to vitamin C in supplements, in which case it would have been a manufactured product with added excipients.

I instigated several tests for her, one of which was based on analysing a sample of her hair. This involved chemical analysis for the level of minerals present, both essential and toxic. Hair is essentially strands of protein. This protein is, as usual, made up of strings of amino acids, one of which is cysteine. Cysteine is present in unusually high amounts in hair and contains the sulphur that gives hair the smell of bad eggs when it is burnt. This sulphur also readily attracts and attaches to minerals and this fact is made use of in this test. Her hair showed extraordinarily high levels of lead, which was the clue I needed.

The symptoms of lead toxicity, as listed in a book that I had at the time, did cover many of her symptoms, and did, at least somewhat, overlap with the symptoms of MS. I suggested that it was possible that every time she consumed vitamin C it was helping to mobilise lead that could have become stored in her tissues. We started a program of chelation aimed at safely removing the lead from her body in such a way that it was no longer able to trigger the symptoms. Gradually her health improved. Further research, and questioning as to the source of lead, highlighted the fact that her apartment was on the ground floor of a tall building at a junction of five main roads. These were frequently congested with traffic hold-ups and much belching of petrol exhaust, all of it lead-laden at that time. On my advice, she and her husband moved to a new house in a quiet back street, and this further aided her recovery. MS was soon a thing of the past.

Aluminium

Another toxic metal we were very concerned about in those days was aluminium. WP was an accountant. Although he had recently retired, he still did the books for a few friends but had recently found he was having trouble with his memory and had to resign. I knew he drank tea, coffee, and alcohol, but when I questioned him he admitted to not drinking much if any water. Some brains have shown up as dehydrated on autopsy so I was in the habit of asking people to drink at least three pints of water a day. He tried this and found that it solved the problem.

This led on to IM, who had retired early to write a book on the history of music. She started well, but had then found that her memory was fading. She would read a page, formulate how she wanted to include that information into what she was writing, then find that she had already forgotten what she had read. Dehydration wasn't the problem for her – it turned out that aluminium was. Testing showed her to have a very high level of this mineral both in her tissues and in her lifestyle. That is to say, all her cookware was aluminium, as were her kettle, coffee percolator, and teapot. She had an arthritis remedy that contained aluminium, loved maraschino cherries, baked cakes for the family using baking powder which included aluminium, used a lot of salt, which had aluminium as a free-flowing agent, and more. When all this was combined it was an overload.

I suggested that they replace all their aluminium kitchenware with stainless steel or some other alternative. She should replace her antiperspirant with an aluminium-free deodorant, and eliminate all the other possible sources of aluminium that I had identified – this was 1980 and the dangers of aluminium were less well publicised then. She was dismayed when I told her what I advised, and her husband thought it was all a lot of nonsense, saying "she is just getting old". However, she put this plan into action, but only bought two replacement saucepans because of the expense. The result? Her memory improved, the book-writing took off, and her husband fretted even more about both the expense and the limitations put on her cooking by the changes. Eventually he insisted she go back to using her aluminium cookware. The aluminium must have gone back into her food and her memory failed. She felt she could not go against her husband's wishes and the book never did get written.

It is rarely a case of 'one strategy solves all similar problems'. Each of these strategies worked purely because the cause had been identified and eliminated.

Carpal Tunnel

Another client was helped in an unexpected way. She was married to a diplomat, a position that meant they changed their home every year or two, and that she frequently lived overseas. However, she had been in the habit of coming back to Sydney for a short period every couple of years. Her wrists were the problem. Carpal tunnel syndrome – oh, how the medical world does love labels, preferably Latin ones. The name 'carpal tunnel syndrome' essentially means a problem that results when the cluster of nearly round bones in the wrist that make up the carpal tunnel, become inflamed. When they are pressed onto nerves that work their way through the gaps between the bones of the tunnel, the pain starts. As the nerves succumb to the pressure of misaligned bones, they become further inflamed, and progressively more painful.

A book available at the time covered the benefit of vitamin B6 in this and related problems, ones that we now generally call 'repetitive strain injury'. I suggested she take an excellent product, available then, though not now. It contained Vitamin B6, magnesium, zinc and manganese. I further suggested that she top it up with even more vitamin B6. This was readily done as it was before the false scare about high doses of vitamin B6. This did the trick. Instead of her regular biannual operations to release her wrist bones, she took to sending me 'thank you' cards at the times she would otherwise have been booking a hospital visit.

The vitamin B6 story is worth mentioning. Sometime after this, if I remember correctly, *The Lancet*, a British medical journal, presented two apparently independent reports (they were actually by a mother and daughter team but having different surnames so they appeared independent). The paper described the apparent neurological toxicity of high-dose vitamin B6. Whereas we were used to having tablets available with up to 250 mg of vitamin B6, they were now reduced to 50 mg or less. We were appalled. It became very difficult to help people with carpal tunnel syndrome like my client above. It was also very difficult to help a further subgroup of people who were schizophrenic (the cryptopyrolurics) of which more later.

Myasthenia Gravis

Another woman came in complaining of very painful muscles, mostly but not exclusively in her legs and arms. "I've been to doctors and they can't seem to help. Can you? The worst of it is, they don't seem to know what is wrong." I made several suggestions and then suggested that she see a local doctor who I thought could help. I could refer on, as was the case in Australia, and request what I wanted them to do, what tests to run, or an appropriate specialist to suggest. Australia had its Medicare System, which was only partially comparable to our UK National Health Service, with one advantage that I made good use of. More of this later. There was also much more respect for naturopaths there than here in England, so greater communication and interchange of ideas and facilities was possible.

This client came back to see me a few weeks later looking much happier. She was thrilled. "I have found out what it is that I have. Now I feel I can make progress." "Oh yes, what did he say?" "It's myasthenia gravis." She smiled at me in triumph and relaxed. But I pointed out that the name simply meant she had a 'grave muscle disease' which we had known all along. The love for Latin names is amazing. It seems that they somehow provide the medical approach with an unearned authority and mystique. She looked slightly deflated by my explanation but could also report on some improvement following my other suggestions to her.

Medicare v the NHS

Medicare was, I thought, a system that had much to recommend it. Every medical procedure had a 'Medicare rate'. A consultation might cost $50, a longer consultation with a specialised consultant might cost $100. As a client, you paid your bill, got your receipt and claimed the Medicare rate back from the government. You were free to consult any doctor you liked, having established both their charging rate and their professional speciality. If your doctor charged more than the Medicare rate, you could claim the Medicare amount back. If you had private insurance, you could send off your receipt covering the rest of the bill to your private insurance company for reimbursement for the difference. People who did not have the spare funds to wait for their Medicare repayment could go to a doctor who 'bulk billed' at the basic Medicare rate. This meant that you signed their form and they simply claimed the amount directly from Medicare.

I felt that this system had several advantages over the NHS system. It showed people that health care was not 'free', that it had a cost, a price, and a value, and that this should be respected. It also meant that, unlike in the UK, even people who paid for private insurance did get some benefit from their medical tax that had gone into Medicare. It also offered many levels of flexibility.

Restoring Homoeostasis

Several things became very apparent to me during my first years in practice. Many of the problems that I had to deal with did not need a chemical drug with toxic side effects. Many of the functional errors experienced by my clients could be corrected by restoring homoeostasis. This meant, firstly, providing the body with all the nutrients it needed and, secondly, eliminating as far as possible, all the toxins and harmful environmental compounds to which the individual was exposed. In this way it was frequently possible to restore normal function without generating any toxic adverse effects.

Over the years I have developed ever-increasing confidence in the naturopathic approach to restoring good health, and in doing it in such a way that there are few, if any, toxic side effects. In addition, this often led to more, and sometimes unexpected, positive side benefits. This was in contrast to the medical approach of treating problems with a medical drug that almost always has one or more, usually many, toxic or harmful, and sometimes unexpected side effects. First 'do no harm', or 'primum nil nocere', or 'non-maleficence', is meant to be the basis of the principal precepts of bioethics. It reminds us, naturopaths and doctors alike, to consider the possible harm that any intervention might do. Unfortunately, and inevitably, all doctors prescribing medical drugs do risk doing some harm. Their rationale is usually "oh well, the side effects are only minor, (this is not always the case), so don't worry about them". Doctors call them side effects, never toxic effects, though they generally use the term 'toxic' if a naturopathic client of ours gets even a minor reaction to a nutrient or similar natural product.

In addition to lecturing at the full-time course at the NSW College of Naturopathic Sciences from which I had graduated, I was also asked to give many individual lectures at other, smaller colleges. One of these taught just Herbal Medicine, one was a college focusing on advanced nutrition, that folded after a couple of years. I was also asked to talk at various special interest groups, such as 'Parents without Partners', mothers' clubs, coffee clubs, and more. Often they asked for a talk on a specific topic, at other times they left the title up to me. Increasingly, on these occasions, I started talking about 'Restoring Homoeostasis'. Some years later I began using the similar but improved title or byline, 'Restoring Health – not Fighting Disease'.

Itchy Heels

A new client came to see me complaining of exhaustion. He had a high-pressure job with long working hours, and on top of that his wife had recently delivered her first baby and she too was working long hours and struggling to cope. I thought, of course, of adrenal exhaustion and prescribed a broad B complex, a vitamin B supplement with a generous additional amount of calcium pantothenate, (vitamin B5) plus vitamin C. Three weeks later he was back, delighted with his improved energy but also thrilled to tell me that his heels had stopped itching. Itching heels? He had not told me about that. He explained that he had not thought to, he had assumed that some sort of cream would be needed and had been trying several, though with little success. Some literature research that evening showed me that not only was itching feet a recognised problem, but that it had sometimes responded to increased intake of pantothenic acid, vitamin B5.

I love it when what we do not only helps with the problem which the client had presented, but also with other issues that have not been mentioned. This is an important benefit of 'restoring homoeostasis', or normal function, rather than 'treating a symptom' as is done with most medical drugs. We rarely have a remedy that works on only one aspect of the body. Most of the supplements, nutrients, and plants that we use are such that they can all react together on a particular tissue. Vitamin C, for instance, is not just a treatment for the common cold, a deficiency of it can lead to joint problems and bleeding gums, even an increased rate of metastasis in people with cancer. These are all problems with a connection to the health of the connective tissues.

Unique Metabolic Needs

Initially most of my clients had fairly straightforward health problems, or so it seemed to me at the start. Skin conditions, arthritis, candidiasis, allergies, fatigue, headaches, sinus problems, digestive upsets, cystitis, and menstrual problems. The clients that I generally found most challenging, and therefore interesting, were the ones that came with a variety of symptoms and no named disease. The challenge then was to build up a picture of the symptoms and focus on differential diagnosis, gradually working down to the real core of the problem. This was often, however, not so much a named disease (beloved of medical doctors), but a damaged, unhealthy, deficient, or toxic lifestyle or diet. From there, one could start at the basic level and determine their best diet. This is done now by determining and applying a person's metabolic type or 'Unique Metabolic Needs' (UMN) and building upwards to restore optimum health. This is a routine strategy that I have followed since this time. Hence, we are back to 'treating the person', not the disease. Several people with similar symptoms may respond to entirely different protocols.

The rigid thinking, 'one size suits all', or 'if it works for some it should or will, work for all' has frustrated me throughout my career. It is an attitude that still remains in spite of all we have learnt in the last many decades. An early example comes from the early 1920s, and a current one, in the 2020s, will serve to emphasis this.

William Hay, working in New York between 1910 and the 1920s, developed the Hay Diet. After suffering acute heart failure, he was found to have high blood pressure and nephritis. At this time the prognosis for such a problem (Bright's disease) was poor. In an effort to improve his health himself he started to experiment with different diets. Then, as now, one of the first things people think of in such situations is to go on a vegetarian diet (often unwisely, but this is another story). He added to this by giving up cigarettes and coffee, then choosing to eat only one meal a day. He went on to experiment with many dietary styles. Eventually he came to believe that different food groups (protein-rich, fat-rich, and carbohydrate-rich) should be eaten separately. He claimed that this was because carbohydrates are digested in the mouth and need an alkaline environment for the carbohydrate-splitting enzymes (amylases) to do their work, that protein-rich foods need the acid environment of the stomach to activate the proteases (protein-splitting enzymes that catalyse the breakdown of proteins) and that fat-rich foods need the bile, homogenising agents and lipases (the fat-splitting enzymes that catalyse the breakdown of fats or lipids).

As has happened before, a given result may encourage its developer to claim an incorrect theory for the results they observe. That is what happened with William Hay. In fact, the body is very well designed to digest all three types of foods in the same meal. Carbohydrates are prepared in the mouth for almost full digestion there if thoroughly chewed. If they are not properly chewed in the mouth, carbohydrates can a least be partially digested in the mouth, where they are broken down from large complex carbohydrates to smaller complex carbohydrates, the process being completed lower down in the small intestine. They may even be broken down to disaccharides in the mouth, though not down fully into their glucose monosaccharide.

It is worth noting here that the term 'digestion' is properly used only for the breakdown of food, and that 'absorption' occurs when the digested broken-down food products are absorbed across the gut lining and then into the body, usually via the blood stream or via the lymphatic system.

Proteins are 'denatured' in the very acidic conditions of the stomach into peptides and polypeptides, which are still chains of amino acids. They are then broken down into amino acids which are finally absorbed, also in the lower digestive tract

Fat-rich foods, in like manner, are prepared for eventual digestion in the duodenum, by the homogenising action of the bile from the liver. At this point it all comes together. From here on down, the smaller carbohydrates are digested down to disaccharides, which are further broken down to monosaccharides by agents in the intestinal walls. The proteins are broken down to amino acids, and the large fatty molecules are broken down, mainly to di- or mono-glycerides, all – and this is the key point – in or near the duodenum and small intestine and *all together,* in so far as they do not significantly interfere with each other, *in the same environment.*

There really is no need to follow the 'non-combining food' ideas of William Hay. It worked for him with his unusual problems. But it is not a universal truth, although some people still adhere to his ideas. If it works for you, then follow this regime, but do not suggest that *everyone* should do it. There is no need, and there are many disadvantages.

In a similar manner today, people are discovering the benefits of a ketogenic diet. This works wonderfully for those with particular metabolic needs. It does *not* work for all. For other people it can be a disaster. I see this so many times in my clinic where I focus on supporting people with cancer, that it dismays me. Treat the person, not the disease. And this starts with determining their metabolic needs.

I have digressed from the autobiographical story here, but treating the person rather than the disease is so important, and this is as good a place as any to expand on my thinking on the subject.

Rapid Healing Tibia TM

Early one morning I heard a shout from TM. I rushed to the bathroom and found him curled up and in great pain. Between us we got him out to the car and down to the local hospital. It turned out that somehow he had broken his tibia, the major bone in his lower leg, often called the shin bone. As was the usual procedure in those days, his whole leg was put in an extensive and hideously uncomfortable plaster cast. He was told to return after six weeks when it would be x-rayed again and they would be able to tell him the extent of the healing that was still needed. They would then give him an estimate as to how much longer it would be until he could have the cast taken off. He was given crutches and told to "be careful". He struggled. He hated the crutches and the need for them.

I didn't think much of the medications he had been given and so replaced them with a calcium-rich supplement. He loved meat and had no inclination to be a vegetarian and so, based on his metabolism, calcium did seem to be the best option. It is not so for everyone. I also gave him various low-potency homoeopathic remedies for shock and to encourage healing. After only four weeks, instead of the requested six, I suggested he go back to the hospital and ask to have his leg re- x-rayed. He demurred, saying he wasn't supposed to go back for another two weeks. I repeated my advice and suggested he admit, when he got there, that he might have made a mistake as to the date, but to ask if, now that he was there, he could have an x-ray done anyway. This might not have been possible in the UK NHS, but it could be done in Australia's more flexible Medicare system. A somewhat reluctant young doctor agreed to do this premature X-ray, as he thought it.

When he reviewed the result, he expressed his surprise at the rapid rate of healing. It had healed so rapidly, in fact, that he had taken the plaster cast off there and then after only four weeks rather than the six-plus weeks that had been expected. TM, naively and meaning to be helpful and informative, had then said to the young doctor, "Perhaps it's due to the calcium tablets and other nutrients I've been taking." However, this was met with a casual brush off from the young and super confident doctor: "No, that could have nothing to do with it. In fact, you're lucky, those calcium tablets might have given you kidney stones." Talk about the wastefulness of scattering seeds on barren ground.

Doctors Are Really Lucky: Medical methods v the Naturopathic Approach

While I was studying the basic naturopathic course, I had thought that doctors were really lucky. They already had the full knowledge of anatomy and physiology, of pathologies and differential diagnosis and other medical issues. All they had to do, if they wanted to become naturopaths, and I couldn't imagine a more appealing goal, was to learn about nutrition and botanical or herbal medicine. I soon learnt how wrong I was.

I had been fortunate in knowing a number of doctors who were at least sufficiently interested in, or aware and accepting of, naturopathy, that they invited me to sit in on a number of their consultations. I enjoyed this enormously. Eventually I came to realise that, in outward appearance at least, there was little difference in what they did and what we, as naturopaths did. The client came in and talked with the doctor. The doctor reached for the prescription pad and wrote the names of the medications that were being prescribed, and the client left to go to a pharmacy and have the prescription filled. On many occasions and in a parallel manner, the naturopath too, in those days, reached for their prescription pad and wrote the names of the nutritional or herbal products that they are prescribing. These could then be purchased either from the practitioner or from a health food shop or similar.

It gradually dawned on me, however, that there was a seismic chasm between the medical philosophy ('take a pill for an ill and risk the toxic effects') and the naturopathic philosophy ('restore normal function or homoeostasis'). It was worth exploring. It was beginning to seem to me that there was, and should be, much more to naturopathy than this. By now it was probably about 1983. My ideas were developing, and naturopathy itself was at an exciting stage of growth. I was not only learning and applying facts, but exploring the concepts and philosophy of this new subject, as we all (I assumed) explored the subject and shaped its direction. However, my early training in chemistry, particularly inorganic and analytical chemistry, had shaped my initial thinking in science. It was thus to me a fundamental and automatic strategy, that if something was wrong, I should endeavour to fix it, to restore it to the way it was meant to be, not to try to beat it into shape in some other way.

Fortunately, I have been blessed with good health. I had the usual childhood problems of measles, German measles, chicken pox, and whooping cough – there was no routine (or very little) vaccination system when I was a kid. Other than this I don't recall having had much to do with doctors, as a child, and even less once I was a young adult. Certainly, from the age or twenty-five, when I was back in London and taking an interest in amino acid chemistry and protein balancing, and in nutrition at Queen Elizabeth College, my first thoughts were always focused on how to restore normal function.

'Homeostasis is a property of cells, tissues, and organisms that allows the maintenance and regulation of the stability and constancy needed to function properly. Homeostasis is a healthy state that is maintained by the constant adjustment of biochemical and physiological pathways.' RXList

There is much more online for further knowledge and for references.

Aunt and My Low Income

By this time, it was more than ten years since I had been in Ireland to visit Aunt. While I missed her greatly, my life here in Australia was very full. I would have loved to visit her, but the real problem was the cost of the airfare and my limited income. I had just been covering my costs ever since I left South Africa and this did not look like changing significantly. I put little importance on a good income, so this did not bother me greatly, but I would have loved to see more of Aunt.

We continued to swap our weekly hour-long audio tapes of course, keeping up with each other's lives. To me they were a lifeline of warmth and affection, support and approval. Her life had become prescribed by a marriage that, although wonderful, did revolve almost entirely round her husband's needs and preclude her from developing her own interests. She had moved from London to Ireland, catering for his need for early retirement and a more tranquil life in the open country rather than in London, but she missed much of her London life. As such, she told me, she lived somewhat vicariously through what I was doing. She had been thrilled by my graduation and was intensely interested in all the stories and case histories I could share with her – anonymously of course.

Cats and Nephralbin

There was one time, however, when she asked for help. She had three cats, which she totally adored, mother cat, daughter cat, and son cat. One by one they went into kidney failure. First the mother cat, then a year or two later, daughter cat. She told me about this, but too late for me to do anything. However, I persuaded her let me know if son cat developed signs of kidney failure. About a year later he did, and I immediately sent over a bottle of a Reckeweg remedy named Nephralbin. As soon as she received it, she started putting a few drops in his drinking water. His health improved almost immediately after that and all was well for a while before he went downhill again. For some reason that only she can fathom, she had let herself run out of it, then told me, then waited until the next bottle arrived, and then worried at how unwell he had become. But once she was giving him the remedy, he picked up quickly yet again and all was well for a while. Then the whole cycle repeated, and I would send another bottle. I never could persuade her to keep a bottle on hand. In this way we kept that third cat alive and well for two more years, much to her delight.

I suspect that she was thinking along allopathic medicine lines: 'Take the remedy and you are cured, there is no need for ongoing prevention', instead of naturopathic lines that involve doing whatever is needed to maintain good health.

Physical Activity

I have always been very physically active. At my various schools I had played all the sports that were available, playing in and often captaining most of the teams. At Imperial there had been the trip to Delft University where I had played on about eleven different teams. I had also won colours in tennis and squash – Imperial College Purples instead of Oxford or Cambridge Blues. Then there had been the decade or more of very active field work with mountains to climb and hundreds of samples to collect and carry. Back here in Pennant Hills (Sydney) I had done an almost ridiculous amount of work in my garden and looked after my goats and chickens. With TM came more hens, plus ducks, and guinea pigs. We also both played squash once or twice a week with his friends at Macquarie University. Squash or tennis, I loved them both with a slight preference for squash. It took less time, was a more energetic workout, and gave the whole group of us time for dinner afterwards in a local Chinese restaurant.

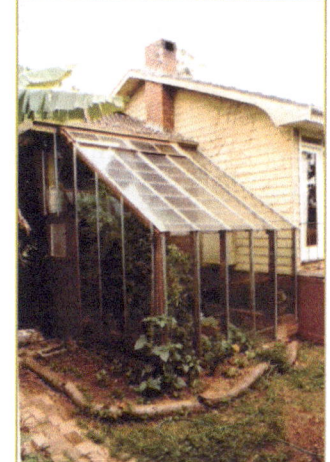

As if we needed more exercise, TM and I had built a greenhouse lean-too in our carport. It was made of wine bottles. No, we didn't drink all the wine – had we done so I doubt the wall would ever have been built. We collected the bottles, and where possible the corks, from local restaurants, and stuck firmly to only two sizes of red and white burgundy bottles.

By the application of judicious spacing of these we could keep the wall regular, steady and straight. Each bottle had to be cleaned and the label removed. It was time-consuming. We wanted the wall of water-filled bottles to become a heat sink, storing up the warmth of the sun from the day and, we hoped, giving it back out during the evening. This meant that all the bottles had to be filled with water, then corked, then laid in place. All went well for many months after the wall was finished, until the occasional bottle could no longer take the strain and 'popped its cork'. At this point, of course, the bottle was lying on its side, embedded in the wall, and so could not be refilled. Nonetheless, we grew some mighty tomatoes in this greenhouse.

We also grew a row of excellent aubergines. At least they were excellent until I noticed pests, of some forgotten variety, on all of the plants. I put a calendula plant at one end of the row. All the pests took off at speed to the other end of the row. I put a calendula plant there too and the pests immediately rushed to the middle plant, and stood, confused, wondering where else they could turn for safety. I dug this middle plant up, burnt it, and was glad to see that that had solved the problem.

Plants, Animals, and Organic Compounds v Petrochemicals, Manufactured, and Industrial Compounds

You can divide the world into groups depending on the criteria you use. In relation to health and the way the body functions, there is the group of compounds and substances that occur naturally in plants and animals. These consist mostly of carbon, hydrogen, and oxygen, and often with a significant amount of oxygen. Then there are all the compounds that come from petrochemicals, and those that are synthesised by various manufacturing processes. There is no absolute certainty in this, but those in the first group, compounds coming from plants and animals, are quite likely to be compounds that can be metabolised, or broken down either successfully or without significant harm, in the human body. Certainly, some can be toxic compounds, but only a few. On the other hand, remedies or medicines derived from petrochemicals or by manufacturing processes starting from a variety of manufactured compounds, are less likely to be broken down safely and eliminated from the human body by existing biochemical pathways, and are more likely to be toxic and cause harm.

Thoughts along these lines set me thinking ever more firmly along the lines of, whenever possible, restoring homoeostasis, giving the body compounds it could use or metabolise rather than ones it had to fight or protect itself from. When you are working as a naturopath, this is not really so difficult to do. Naturopathy is essentially about restoring optimal and good nutrition and the safe use of plant extracts.

Collapsed Lung

Not long after this, a woman came in asking what I could do to help her husband. He had been in hospital and both lungs were collapsing. Every time they thought they had repaired the problem (I didn't have any more details than that) he would try to get up and leave, cough some more and fall ill again. I put together a combination of the herbs that I thought might help. As I recall, they included coltsfoot, red clover, pleurisy root, comfrey, and horehound. As I had from the start of my career, I loved having these tinctures and being able to blend my own combinations. Two days later a chap came in and asked for "more of that lung remedy please". I was keen to know more.

"Oh good, how is he?" was the obvious question, "is he improving at all?" I was not that confident, but I did figure I had used the best of the herbs I had available. "Oh, fine, it's me actually, I got better almost as soon as I took your mixture."

What a lovely result and what good feedback for me.

---

[i] Knud Asbjorn Lund, *Understanding Our Fellow Men,* New Knowledge Books, 1958, 1971.

Chapter 13

Beacon Hill, Disastrous Fire

S oon after we had completed the green house, TM left for a three-month study course in Gottingen. I joined him for part of that time and was particularly impressed by the friends of his who had invited us to stay. With only two rooms, each about ten feet square, and a small kitchen, three floors above the ground, they managed to grow a significant amount of their food, especially herbs, leafy vegetables and tomatoes. They had developed a lot of ingenious ways of growing plants up their outside walls, and more. I got many ideas from them that I have used in later years and in different forms of accommodation.

TM then completed his thesis and accepted a job in algae research in Dee Why on the east coast of northern Sydney, about a ninety-minute drive east from us in Pennant Hills. It was clearly time for us to move. We bought a wonderful 'old' sandstone farmhouse. It had the double advantage of being both very much closer to where TM had just started his new job and additionally closer to my own office in Cremorne. I thus reduced my travelling time from an hour each way to twenty minutes each way.

Just after the Second World War when I first passed through Sydney on my way to New Zealand as a child, the property had been a 60-acre farm. By the time I bought it, it was on the usual small quarter-acre block. Gardening time was anyway now limited, work was truly taking over, and any remaining aspiration to having a smallholding had faded. The house (Beacon Hill) was made of hand-hewn blocks of sandstone and had wooden floors and wooden ceilings about 12 feet high, and I loved it. Australians thought it really old, but it was only built in 1910.

With the help of countless friends, we moved our possessions, a relatively simple procedure, and our plants, pot plants, compost and more from our organic gardening activities, a process that demanded several trips. I would have loved to take the greenhouse we had built from empty wine bottles, but that was not practicable. We swiftly settled into the delightful new house and life returned pretty much to normal, with one exception. Now that the garden demanded very little time, I was able to focus more on research and writing.

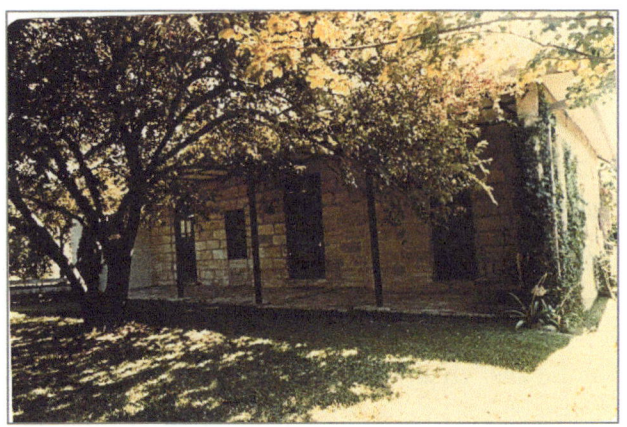

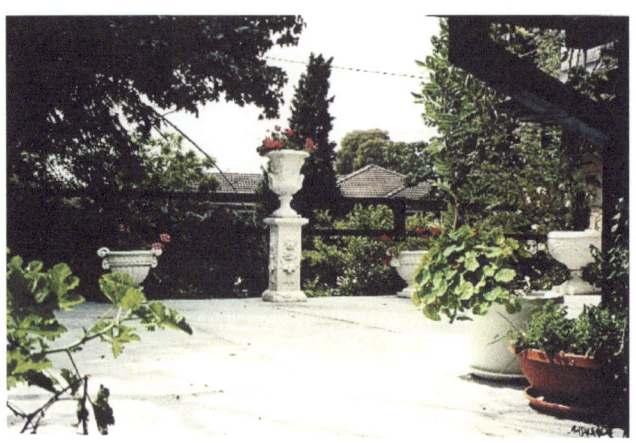

Writing

Sometime after I had started writing articles, initially with reluctance and rapidly with increasing enthusiasm, Allen and Unwin, publishers, asked me to write books for them. Again, I demurred, saying that writing articles was one thing, but that writing entire books was something else altogether. In about 1981 they had asked for six books in the next six years, but I was immensely busy with all my other activities as I built my professional life and the practice, so it took me six years to write one book. They published this under the title of *Living with Allergies*. I had, of course, been working with allergies and food sensitivities almost since the start, so it was hardly surprising that my first book was on this subject. I dedicated it, of course, to Aunt, as I do this one. I filled it with a variety of case histories and strategies for both detecting allergens and avoiding them. I formulated diets with reduced chances of causing problems. It was an almost inevitable choice of subject as it was one of my main focuses of work. The writing wasn't as difficult as I had thought.

The next year I wrote a segment called 'Offsetting the side effects of the pill' for a book called *Love, Sex and Fertility*, edited by Barbara McGregor and published by Wellspring Publishers, 1987. Such was my enthusiasm that by then I was thinking I was ready to take on the challenge of a second book on my own, but there was to be a delay due to all else I was being asked to do.

Stomach Ulcers

Martin came to see me because of the acute and agonising stomach attacks of pain he would get during the night. The pain would start at about eight o'clock and gradually build up to a crescendo by about two or three in the morning, then subside. If the pain became unbearable, he would go down to the local hospital, not far from where he lived. Sometimes he would be given painkillers, sometimes other drugs, and at other times antacids, all to no effect other than the production of toxic side effects. He persevered with them because he considered them to be less painful than the full-on attack that would develop if he did not treat the problem. He told me that he had had many tests and no cause for the pain had been detected. It sounded to me as if he had an ulcer, but he was told that none could be found. There seemed to be no other help to be had from the doctors he consulted. I still thought it sounded like an ulcer, so I decided to treat it accordingly, knowing that my naturopathic approach would not cause negative toxic effects even if it did not solve the problem.

I suggested that he have handy some slippery elm powder and some aloe vera juice. I advised him to make sure that the slippery elm powder was just that, and not 'slippery elm food'. The latter was commonly available in Sydney at the time and usually consisted of about equal parts of slippery elm powder, milk powder, and wheat flour with added sugar. I had many clients with either milk or wheat sensitivities and so had become used to warning clients not to use it.

I advised Martin that the moment he felt the slightest pain starting, which he assured me he had become adept at recognising, he was to mash a teaspoonful of the slippery elm powder into a quarter of a banana. The banana is mucilaginous as is the slippery elm. They mix well together and, what is also important, provide a reasonably pleasant-tasting mix. He was to eat that and then to sip organic aloe vera juice in tiny amounts, taking in so little each time that it didn't stimulate a swallow reflex. The aim was to have the juice trickling slowly and almost continuously down his oesophagus, and hopefully over the areas where the pain started. I was still working on the assumption that there was a break in the stomach lining, possibly so small that the scan had not been able to detect it, and that what I was giving him was firstly a 'bandage' in the form of the slippery elm covering the hole that I presumed was present, and secondly, to stimulate healing with the aloe vera juice.

A few nights later he phoned me up to say that the pain had started and to confirm what he should do. I repeated the instructions and told him to phone me if it continued to get worse. I heard no more until the next morning when I phoned him. He told me that the pain had indeed started and built up, but more slowly than usual, and had stopped sooner and long before he needed any painkiller. We adjusted the procedure slightly, and from then on he had only a few minor episodes. The minute he got the warning of the start of the pain building up, he took my prescription. The pain would rapidly diminish in severity, and very soon in frequency until he was able to report that he had gone for a month with no problem. I continued to assume that he had had an ulcer, but I imagined it to be more the shape of a vertical hole through the stomach lining, thus with little to show on the surface other than in the shape of a flatter ulcerated area.

Put simply, the stomach wall can be thought of as made of a protein and a muscular wall with a protective mucous lining. It is *expected* to house the very strong acid that is required for the denaturing of the protein foods. This denaturing involves altering the nature and structure of the protein-rich foods so that they can then be attacked and broken down further on in the digestive tract. This latter part of the process is aided by specific enzymes from the pancreas that break the protein down to individual amino acids in the duodenum and small intestine, from which they are absorbed.

This acid is hydrochloric acid and it is so strong that it is perfectly capable of digesting your thumb if you were foolish enough to dip it in. It could certainly digest the muscular stomach wall. To protect this there is the mucilaginous lining to the stomach that is unaffected by the acid. The acid is prepared within the stomach lumen, from individual atoms of hydrogen and chlorine, in the form of positive hydrogen ions and negative chloride ions. Each of these is propelled from the appropriate cells of the stomach wall and then through the mucilaginous lining. They only come together (effectively in pairs) once they are each safely through the protective layer and can safely form hydrochloric acid within the lumen or open space of the stomach.

This is a clear example of where the naturopathic approach of restoring normal function is far better and safer than providing a medical drug that is simply designed to neutralise the suspected acid, but not solve the problem.

Throughout my fifty years in practice, both as a nutritionist and a naturopath, I have remained frustrated by the absurd thinking of doctors and pharmacists who insist on providing antacids to people with acidic-like pain in the stomach. It is worth repeating, the stomach is *meant* to be acid. Its contents are *meant* to be acidic. You *need* this acid to prepare the stomach contents for their proper digestion. What you *also* need is an intact stomach lining. This is not likely to be created by antacids. What is more likely to happen, if these antacids are used frequently, is a build-up of improperly- or badly- or semi-digested stomach contents, possible inflammation, and probable pain. The most likely benefit from purchasing and swallowing antacids is to the pharmacist's pockets as they sell unhelpful 'remedies' to the endless need of the poor sufferers. I say endless, because far from providing a long-term solution, these antacids are likely to interfere with good digestion and absorption.

About this time I learnt that, at great expense, some equipment had apparently been brought out to Sydney from the UK designed to actually measure the amount of acid in the stomach of poor ulcer sufferers. Unfortunately, I only learnt of this at the end of the trial. In total frustration, and after all the patients who had been offered the test had been tested, the equipment had been packed up and was being returned to the UK. Contrary to expectations, *none* of the ulcer sufferers had been found to produce an excess of stomach acid under whatever circumstances they had established.

There was more frustration, mine this time, because not once had the research team looked to see if they could find people who produced too *little* stomach acid. I anticipated then, and now, that they would have found them, had they looked. Unfortunately, I did not work in that hospital, I did not have a research grant, and I was too late to add in my own suggestion for further research. I thought then, and still think, that many people with stomach pains are suffering from too little stomach acid and compromised or poor protein digestion which then leads to inflammation, a damaged stomach lining and other reactions.

I do mean here true stomach pains, pains over their stomach, not indigestion pains over their middle or lower abdomen, to which many people are actually referring when they say 'stomach'. It is certain that these pains can often be stopped by supplementation with tablets containing hydrochloric acid and proteolytic digestive enzymes, both of which aid digestion.

At this time less was known about Helicobacter pylori, also known as Campylobacter pylori, a gram-negative, spiral bacterium, now thought to penetrate (screw its way into) the mucous lining of the stomach, and trigger infection. What I do know is that any of my patients who complained of stomach pains and followed my suggestions were soon pain-free.

Failing to 'See' or Correctly Label the Internal Organs

I was spared another possible frustration in an entirely different way. As naturopaths we had good lecturers and wonderful diagrams of the internal organs and workings of the human body, but we had nothing to work with, no cadavers to cut up or inspect, no chance to 'see the real thing'. It is clear from some of the text books that although most diagrams of the stomach make them look all much the same and of nearly standard size, this is not a true reflection of reality. Roger Williams, in his book *The Wonderful World Within You,*[i] shows diagrams of about fifteen different stomachs of entirely different shapes and sizes. Imagine a pair of brothers. We can call their 'owners' Peter, who has a very small stomach, and Paul, a large stomach. Peter will soon be called a picky eater and Paul will be labelled greedy. Their mother is frustrated with the ongoing battle to get them both to eat their meals, of the same size and at the same time, and finish them.

It is lunch time and food is put on the table.

Mother: "Now eat everything up, Peter. I'm tired of you leaving half your food and then coming back in the middle of the afternoon and asking for more, just after I've cleared everything away."

Peter: "Yes, Mum," and he means it. He really does. He sets to with a will, determined for once to eat as much as big brother Paul, and as quickly. But as ever, his stomach is full by the time he is only halfway through, and he is finished.

Mother is annoyed yet again: "Good heavens, Peter, can't you finish it, just for once. If you don't, you will just have to get some bread and jam to fill up on later. I am not cooking more if you don't finish your meal now."

By mid-afternoon poor Peter is hungry again. He braves his mother's wrath, asks for more food, gets given bread and jam or some such, and as a result is both unhappy and undernourished. He probably also develops eating issues, largely emotional. Paul, perhaps to show his prowess at eating an adult portion, possibly due to the boredom of sitting there while poor Peter continues to try to eat just a little bit more, may develop a habit of overeating and the possibility of developing obesity in later years.

Feedback

I was, in those days, writing articles regularly for several magazines each year, often monthly, and looking for new topics. Case histories were popular, but one of the problems with them was that frequently I didn't know the end of the story. People would come in, tell me the problem, get help on their treatment and then just disappear. They would come back if they still had problems, but if their symptoms all went away, the first I was likely to hear of it was possibly some years later when they returned with a different problem.

I would ask: "How did you get on with the so-and-so that you consulted me for a couple of years back?"

"Oh, that was fine, everything cleared up after I did what you suggested, thank you."

I am always delighted for them, but am generally left wishing they had thought to tell me without having to be prompted by some other factor.

Fibroids

RM was different. The mother of three children under twelve, she had seen me a few times, usually about one of the children who she preferred to have treated naturopathically than medically. This time it was for herself. Her sister brought her in, explaining that she had wanted to come sooner but had not been able to get out of bed. She had been bleeding heavily, vaginally, for about six weeks. Her gynaecologist had told her she had a very large fibroid and should agree to an immediate operation and hysterectomy. She argued that she wanted to avoid the hysterectomy if at all possible, and she wanted to see me instead and find out what I could do. She had bargained with the gynaecologist and they had finally compromised and come to an agreement. She could see me, but if that did not resolve the problem within six to eight weeks, she would agree to the operation. She really liked the gynaecologist, who had seen her through three childbirths, and she had great faith in him, but she was also very keen to avoid an operation and to continue to rely strongly on the naturopathic approach to health care. She made a forward appointment with him as they had agreed, and then came straight to me for help with her treatment.

I wasn't, at that stage, too sure what to do about fibroids, and this was certainly the first major example I had worked with. However, I had been having good results with a number of homeopathic products in the Reckeweg range, a range of 75 low potency plant remedies. I decided to start with them. I used R 28. I also made other suggestions to her in relation to diet and lifestyle etc, and to detoxing. Imagine my delight when, at the end of the allotted period she came back to see me and to tell me that her bleeding had stopped entirely, almost as soon as she had started on my program. In other situations, it might all have ended there and I might never have known the outcome. She was 'cured' in her own mind and had no need to do anything more. However, due to her promise to her gynaecologist she had gone back to see him, been examined, and told the bad news that she now had two fibroids not one. The good news was that instead of the one being the size of a large grapefruit, they were each about the size of an orange pip, and that he was sure they would both soon disappear entirely, as indeed they did.

Liver, Digestion, and Foot Reflexology

Another unusual diagnosis with a surprising outcome involved a man who had come to see me about his indigestion and abdominal bloating. He had been keeping his hand at the bottom of his abdomen while he had been explaining about the gas and discomfort he was feeling. When he stood up, he staggered slightly and commented that his right foot was painful. I asked to see it, pressed a few points until I found the spot that was really tender. It was his liver spot on the reflexology chart, and I was able to say that his problem was NOT intestinal bloating but trouble with his liver, which fortunately I was then able to treat.

Iridology and Constipation

TR provided another unsuspected diagnostic tool. She was experiencing frequent and debilitating headaches. By this time we were sitting nearly side by side and I took a close look at her. Around the pupils of both eyes, the inner circle was a solid yellow. This suggested to me constipation and a toxic bowel. I asked her about bowel movements. I was not surprised when she said she usually 'went' once or twice a week instead of the desirable three times a day (at least if you are eating three meals a day). Once we sorted out her constipation, her headaches stopped.

Watching Operations

I was by this stage really wishing I could watch an operation, or even an autopsy – anything to actually *see* inside the human torso. Here I was lucky. A very good friend was a doctor and also a lecturer at the college where I too taught. One day she invited me in to watch an operation, if I was interested – Of course I was interested. It was a small local hospital, otherwise this might not have been possible. We both arrived, prepared, and 'scrubbed up'. I was introduced as a colleague and medical biochemist, both true, and I was told to maintain near silence, say little, and not ask questions. I obeyed this firm instruction in fear of losing this amazing opportunity. We went into theatre. The patient was brought in on a trolley, still awake and able to chat with the surgeon. She was to have an ovary removed. I never learnt why.

"I know you will take good care of me, won't you, Doctor?"

"Of course I will," he assured her, and there did seem to be a good level of trust and friendship between them.

Two other medical students then came in and were destined to watch the operation, presumably as part of their course work. The operation proceeded and I remained rooted to the ground, leaning over as much as I dared, fascinated by all I could see. At some point, it seemed, the surgeon moved from friend-of-patient mode to professor-demonstrating-his-prowess to two students and two visitors. He started to lift out the small intestine and showed us its length, then moved the small intestine aside to show us the uterus and other organs. Finally, one of the students asked where the appendix was.

"Here." The surgeon hooked it up, lifted it out and said, "Might as well remove that." And he cut it off then and there and sewed up the end of the colon.

I was horrified, and sorely tempted to remonstrate, but it was hardly my job. Fortunately, the male student intervened and asked why that had been done, to which the surgeon replied, after some slight hesitation, "Well, if after the surgery she does have right-sided abdominal pain, we will know it is not due to a problem with the appendix." I remained horrified and could only think of the opportunity for toxaemia and of possible leakage of colon contents into the abdomen. I have, rightly or wrongly, had diminished trust in surgeons ever since.

The same friend was able to have me invited into a second operation soon after that, but one that she could not attend herself. This was to be a lumpectomy for a woman with a breast tumour. Again, I scrubbed up. This time I was asked if I would like to assist. Of course,

I would! Honesty, however, determined that I protested, if only mildly, saying that I was not really experienced in this department. However, I was soon drawn in and involved. I suspect they were somewhat short-staffed. I was given forceps (I think) and asked to hold this, then let go, then hold that. There was a good deal of relaxed banter and discussion. Someone asked, having seen the size of the tumour, why a lumpectomy was being done when clearly a mastectomy was required. "She has already had her right breast removed. She was pretty upset about that. I don't think she could handle the loss of both of them. We don't think she has much chance anyway."

This was back in about 1986. I cringed slightly, having read of people who had been able to hear what was being said around them, even while under the anaesthetic.

That operation was followed by a male lumpectomy, which, by comparison, was obviously less interesting, though I was interested to hear the surgeon's comment. "These tumours in men are much rarer than breast tumours in females, but possibly more dangerous."

I was very grateful for both opportunities. Observing the inside of the torso had been hugely fascinating, and I was only sad that I had no more such chances.

Arthritis

I enjoyed working with people with arthritis and hoped to be inspired and learn something useful as I listened to a radio interview while driving through the rush hour traffic to work one morning. The interviewer described the arthritis specialist in glowing terms. He had done seven years of medical training, x more years of surgical training, then y more years of training in arthrology. She was clearly impressed with his credentials and the duration of his training. He, in turn, outlined the different types of arthritis, named them, described them in some detail, and held positive hope that a lot of new developments were becoming available and that much could be done for people suffering with the disease.

After the interview, listeners were invited to call in with their queries. And in they came, questions about all sorts of locations of arthritis, all sorts of types of arthritis, and all sorts of symptom pictures. I listened with bated breath, hoping to learn from the answers more of what could be done. Imagine my disappointment when I heard his answers. They were all essentially the same: painkillers, anti-inflammatory drugs, or surgery, or painkillers, or surgery, or anti-inflammatory drugs, or pain killers … and so it went on.

It seems they had been learning more and more about arthritis in descriptive terms, but with little progress in the development that was of any help for the client. As I write this, back in London and several decades later, focused on cancer, I find myself comparing it to this latter disease. As if by coincidence, while I have been writing, there has just been an announcement of a new research direction in the even earlier detection of cancer. So they can detect it sooner, but there was no mention of any improvement in treatment or treatment outcomes, little benefit to the client, at least for a few years, and no real understanding of the causes and how to correct them. It does seem as if much of medical research continues to be aimed at developing more use of medical drugs, than in correcting or curing the initial problem.

I revelled in every aspect of the mix I had created within the range of my professional interests. I loved researching all the technical information as it came out. I loved turning this information into articles that I could write up. I also incorporated it into the lectures I prepared for the students. By this time my part of their course consisted of giving them two hours a week of biochemistry (Year 2), two hours of general nutrition and macronutrients (Year 1) two hours of basic nutrients, dominantly vitamins and minerals (Year 2) and two hours of nutritional therapies (Years 3 and 4). This gave me both time and ample opportunities to expand the content each year. Naturopathy itself, and the material encompassed in the course, was also expanding rapidly at this time.

Throughout my career I have continued to maintain this blend of (a) consultations with clients, (b) lecturing to both students and post-graduates, (c) writing both for the general reader and the more technically minded readers (d) the overall development of the natural therapies in general, and their place in our society and (e) the supply, mostly via the shop and the practice, of the products that could best contribute to health.

Fighting Back

It seemed to come almost out of the blue, but suddenly it looked as if the Big Guns in the form of Big Pharma, although we didn't think of the pharmaceutical industry in those terms back then, was about to destroy our profession, industry, and business. This was the time of multivitamin therapy, orthomolecular nutrition, and orthomolecular psychiatry. We used generous doses of all the nutrients we had. In those days we did not have the vast range of more subtle products, ones with potentised ingredients, and those made from a multitude of organic food and herbal powders.

We were abruptly told that the most of any nutrient that could be included in any nutritional product was to be the RDA (Recommended Daily Allowance) level. I forget the exact wording, but at that time it was something like: the RDA was the amount of any nutrient, in the opinion of the Board, needed to prevent overt signs of deficiency of the nutrient in the majority of healthy people. 'Healthy people' were defined as those in robust good health of mind, body, and spirit. We picked that one apart.

'The Board' was made up largely of a group of people with little interest in or knowledge of good and supportive nutrition. It included pharmacists, people from the food industry and similarly disinterested people, the majority of whom had little interest in improving the food quality or the health of the nation. 'Overt deficiency' meant we would only be allowed to give less than 2 mg of vitamin B1, barely sufficient to prevent Beriberi. The RDA for vitamin C was 75 mg. That might have prevented scurvy but was going to do nothing for people when they got colds or developed the flu. The majority? Well, what about the minority of people (theoretically that meant up to 49%) who ate the average junk food diet of the day. Clearly health issues would increase.

The natural health industry got itself into action. All the health food companies, all the health food shops, and many of the key practitioners whose practices could be decimated by this legislation, got together. Blackmores, a major supplier in Sydney at the time, and Barbara McGregor, one of their key people, set about the plan. Thousands of 'protest' kits were prepared. Cardboard flat-pack boxes were designed in the shape of small posting boxes for the protests. These were given away to every retail outlet and every practitioner's office, every gym, and more. Forms and letters were printed, making it as easy as possible for people to either add only their name, or the name of their MP, or to go further, and write their own comments. People were also encouraged to write their own individual protest letters. Barbara, who is still a good friend, was heroic and dynamic in spearheading the whole project.

So often I hear people say, "What is the point? If I am writing to my MP, I am just one person with little clout." However, at that time the general acceptance was that for every letter that an MP received, they should assume that 500 other people felt the same way but had just not got round to voting, writing, or protesting.

We finally had 120,000 letters to send to Canberra, suggesting that 60,000,000 million people were protesting. The population of the whole of the country was only 15.76 million, so this protest represented about four times the country's total population. This was in fact a huge protest, even allowing for the fact that we had made it as easy as possible for people to protest. That legislation was soon dead in the water. So never think that you are just one person and hardly count. Each protest can be a lot more effective than you think.

Calamity - Disaster - FIRE

I am amused by the thought that (according to a friend from many years ago), the Chinese symbol for 'crisis' is closely connected with their symbol for 'opportunity'. Whether or not this is true, I like to believe it. This was doubly important one evening about this time. The phone rang at 11.30 that night. I was asleep, so TM, the night owl, took the call. I woke and could hear most of it through the open doorway: "What is it? What happened? When was this? How bad is it? We'll be there in twenty minutes." This did not sound good. I was up and dressed in a flash and we headed off for my practice, office, dispensary and shop. There had been a fire, but we knew little more.

As we pulled up in the parking space at the back of the building, we could see obvious signs of burning at ground floor level. Then I could see that the upstairs windows were blackened and either open or broken. In my distressed state I wasn't thinking too clearly, but I do recall thinking that I had been in the middle of marking the biochemistry exam papers and had left them on my desk. I hated both setting and marking exam papers, routine chores that came every term or semester. Perhaps this fire meant I wouldn't have to do it? Small comfort.

The fire brigade was in full control when we arrived, but the fire, although out, was still smouldering. It seemed someone had come in via the back door and lit the fire at the bottom of the stairs. These had acted as a funnel and drawn the fire up the stairs as well as across the entire lower floor. From there it had spread both throughout the shop to the front, and backwards to the dispensary and books section, and then upstairs to all four rooms. Appalled, we hung around and asked questions, but learnt little except that there was clearly nothing we could do. In fact, we were told that technically the fire brigade now 'owned' the building, and could do what they liked with it. In real terms, this left them free to pull down a wall or break out a window if they deemed this necessary for firefighting or safety reasons. It seemed they would control the building until they were sure there was no further danger and then lock or board it up. I could return in the morning. Unfortunately, this had happened on a Wednesday, the day we had had almost all our deliveries for the next seven days. This led to two problems for us. Firstly, all the newly delivered products were now fire damaged, increasing the loss to a full week's turnover, and secondly, there had been a large amount of carboard and paper, left from the unpacking, that had clearly fuelled the fire and given it a head start. If only the arsonist had struck on Tuesday, I would have saved the value of a whole week's sales. But apparently, according to the firemen's local gossip, he had set two fires in shops about five miles away the night before.

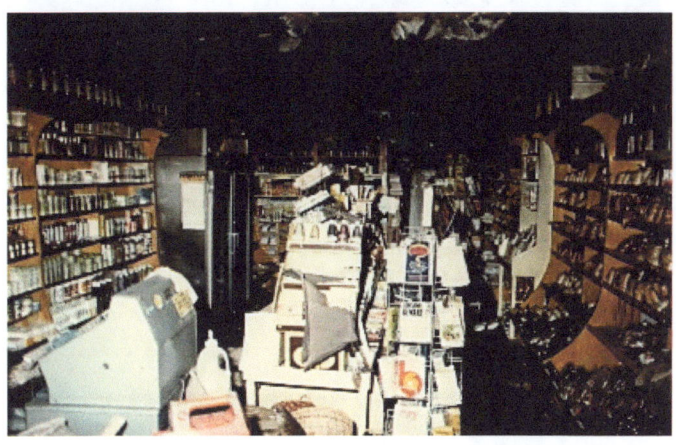

Home, sleep, worry, agonise, plan. Hope? Not much. The next morning we phoned around. I had a great and extensive group of friends. They were all marvellous. A chiropractor colleague two miles away offered me a spare room in his practice which I could use if I wanted to continue to see clients, which of course I did. I was duly grateful. Max, my practice manager at the time, was wonderful and arranged to collect and answer the calls while I threw myself into the physical activity of clearing and sorting, activity being my best antidote to the crisis. Friends arrived with cars and we piled all the usable stock into them to take home to Beacon Hill and then offer them as a (literal) fire sale. Most of the damage was smoke damage to the labels. All the packaged goods had, of course, to be abandoned. All the books for sale could be saved and sold off at a discount. All my office material and my library from upstairs was taken either home and stored, or to the chiropractor's office so I could continue to work. I organised a new phone line. There were no mobile phones in those days.

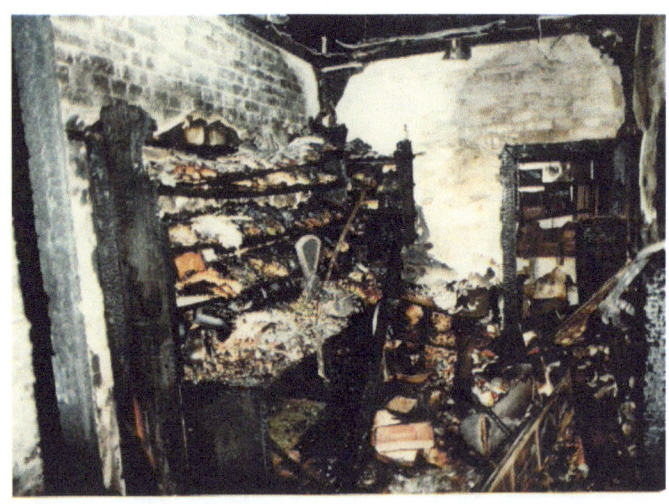

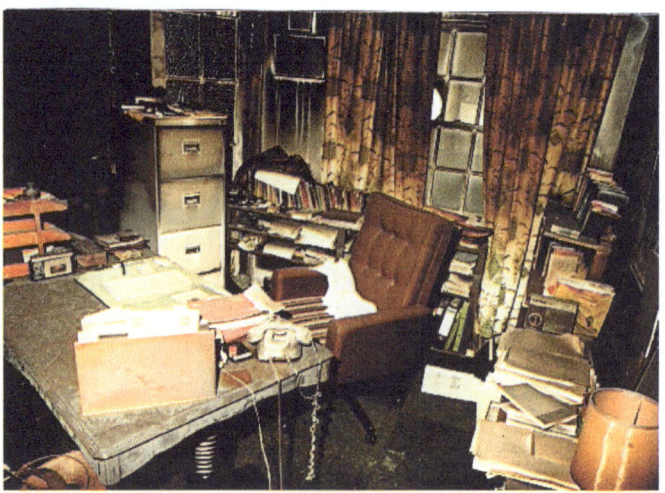

What was I going to do? I didn't occur to me to give up and close shop. My home, heart, and dreams were tied up in these premises. I didn't think twice. I would clear it up for a start, salvage everything that could be salvaged, have fire sales of everything I could sell. Every last cent had to be retrieved. There were no spare funds and now there would be no income. I had to let the junior staff go as I was told it would be at least three months before the building could be used again, even if I did want to restart the business – which of course I did.

For the next four months or more I worked from dawn to dusk. Initially it was grimy, dirty, smelly work. There was an unbelievable amount to do. With the help of many wonderful friends coming in in shifts over the next few days, somehow things did get done. Eventually everything that could be retrieved was stored, either at home (luckily, large enough to absorb it) at my new and temporary office, or in a separate brick storeroom that I had at the back of the main shop building. Its entrance was only to the outside world and not via the shop, and as an entirely brick building it had not been affected by the fire. This was fortunate as it already contained a significant amount of very costly stock. At that time I was the Australian importer of the Weleda ranges of toiletries, cosmetics, and remedies and I imported and supplied a number of shops as well as individual members of the Anthroposophical society, hence the holding and storing of a wholesale quantity of stock. In between these jobs I phoned all my clients, explained the situation and gave them my new phone number.

MX, the second of my senior assistants, was a huge help in all this. My first senior assistant was ML. She was a gentle person and a very good friend and gave me wonderful support. She was also a nurse and a masseuse, and a delightful person to work with. That was until she had to tell me that her live-in boyfriend was being charged with drugs. I was horrified, then even more so when it seemed she was now taking drugs herself. I offered her all the help I could, but also, of course, had to say that I could no longer employ her, not with the risk of her bringing drugs in, or using the shop as a pick-up point.

MX was equally wonderful, in a very different way. She was very efficient and hugely thoughtful, proactive and competent. She dealt with all the changes following the fire in a way I could never have matched. She and her friends helped with the clear up. She then masterminded the resurrection. She seemed to know just what would be needed, what to order in the way of new flooring, new shelving, new till, new scales. She also knew and advised on the best colour schemes and materials to use. I was grateful beyond words. Later, she fell in love with a policeman who took her to live 'way out west' in Broken Hill. I was delighted to see her so happy, but immensely sad to see her go. She had become a good friend and had been an amazing help through the fire and other times, Imagine my delight in 2020 when I received an email from her after she tracked me down online.

I had only three senior assistant-receptionists throughout the years that I worked in Sydney. I had others, of course, who assisted them, and they tended to vary more often.

The building had to be given over to the company that would clear out all the 'rubbish' or everything I didn't think could be saved, and then had to be surveyed for safety. The staircase was badly damaged but could just about be navigated. All the upstairs floorboards were charred and would need to be replaced. In some places there were gaping holes to the floor below. The salvageable furniture was removed, as was my four-drawer metal filing cabinet, once it had cooled down. Amazingly the contents were not burned, though for months afterwards, every time I opened a file, a confetti of scorched and burnt bits from the edges of pages would float gently out. All this time I still had to work, seeing clients in my new office, lecturing at the college, and on top of that, planning the restoration with the help of MX.

There was almost no money for this reconstruction. I had been underinsured. I had not thought to have the insurance company cover the cost of rubbish removal and the many other hidden costs they don't tell you about until you read the very small print after the event.

And the exam papers? The tops ones were dark brown and all but burnt to a crisp, but the black writing was just legible, and in time I got the marking done.

I coped, somehow I coped. My friends were amazed. I think I only did it by immersing myself in everything that had to be done, and not thinking too much beyond the next task.

Two months later there was another crisis. While I was working in my temporary office, a friend had walked past the premises to see how the rebuilding was going. He rang to tell me that the door to the back brick storeroom had been broken open and everything in it had been taken. Thousands of dollars of stock, both the newly imported Weleda stock and whatever salvaged stock that I had stored there. All I had left that was in pristine condition, had gone. Shock. I phoned TM with the news at his university about an hour's drive away and then drove to the premises. The storeroom? I looked in. There was absolutely nothing to see. Worse, there was nothing I could do. Nothing to get stuck into. I could only stand and stare. I collapsed like a burst balloon and sat in my car and sobbed until TM arrived. I was worn out with exhaustion and worry, and this was just the last straw. It was the 'nothing I could do' that was the real last straw, nothing I could do to retrieve or rebuild. Worst still, I had thought we were over the worst and heading for a rebuild. Now I had this to add to it.

As part of the resurrection, I decided to buy a fireproof filing cabinet – once bitten twice shy. I asked the salesman if the new one I was buying would survive a fall through the floor to the level below, so I could use it again if necessary.

"I wouldn't worry about that," he advised. "For all the businesses that go through what yours has gone through and try to restart, eighty per cent of them fail. It's hardly worth the bother." It had never occurred to me to give up and do something else. I have no idea anyway what I would have chosen as an alternative. I could not imagine life without the Natural Gourmet and Pharma Natura. They were my home. They were the place where I truly belonged, the place from which all the activities that were important to me took place and from which they radiated: my consulting room where I met with clients, the shop from which I advised customers, the articles I wrote and sent out to the magazines, my library from which I prepared the lectures that I took out to the various lecture venues. Everything I had, effectively my whole professional life, had been invested in this building and business.

Eventually, however, everything was renewed or restored, and we set about rebuilding our customer base. We traded at a loss for about four months until people gradually learnt that we were back in business again, then, thankfully, we moved into profit. That was, of course, an enormous relief.

"Would you work if it wasn't for the money?"

I recall a time in Perth when the discussion with a couple of friends involved what each of us would do if we (somehow and magically) could continue in our present lifestyles but were not required to work for anything or allowed to do anything for money (all would be found). Most people said they would choose their current hobbies, or a life of relaxation. I realised I would choose to continue doing exactly what I was doing at the time, exploring the geological world around me (as I was doing when this discussion took place) and learning more of its underlying chemistry. I had loved the field work and travelling. In addition, chemistry is such an amazing subject, it can be applied to so much.

Now, as a naturopath, I was certain that I would continue to work as I had been doing. I thought in terms of how lucky I was to have a hobby that paid, if not a huge amount, at least sufficient to live comfortably. I could also go to bed each night feeling I had helped several or more people, either to improved health or enhanced studies. I could also wake up each morning, consider the day ahead, and look forward with enthusiasm and excitement to what I would be doing. I would keep doing it even if it didn't improve my income and lifestyle. So yes, on that basis, I was of course going to rebuild and go back to what I had been doing before the fire.

People still ask me, nearly fifty years later, why I don't retire. They say such things as, "You have the money, you could sell up, you could relax, and do things that you enjoy." To this my response is always the same "I am already relaxed (though I agree I could be a bit more so) and every single day I am doing things that I enjoy, that excite and interest me, and that I value. I cannot imagine a better life.

However, that dismissive pronouncement from the salesman selling me my fireproof filing cabinet did contribute to a daunting launch of our new incarnation. The first six months had been touch and go. I had steadfastly refused to think about failure or going broke. I could, at the start, have broken the lease as the property had become uninhabitable, but I had already agreed to continue it. I would have to keep paying the rent no matter what I did. I couldn't sell it, there was nothing to sell, no business and no material assets.

Looking back as I write, I am not sure how I managed, either financially or mentally. Head down, I battled on, just managing to pay all the bills at the very last moment. Then suddenly business began to pick up as people discovered we were open again. We were off and running once more.

The 'challenge'? It had certainly been that. 'The 'opportunity'? I now had wonderfully designed, if economically built, new premises, both upstairs for the practice and my office, and downstairs for the retail and dispensing. Ultimately, this had definitely been an opportunity and I fully intended to see what I could make of it.

Fred

Fred had been coming to some of my evening lectures at the Naturopathic College. I was curious to know what he wanted when he asked if he could visit me in my home one evening the following week. It was, indeed, an unusual question, but when he arrived, he presented an opportunity that seriously interested me. He had been an alcoholic for some years and had then gone through the entire protocol of Alcoholics Anonymous (AA). He had been very successful and was now one of their instructors. He said that it had occurred to him, week after week as he listened to my lectures in general nutrition, that nutrition could play a significant part in helping some of his clients to get over their alcohol addiction. He pointed out that he and I had complementary skills and we could work together. I would provide nutritional advice and he would work on their Twelve Steps program. After some discussion and planning, a scheme was evolved.

For the next year or so we had an alcoholics' clinic every Monday. We used two of my offices upstairs on the first floor. Fred introduced the clients and brought them in to see me. I went through their diet – usually laden with sugar and coffee as they struggled not to succumb to having an alcoholic drink. Gradually we managed to improve their diet and had them taking a variety of supplements. These included key minerals such as chromium and vanadium, and many of the B group vitamins. The client would then go back to Fred's office while I saw the next client. Fred talked them through the AA Twelve Steps and encouraged them to follow their nutritional program. Somewhat to our surprise we were amazingly successful. In fact, we were one hundred per cent successful except for Steve, who continued to insist he wasn't an alcoholic but who continued to come along most Mondays nonetheless. He was a large imposing man who chose to flirt instead, saying he only came to see me, though patently that was not the case. Clearly, he kept coming due to some internal drive of his own.

I was careful to manage these clients' blood sugar levels and deal with any food allergies, of which there were many. Throughout, they all benefitted from more nutritional guidance and for the whole time they stayed with us they all improved enormously. Steve kept coming, still insisting that he wasn't an alcoholic. I did not argue with him, just kept inviting him to come back each week, which he generally did.

To my great sorrow, about a year later, Fred developed a melanoma on his right arm, a big one. He dropped out of the counselling and our clinic work also dried up. This was some years before I started to specialize in cancer, but I did what I could. Fred insisted he was improving, although to my eyes the melanoma seemed to be growing. He was writing a book. "Once I am over this," he kept saying, "I am going to write a book on the terrible ways that doctors treat you when you have cancer." He visited us, TM and me, from time to time for a chat, sure he was getting better. Sadly, some months later we learnt that he had died.

Two years later I was surprised to see Steve in my waiting room. "I'm not really here to see you," he said. "I just have to tell you something. I always knew I was an alcoholic, but I wasn't going to acknowledge that to other people until I was cured. I kept coming to see you because you didn't spend any time trying to make me admit that I was one. Instead, you simply talked and guided me where you could. It is over a year now since I have had a drink and I am not going to go back on the alcohol." I was delighted. My only sadness was that Fred was not with me any longer and I could not share the information with him, though perhaps, wherever he is, he possibly does know.

AK, MI, Cancer

At this time I was willing to accept clients with any form of health problem, confident that I could be at least of some help to them. But I wasn't sure about cancer. Like most people who knew relatively little about it at this time, I found cancer a somewhat scary subject. I had also been told that we were not allowed, legally, to treat either it or diabetes. I was aware that with most other health problems you could try things out. If one diet, nutrient, or herbal regime didn't produce the desired results you could try another one, or a modification of it. With cancer, I thought, time was against you. It would be important to plan things correctly, right from the start. If people wanted to come to me for cancer care, and very few did in those early days, I generally chose to leave well alone, or referred them on, usually to one of the orthomolecular doctors. However, there was one exception to this.

AK, an excellent and innovative Greek doctor, was also a nutritional enthusiast. He had moved from Sydney to the Australian outback a year or two earlier and become the 'local' doctor to an area larger than any county in the UK. Each year there would be a gathering of the Aboriginal families, those who worked on the great sheep and cattle stations or at the house of each of the sheep-station owners. The general health of all would be seen to as required, and the next group of children would be vaccinated.

When Archie first arrived, he learnt that every year many of the children died soon after being vaccinated. He was keenly aware that the Aboriginal families, who comprised most of his clients, were probably not very well nourished. The only 'shop' on the sheep stations would generally be in a hut run by each of the various 'station' owners, spaced often a hundred miles or more apart and serviced by a weekly supply truck. Most of the food was highly processed, tinned, and packaged convenience foods. Baked beans, cereals, white bread and jam, were common staples. Each year children of specified ages were vaccinated. Archie was horrified when he learnt how many of them died soon after their vaccination.

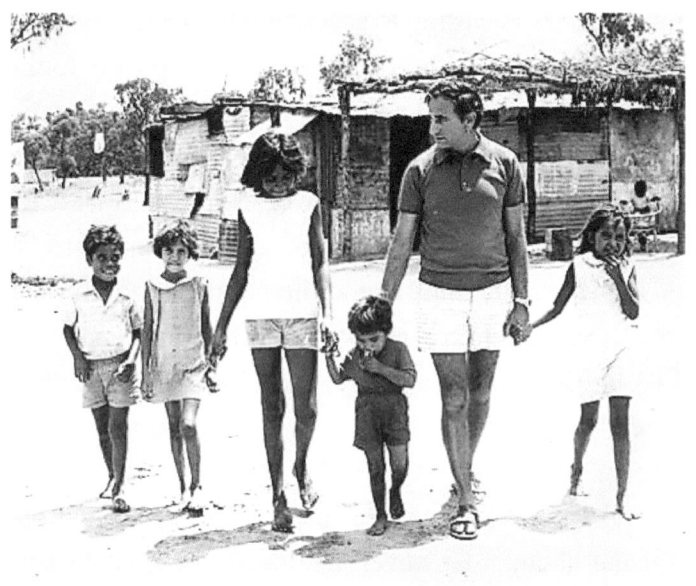

When he arrived, he was quick to recognise scurvy and several other signs of nutrient-deficiency and initiated a practice of giving the children intravenous vitamin C and other vitamin supplements prior to vaccinating them. In the following two years, not a single child died. The improvement continued, and in this way he was able to save many lives. In spite of this there were dissenting doctors who criticised his work and what he achieved. In fact, so many of the medical authorities were annoyed that there was talk of him losing his medical licence, presumably for using 'non-standard procedures'.

But if you never do that, if you never research and explore or follow developments as they are happening, even if novel, how can medicine progress? I was sad to learn of his death in 2012.

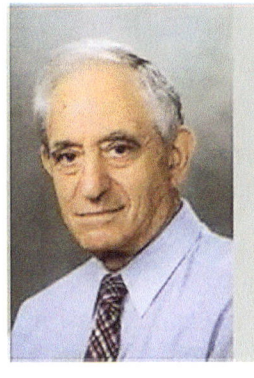

"I found the whole vaccine business was indeed a gigantic hoax. Most doctors are convinced that they are useful, but if you look at the proper statistics and study the instances of these diseases you will realize that this is not so."

– Dr. Archivides Kalokerinos, MD

Shortly before he left Sydney, he had referred one of his clients to me with forceful instructions that I was to take on MI as a client as he, Archie, didn't know who else to refer him to. I insisted that at this time I did not see people with cancer and was not experienced in it, but Archie was a very persuasive man. MI duly came to see me. He had extensive and systemic lymphatic cancer. That is all I recall of the diagnosis except that he had been told he had only four months to live, at most. He had also been told that it was a toss-up as to whether his heart condition or the cancer would kill him first. His doctors had told him there was nothing more they could do for either condition.

Without the internet or ready access to conferences close to home, we had to rely on books. And books, by their very nature, are almost always a year or two out of date by the time they are published and widely distributed. I had a couple in my library: Dr Richard Passwater's *Cancer and its Nutritional Therapies*[ii] which had just arrived at our wholesalers, and a colleague in America had sent me

Bruce Halstead's *Metabolic Cancer Therapy*[iii], a 1980 Golden Quill Publication. The first book covered the vitamins plus selenium and laetrile, but nothing much else. The second book, though only a mere twenty pages, I found far more interesting and useful. It covered, but only in brief: mental health, aerobics, nutrition, hydrotherapy, laetrile, benzaldehyde, enzyme therapy, DMSO, Vitamins A, C, and E, minerals selenium, germanium, and zinc, detoxification, oxygen colonics, coffee enemas, enzyme enemas, high colonic enemas, electromagnetic therapy, and hormone therapy. Frustratingly, each paragraph was only a single sentence on each topic, which left much to be desired. However, it did give me topics to research further as and when I could. The last couple of pages finished with dietary recommendations and a couple of 'low-stress' vegetable drinks and smoothies.

I now know that there was a lot more available at the time in America, but probably only known to a small handful of people dispersed throughout the many states. I was lucky to have even this tiny booklet. The last six suggestions were not available to me in Sydney, nor was germanium, but the rest I could employ.

When MI came in to see me it was obvious that he was very unwell, thin, grey faced, and very shaky. His heart was so bad he could barely walk to my office and he collapsed on the chair at my desk. He started off by saying, "No herbs or homoeopathy, none of that wacky stuff and nonsense." This was not a good beginning, but I had to remember that he had come from a medical doctor, not via a naturopathic referral. During the following weeks I did what I could. There continued to be much that MI would not do, and I passed swiftly over these things. There were also things I could not access. No one, for instance, was importing the pancreatic enzymes into Australia at this time. But he would agree from time to time to change his diet, take one or two nutrients, buy organic on the rare occasions he could find it, and eat apricot kernels.

When he returned for his second consultation there was an obvious, if small, improvement. He said he did feel a bit better and posed a cautious question as to the use of the other nutritional supplements. He left with a small package of them. Some weeks later he said he felt yet more improvement and asked about herbs, for he thought that, unlike homoeopathics, at least there was some substance to them and they might be useful. I gave them to him, and there was indeed a further improvement. In this way we continued. As his confidence grew, so did his willingness to take more 'exotic' (as he thought them) remedies, and so his health improved still further.

I was crossing my fingers and hoping for the day when he would accept homoeopathic remedies from the Reckeweg range. There were two products that I thought would help his heart a lot. When the time came and he was ready to be even more adventuresome, I assured him that, although they were potentised, and so technically homoeopathic, they were still only low potencies and that there was still some of the original substance left in the preparation, even if, to his way of thinking, very little. So we carried on. He had by this time well out-lived his predicted four months. His heart was stronger and he could go for walks.

Even his oncologist was surprised, but pleased, with his survival, and in time he reduced the monthly check-ups to four times a year, and six months later announced himself bored with MI as a client as there seemed to be nothing to study. By then, MI was dropping in to see me from time to time, probably more for a chat and reassurance than anything. His own mental attitude was terrific. At one point he said to me, "I'm too busy learning hydroponics to have time to think about having cancer." By then he had moved way out into the outback himself. The soil was sandy, there was no rain and little chance of gardening organically. As a result, he had settled on learning about hydroponics, such was his newfound confidence and determination.

During all this time I had a full schedule. I continued to lecture for up to eighteen hours a week, I saw clients four days a week and on Saturday mornings, and read, researched, and wrote in every spare moment I could find. With no internet, I sometimes spent Saturday afternoons in Sydney University library, even though there were no journals there that held a great deal of interest.

As I write this and look back on the schedule, I am amazed at it. Yet I know that at the time it did not seem excessive. I loved all of it, and revelled in everything.

Many of the anecdotes relating to my professional time in Sydney I wrote up each week and kept them as *Notes from a Naturopath*, making them available on my website, which is why they are not all repeated here. https://www.xanddriawilliams.co.uk

---

[i] Roger J Williams, *The Wonderful World Within You: Your Inner Nutritional Environment,* Bantam Books, 1977

[ii] Dr Richard Passwater, *Cancer and its Nutritional Therapies*; Pivot Original Health Book, 1978

[iii] Bruce W Halstead MD, *Metabolic Cancer Therapy*, Golden Quill Publishers, 1978, revised 1980.

Chapter 14

The Later Sydney Years

A year or so after TM had completed his research and been working for the company that had necessitated our move to the sandstone house, we learnt that he was to be transferred to the company's office in Perth, Western Australia. Would I go too? It was a very difficult choice. I loved my life in Sydney, the career and place in it I had built. I loved my clients and had built up a range of contacts and friendships. I could perhaps have rebuilt it in Perth, but I already knew Perth from when I had lived there. It was very much smaller than Sydney, and with far fewer opportunities, at least for me and in my profession. I recalled, with a measure of remembered frustration, the problems of finding most of the things I wanted which, once again, would have to be ordered 'from the Eastern States'. TM and I were tremendously good friends, 'buddies' to use the Australian slang. We lived together wonderfully comfortably, ran our parallel lives and shared countless interests, but was that enough for me to sell up and leave everything I had created in Sydney over the preceding fifteen years. In the end I had to decide that it wasn't.

Best Break-Up

We had what must have been one of the best possible 'break-ups'. We had bought this sandstone house equally and so we got the estimated value from three estate agents, divided the average in half and I bought him out. Then came our possessions. We were very clear as to what had belonged to each of us prior to our coming together some years earlier, and these, of course, we each kept. The things we had bought jointly since that date we collected together in our very large living room. Then it began: "I love this and would like to keep it, but I know you like that and you should have it, even though I also like it". Or, for a while, we took turns in choosing, then we repeated similar comments. We both adored Asian cooking. TM was wonderfully good at it. In fact, he was a wonderful cook, period, and loved doing it. I was going to miss all the excellent meals he had prepared with great frequency. We both loved the book on Asian cooking. In the end he allowed me to keep it, which I did for about ten years, but when we met up again in London, I decided it was his turn to have it. At the end of this dividing-up process we were left with a small group of items, about which we did argue. "You have it", "No, you have it". Neither of us wanted any of this residual pile. Having completed that we went out for dinner and wondered why we were splitting up.

Business as Before

Once the business was re-established and on a firm footing after the fire, my life continued much as before, although of course without TM. I was working in the Sydney practice, lecturing mostly at the NSW college, writing monthly articles, and doing occasional television interviews. The garden at the sandstone house was too small to fully occupy my weekend, so now that I was once again living on my own, I also had time to spare. I knew no one with whom I could play squash and so took up playing tennis again instead, and loved it. That was putting it mildly. I started having coaching lessons for an hour at seven o'clock every morning before work, then at the age of forty-four, I started playing in competitions as well as socially at weekends.

The building that housed my shop and the practice was situated on the main road in an area of Sydney running along the north shore of the harbour. A short ferry trip close and parallel to the Sydney Harbour Bridge, and facing the Sydney Opera House, took me into the heart of Sydney centre when I wanted it. Otherwise, I drove. My building backed onto a smaller back road, and had behind it a tiny slip of garden, one banana palm tree and a generous area for parking my car.

I reversed out one Saturday afternoon, after we'd closed up, and swung the car round, ready to head for home. Then I realised that in the house across the back street, exactly opposite the back of my building there was a 'for sale' notice on a small semi-detached bungalow. On the spur of the moment, and with nothing on my mind but my hair, I stopped, and walked over to it, thinking to explore. This was more out of curiosity than anything else. Two Asian men were talking with the estate agent, so I had a look around, stood by them for a while, and then heard them making arrangements to meet up with the possibility of completing a sale during the following week. I mentally shrugged and started to walk away.

"Can I help you?" The estate agent obviously wasn't going to miss a chance.

"No, no, I was thinking of buying this house, but it seems you now have a sale". I wasn't really sure what I had been thinking, but I certainly did like the house, and the price was both reasonable and affordable. The fact that someone else might have decided to buy it had focused my mind as to the benefits of buying it. It seemed that my habit of purchasing properties on a spur-of-the moment basis was going to continue. Or perhaps this was another of those serendipity moments that had helped to guide my life

There was an excellent financial loan system available in Sydney in those days. I had taken out a mortgage/loan to pay TM for his half of our sandstone house when we split up. Though called a mortgage, it was unique in that it was more like a monstrously large overdraft. Anytime I had some money 'to spare' I could put it into the account and reduce the amount of the loan, but I could also take it out again as needed. Ever since I had been thirty-three, I had worked for myself, with no regular or fixed income. My income rose and fell in relation to the business or the practice, so this system suited me perfectly. Learning to survive at the age of thirteen on a mere thirty pounds a year to pay for everything I needed beyond my bed and board, had bred in me the habit of spending money carefully and never squandering it casually or needlessly. As such, slowly and steadily I accumulated money rather than actively saved it. When this account grew sufficient for a deposit on the next property, I was able to make the next purchase. In this way I bought several properties which I then rented out.

Purchasing this house would have a number of benefits. It would mean that in time, I could sell the shop. My practice and its contribution to the activity of the shop were an integral part of the latter, its success and its turnover. This meant that to sell the shop profitably I had to show that I would continue to support it and contribute to its volume of sales. With a practice a few yards away, it would be clear to any future buyer that many of my clients would continue to move over to the shop to buy the majority of the products they wanted. Moreover, I actually was ready to sell the shop. Although it had been a great start into the profession, it had served its purpose for me. It had been great fun to run and a pleasure to work in, particularly in relation to the people I met there and talked with. But it had run its course. I realised now that it would be a relief to have that responsibility removed and leave me free to focus more fully on clients, lecturing, and writing.

It would also make it much easier for me to travel more. Nonetheless, looking at this house for the first time, I was ready to walk away and leave it to the others. But the agent was having none of it. Perhaps he saw a greater enthusiasm in my eyes than in theirs. I continued to sound positive. I arranged to meet up on the Monday and sort out details, provided I had a clear field – which he promised. I didn't want any escalated bargaining. I figured I had the weekend to think it all through and do the sums before committing, and drove off home to give it more thought. The thinking went well, I bought the house, painted the inside and let it to tenants. It was easy then to let a property on a monthly basis. I kept it for a year or two, and then made plans to sell the shop and move my business into the house, pointing out to the purchasers of my shop my continued presence at their back door. It was then easy to arrange to take over from the tenants in the house on their monthly arrangement, and orchestrate my move across the road.

The new premises were excellent and ideal for purpose. There was a small garden in front, soon put to herbs, and surrounded by a tiny picket fence – I had always hankered after one of these, though they were a rarity in Australia – and there was sufficient space to park my car.

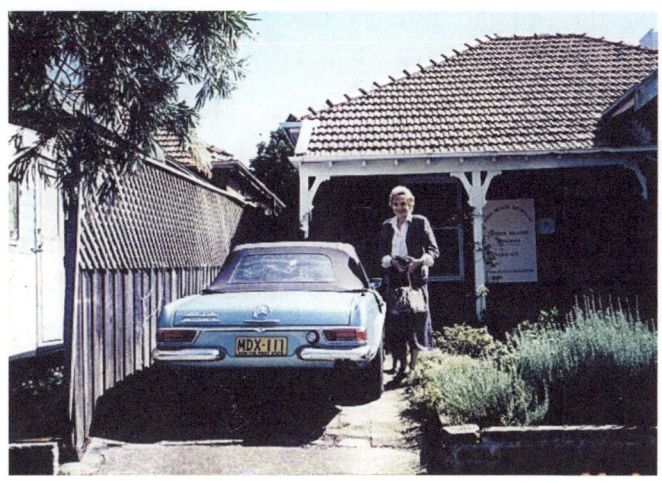

The house was a semi-detached long thin strip, with a corridor running down the length of it. There were two front rooms, originally designed as bedrooms. The front room, bright and sunny, became my office, the next one the admin office and dispensary, though we sold only the items that were 'practitioner-only' lines and could not be sold in the shop across the road without a practitioner. This was a very small part of the business and did not, I hoped, dent the sales going through the shop I had sold. The third room widened out to include the corridor, and would have been planned as the sitting room. I used it as a generous waiting room. Then came the kitchen and bathroom, and finally a fourth room that had been added on and could be used by new graduates, starting their own business, as before. Behind that was a courtyard garden with two huge avocado trees. They were different varieties, each dripping delicious fruits at a steady rate for about five overlapping months of the year so that there was rarely a time when I wasn't steadily provided with them. I wanted butter? No bother, just go out and pick up an avocado, use what you want and toss the rest. Wonderful.

My desk, at the window of the front room, allowed me to get a good look at clients as they arrived and left, and to hear what they said. This was often useful and informative.

By the time of this move I was supported by my third senior assistant, GJH, the final one of my fifteen years in full practice in Sydney. In fact she was the only assistant I had in this new location as the retail side was negligible and I only needed the one receptionist. She was very mature and responsible as well as being warm, friendly, and competent, and was fully capable of looking after things during my absences as, about this time, with a growing income, I was able to start travelling again – six-monthly trips to London, to conferences, and other academic trips to America. I was able to fly to London once a year and spend most of that time in Ireland with Aunt. This was often, though not always, over Christmas and New Year as this tended to be a protracted holiday period in Australia, and the demands of the practice were correspondingly reduced.

I combined these trips with visits to clinics and laboratories across the US. On one trip I went to Trace Element laboratory in Texas, https://www.traceelements.com, where I had been sending hair samples for mineral analysis. I was exposed for the first time to their amazing hospitality, the full southern inflection, their courtesy, and more. They phoned me after my visit, thanking me for coming and saying, in their slow drawl, "We all felt most benefitted by your visit", a phrase that I appreciated and have never forgotten. All the hair analysis was done in the US at that time, though AML did consider setting up for it in Sydney. From Texas I went to Doctors Data in Chicago https://www.doctorsdata.com where I was also sending hair samples for analysis. I was warned that the temperature would be minus 22 ℃. Since I had never experienced anything much below zero,

I was curious as to how it would feel. The reality was something of an anti-climax, as I was met and bundled first into a heated car and then an overheated office building.

On another trip I had been visiting a nutritional supplement company in north-west USA. I was interested in the concept of people having different types of metabolism and so needing different combinations of nutrients, particularly in multi-vitamin and multi-mineral supplements. This was a concept that I have since established as an integral basis for planning protocols for individual clients. The company I was visiting was offering an interesting possibility whereby they would tailor the supplement combinations that I could use in my practice. It was an offer I accepted, and took up when I returned to Sydney.

After a lengthy day of discussions, their nutritionist asked if I would have time to meet up with him the next day for more discussions, and to have lunch. I assumed this was for further technical talk and to visit other facilities, companies, or people, and was a little surprised when he said, as we drove off, "I hope you brought your passport with you". I had, and thought little of it. As ever, my one-track mind was on work and I was far more interested in the technical discussions we were having. Eventually I realised we seemed to be going a long way and queried our destination. To my surprise he had planned a long-range lunch. He felt I could not leave the USA without going north into Canada and British Columbia. Suddenly the typical American homes gave way to the delightful architecture of BC, at which point he became a most informative host, explaining some of the many differences between the two countries.

To my mind one of the advantages of being a general practitioner as a naturopath was the amazing range of problems that I was asked to deal with. It had been that way since I started and was clearly going to continue that way. At the end of one morning, when a client, OP, had just finished his consultation with me, I received a surprise. At that time I had a large table that I used as a desk and he had been sitting opposite me. This was the first and only time I used a table and sat clients so that there was furniture between us. Soon after that I bought a desk and always arranged my room so that clients sat either beside, or better still, at an angle to me. This allowed for much improved rapport and communication. As we finished the consultation, OP stood up, ready to leave, and then stopped. He just stood there, leaning slightly down on his hands, as if waiting for something. I asked him if there was anything else he wanted to say. He assured me that there wasn't and then said, "I'm just waiting for the table to go back down to its proper place."

I realised then that this was a case of disorder of perception, and probable schizophrenia. It was, and so I changed my focus. At the time I had been getting good results with such people by balancing their nutritional chemistry and related biochemical problems. By determining their histamine levels I would distinguish between histapenia (low histamine levels) and histadelia (high histamine levels), rebalancing their nutrients as appropriate, then testing for kryptopyrol. I could then treat these three groups of people with different pre-selected groups of supplements.

This was near the time when Geof Bland became prominent. He used regularly to post out to those of us who subscribed, small tape cassettes with interesting information and interviews with a number of professional colleagues – The sort of thing that these days is done regularly and much more easily via a webinar, Zoom or Skype. But in those days these tapes were nuggets of gold to be treasured and eagerly awaited.

All this time the practice was growing and I was enjoying the work enormously. I had 'fallen' into a career in naturopathy almost by mistake, or more accurately, by taking up every offer or challenge that I had been presented with. This went all the way back to 1966-67 when, on a skimpy research grant I had studied amino acid balancing in an effort to get the best quality nutrition from an economical vegetarian diet for the least money. I thought myself to be very fortunate.

Now a few years later and more settled, I was going on longer trips knowing I could leave the practice in the safe hands of GJH.

When I travelled overseas. I was keen to learn yet more, so I planned a trip to San Francisco for a weekend seminar given by Dr Jonathon Wright and Dr Alan Gaby. The seminar was excellent, the meeting was excellent and destined to lead on to great things. On the Saturday I was queueing in the Hilton Hotel snack bar to order lunch when an American voice from behind said "Do you come from Australia?" (I was pretty sure I hadn't picked up an Australian accent, but it seems I had, or just enough to be recognisable), and "Do you know Dr Archie Kalokerinos?". I assured the voice that I knew Archie Kalokerinos very well, that he was a colleague and great friend and had referred many clients to me, including my first cancer client (MI, chapter 13).

The voice in my ear, in the Hilton hotel sandwich shop that Saturday morning, was that of Dr Robert Erdmann, followed by that of his wife Marie. After a lengthy chat that evening, at the end of the conference, they returned to their home in Palo Alto, and the next day they brought back with them a pile of photo-copied articles for me and a list of names and addresses of the people, companies, and laboratories that I simply had to contact and

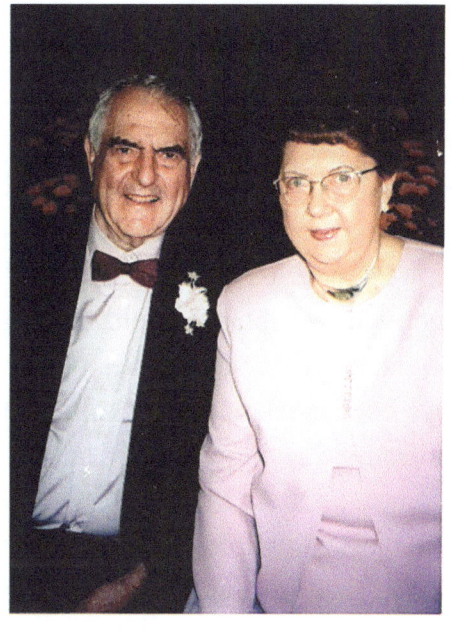

meet in my travels across America. They must have worked through the night. It was like being showered with nuggets of precious gold, which I then explored in the weeks ahead. They were wonderfully generous and enthusiastic and the three of us were destined to become great friends.

Robert specialised in amino acid chemistry. He did urine analysis for his clients and then, working with a company called Jo Marr, prescribed the missing amino acids. This had led to a small book called *The Amino Revolution*. After further discussions, Robert and I decided to combine our experience, his in this aspect of amino acids in clinical practice, and mine in amino acid biochemistry. We planned to write a much lengthier and more technical book on the place of amino acids in nutrition and health. In the meantime, my second book, *What's In My Food*, was in preparation. I had frequently been frustrated by the fact that the nutrient levels of foods were commonly given on a 'per serving' or a 'per weight' basis. If it was 'per serving' it was difficult to compare foods as to their relative merits. Different compilers seemed to have different ideas as to what constituted a 'serving', and they frequently varied in size.

Then I found a book in which the data could be rearranged to show the nutrients listed on a 'per 100 gms' basis. That was a definite step forward. However, it still didn't, to my mind, solve the problem of being unable to readily assess which foods were the most nutrient dense and so most worthy of a place in a high nutrient-dense diet. After all, we don't eat a fixed amount of food per day. Instead, if we maintain a constant weight, it is probably because we are eating approximately the same number of calories per day. Satiety values of foods would have been a better yardstick, but was, of course, difficult to measure and somewhat variable from individual to individual. I wanted tables that listed nutrient densities on a 'per 100 calorie' basis. This is still extraordinarily difficult to find. I also wanted one that spoke of single foods. I had no interest in the nutrient densities of twenty different types of biscuits. I wanted the nutrient densities of individual components of the biscuits, different types of flour, or fruits, or vegetables.

My only computer for some time had been the large and cumbersome desk model in three parts that I had been told to 'boot', and considered kicking. This anchored me to my desk in the office. I badly wanted something more portable that I could take home in the evenings and so continue to work when I got there. All that was then available was a 'luggable', the size of an old-fashioned Singer sewing machine, a great heavy weight and with no battery.

At about this time I was alerted to the imminent production of Pivot, by Morrow. It was arguably the very first, light-weight personal computer. It weighed in at only nine and a half pounds, plus the removable battery, and thus was unbelievably light for those days. It ran for a full hour on its battery – impressive – had 128 K to 512 RAM and two 5 ½ inch floppy disks. The screen, of course, was black and white. To top it off there were two built in 'handles' for the shoulder straps. It cost the then reasonable sum of $AU 1,995. Consequently, I organised a return trip to San Francisco and Robert Erdman and the work on our planned joint book on amino acids. I planned this trip to coincide with the production and delivery to Robert's house of a Pivot.

The computer was wonderful, and Robert and I wrote intensely for three weeks. Later he came to Sydney to resume the writing, and later again, on my next trip to Ireland, I stopped over in San Francisco to continue further. We were doing really well until we hit an unexpected obstacle. The publishers of Robert's first book insisted he could not publish another one on amino acids, even though his was much shorter and very much less in depth, though more popularly readable. We thought that ours would be targeted at an entirely different readership. However, the publishers obviously thought that our book could be in competition, or superseding their book. Robert generously suggested that I could be the sole author of our joint book, but I knew we needed his name attached to it to penetrate the American market and generate sufficient sales for it to be viable. So sadly, that project died. However, many very interesting and mutually profitable and enjoyable collaborations and discussions developed from this.

I returned to Sydney with Pivot, having sat ostentatiously in the airport lounge and on the plane en route, soaking up the curious and (I hoped!) impressed stares of my fellow business travellers as I nonchalantly typed, then flipped up the keyboard and slung Pivot over my shoulder when the flight was called. All of this was a definite novelty in those days. I was, as ever, heavily work-focused, arguably most of the time, and it was a huge step towards further freedoms to be able to sling Pivot over my shoulder each evening and take work home where I could continue to think and formulate ideas.

Soon after I purchased and mastered my Pivot computer, with its enlarged memory (not much by today's standards, but a lot more than my first desktop's 64K), I also came across a program that did list the nutrient content of foods in a variety of forms. The program could be adapted, and I discovered I could find the listings on the desired 'per 100 calorie basis', although it meant a rather odd way of recording it. I immediately decided to turn this into a useful reference book for myself. One of my article publishers learnt of this and asked if I could turn it into a book that could be published. I was delighted to try. It was not a sophisticated program, and the book layout reflects this, but it excited me and served its purpose. After all, on a per 100 gms basis you could argue that you get a lot more nutrients from almonds than from lettuce, almonds being heavy things, but if you consider the relative calorie content, and the relative amounts you can eat of each, the difference between the two is easy to see. On a per calorie basis, both the dark green and the red lettuces are more nutrient dense than the almonds.

Overseas Lecturing

I was delighted to be given the chance to revisit New Zealand. Blackmores asked me to lecture at a conference in Wellington. I was delighted, both at the chance of lecturing, and also at the opportunity to spend a day exploring Wellington itself and drive out to Muratai where I had once lived as a child. However, I only spent one extra day there. As always, I was keen to get back to my office, my clients, and my students.

On another visit across America and to Aunt in Ireland, I was with a friend who was scheduled to give a talk in the Ecology Department of Queens in Dublin. To my surprise, once we had all met up, they asked if I would be willing to give them a talk too. They were interested to learn more of naturopathy and its role and potential in overall healthcare. After that, it was down to the pub for a Guinness. They made up a lively group.

On a subsequent trip, across America, on my way to Ireland and Aunt, I was asked to stop over for a couple days at the John Bastyr College of Osteopathy and Naturopathy in Seattle, Washington. I was particularly interested to learn more of their education standards – the undergraduate naturopathic training in general, but of course nutrition and biochemistry in particular. I was able to combine this visit with a follow-on stop in Portland, Oregon, and give a couple of talks to the Naturopathic College there, and learn more about their syllabus and standards. I was glad to be able to feel that our courses in Australia matched up to their standards.

Most of these trips involved a stop-off in San Francisco to meet up with the growing number of colleagues and friends I had there. Robert Erdman introduced me to Dr Robert Cathcart, who was enthralled by the developing possibility of colour computers and was determined to draw the coloured flags of every country in the word on his screen. His more important work was recognition of the use of large doses of oral vitamin C and the process that he came to call 'Bowel Tolerance C'. http://www.doctoryourself.com/titration.html

As these and subsequent trips came and went, Robert introduced me to many other wonderfully enthusiastic colleagues from whom I learnt a great deal. These included meetings and friendships with many different people, including Dr Abrahm Hoffer, the eminent orthomolecular psychiatrist from Canada, Irwin Stone, known for his first use of ascorbic acid in the food-processing industry, and of course Linus Pauling, probably best known for his scientific obsession with vitamin C. I was delighted with this last as I first knew of him (at least of his work) when I was a chemistry student at Imperial in 1958-61.

About this time I had a call from MC's husband. He and his wife were friends, both chiropractors, living several hundred kilometres west, in New South Wales. The distance was not considered to be of much consequence in this vast continent, greater in size than most of Europe and as large as mainland US. We met up frequently, as they often came to Sydney for conferences, and I had visited with them on more than one occasion. MC had just been diagnosed with cancer. She was flying down and could she come and stay? Of course she could. I knew little of cancer at that time, in spite of having worked with MI (see case history end of Chapter 13) There was little confidence then among my professional colleagues that we could do very much for people with this disease.

She and I talked, she wrung her hands, she wept. We wondered in agonies of indecision whether or not she should have a biopsy. We read all we could find. She wanted to tell no one, to hide away from everyone she knew, hating to be seen out of control or vulnerable, so I had to offer vague reassurances to our joint friends when she stopped attending our various professional gatherings. Without an internet to go to for the latest information, we relied a lot on phone calls to colleagues in the US and on faxes. Robert Erdman, among others, was most helpful. In Sydney, the two laboratories I used that offered 'alternative' options suggested what they could do to help, but they were not primarily cancer focused. We learnt, she acted. She also chose to stay in Sydney, leaving her husband to run their practice inland. Effectively they split up as a couple. Then, as she got control of the situation, she drew away from me too, hating that I had seen her when she felt helpless, hopeless and frightened. Because of this, I suspect, she cut off many people who could have helped her. On our last phone call I gathered from the symptoms she described that the cancer had spread to her colon, and soon after that she passed away.

According to the four Greek temperaments (see my book *Love, Health, and Happiness,* and Ch 14 of this book), we were both cholerics temperamentally, she strongly so, me tempered with a certain amount of a lighter sanguine nature. We maintained, as is often the case, a careful balance of each being seen to be as strong and confident as the other. These may be useful characteristics in practitioners, when decisions had to be made, responsibilities taken, and the clients want to feel we can be relied on and provide some form of security, but it can be most unhelpful, as in her case, when it means you do not like to show vulnerability and do not look for or readily accept, help, and cannot deal with the fact that you are in need. Worst still was that she felt ashamed I had seen her in a vulnerable state and consequently had chosen to stay away from me. I understood the reason although I was saddened by the loss of the friendship.

I continued, of course, to run my full-time practice in Sydney, to lecture at the naturopathic college, and write articles for the magazines. Over the years, and with increasing frequency, I had been asked to be on television programs as and when relevant topics of interest cropped up. Then I was asked, by Metagenics, one of the major and most biochemically oriented nutritional supply companies, to run a post-graduate course in applied nutritional therapies. This involved a weekend each month in Melbourne and another each month in Sydney, and lasted for eight months a year. As I recall, it ran for two or three years. Quite a daunting schedule, but again, I loved it.

By this time I was continuing to make annual trips to Ireland and Aunt, taking advantage of the fact that most people in Australia go on extended holidays over the Christmas and New Year period, often of several weeks. Most of them are too busy having fun to think about being ill, and client numbers dropped. For students, this is their long summer break between academic years, and as a result I was not scheduled to give lectures or run seminars. Being absent did not cause major problems. What it gave me was plenty of time for writing and I frequently wrote a number of articles as a result of the colleagues, clinics, laboratory companies, and supplement companies I visited. While in Ireland, Aunt and I spent most of our time together, walking and talking. But that still left plenty of down time for me, and a number of articles, or book chapters, were written with me propped up in bed, either late at night or very early in the morning.

Choosing the right clothes for these antipodean trips was always tricky. If I left Sydney in December, mid-summer, it was a challenge to wear clothes warm enough for landing in chilly London. In fact, when I started on these travels I didn't have a single overcoat. The most I ever needed in Sydney, in the coldest of winters, was a suit with a jacket which I could wear over a sweater on the rare days when the temperature fell below 10°C. A group of us shared a somewhat shabby overcoat that we swapped around to whoever was going travelling to colder climates. It was a little easier if I left in the June winter.

By this time, I had made a number of friends in London, as a result of the various activities in which I was interested, including Friends of Imperial College, my old alma mater. I have said that whenever I returned to London from my travels, I used to 'hug the lamp posts', such was my affection. That affection had returned. I had no thought to return to live in London, but I longed to have a toe-hold there. As a result, I had bought a small one-bedroomed flat in Chelsea. This had meant that for some time I had been able to rent it out for short lets, a few months at a time, in such a way that I could stay there when I needed it for myself. The downside was that as other people would be using it, I had to make sure that everything personal I left there was stowed away in a basement storeroom during my absences.

On one such trip I had been flying over the US wearing only light clothes, suitable for leaving a swelteringly hot Sydney, knowing that my planned stops were in relatively warm parts of the US and that when I landed in London, a short trip on the Underground would take me to my flat and my store of winter clothes.

As we were flying over Newfoundland and not expecting to land until we reached our destination, we were surprised to hear the pilot saying that we were going to make an unscheduled stop. We were never given an official reason for this but the story went round that the windshield(s) in front of the pilot(s) had cracked or broken. Whatever it was, we came down into thick snow and were bussed from the plane to the airport building. I don't recall why, but I do recall that I was wearing very open court shoes, most unsuitable for the snow drifts. We spent long hours in an unprepared airport with very few shops of interest, little to read, and not much to do.

I fell into conversation with a delightful woman, probably in her forties, most beautifully dressed and elegant, who told me she had terminal cancer and was making what she assumed would be the last trip of which she was capable. She had only months to live, but was looking forward to buying new clothes and making plans. I was impressed by the positive way she was dealing with the problem. At this time, I had had little to do with death, and was very interested in what she had to say. I learnt a lot from her. It was only about six months later that I learnt she had passed on.

By this time I had been in practice as a qualified Naturopath for well over a decade. I had anticipated that my life would continue in much the same way; but thing were about to change.

I was making more frequent trips to Ireland and Aunt and becoming reacquainted with London, and it became a nuisance to keep packing and unpacking my store room when I was in London, so I bought a small studio flat to have a personal and exclusive base there and a place where I could leave possessions spread out, not packed up ready for a sub-let. Consequently, packing and unpacking was not such a chore and I could travel light. I did not let this flat out in my absence. In any case, I was by this time coming to London twice a year and so the gaps between were only about five months.

I continued to write books. The next was a small one entitled *How to Prevent Osteoporosis*, published in 1991. It was requested by

Wellsprings Publishers, who were loosely related to the Australian Wellbeing magazine for whom I wrote a great many articles.

Somehow, Letts Publishing in the UK learnt of my books, *Choosing Health Intentionally* and *Choosing Weight intentionally* and asked to publish them. I agreed.

They also asked me to write a book on stress, that became *Stress, Recognise and Resolve*. Further, they suggested that I should have a publishing agent and suggested three people. Hitherto, I had not felt the need for an agent and had always negotiated directly with the publishers. However, I recognised that they did have a point. I liked SM when I met her, found we got on well and agreed that we should work together. At this point I had four other books in mind: *The Four Temperaments*; *Beating the Blues*; *You are not Alone;* and *Fatigue, the Secrets of Getting Your Energy Back.*

I shared these ideas with SM, when in London that Christmas. She liked them and talked with various publishers over the Christmas holiday period. When I returned from Ireland on my way back to Australia, she was delighted to tell me that she had lined up publishers for all of them. There was a lot of writing ahead.

When I came to London the next time, the Letts' promotional book tour took me, chauffeur-driven by their agent, around a large part of England as we visited an average of three towns and several radio and TV stations, magazine publishers, and bookshops in each. When I then went over to Ireland to visit Aunt, I was also driven up to Belfast. There I saw the effects of the north-south tension for myself. All radio stations, newspaper offices, and other publicity companies were high-risk IRA targets and so security was fierce. We had to go through two or three checkpoint doors to enter each building. Our car, and those of other people as well, was stopped and searched at a couple of check stops just as we were driving through the city centre. Entering the hotel where I was staying was considerably more challenging than getting through modern airport security.

During the next few years, a pattern developed. I ran the practice loving the interchange with clients, then flew to Ireland for Christmas, and sometimes during June or July. I would also plan a trip, usually focused on one or more conferences in the US. At about this time I had sold the shop and moved into the house behind it that I had bought.

I became progressively more interested in problems relating to the digestive tract. The chemistry that goes on there is fascinating. It can also be tested, and then corrected. Progressively I came to realise how important it was to correct any imbalances in that area, in what was becoming known as the 'biome', as a basis for much else that we did. This is so, even though we didn't then have the tests that are available now, in London, twenty or more years later.

And I went on writing. I was glad of the writing schedule. I loved running the practice for the interchange of ideas and experiences with clients, but I wanted more of a challenge, a mental challenge, which is what writing the various books gave me. For the past fifteen years my life had been regimented by the clock. Client appointments of fifteen, thirty, and occasionally sixty minutes, and lecture schedules. I felt a yearning for 'unstructured time'. It became a phrase I rolled around in my brain from time to time. I found a way to achieve this, albeit in a small way.

I would work in the practice or at the college during the week, and possibly socialise in the evenings. Then on Friday evenings, if I had no other plans, I would come home and settle down to an evening and two full days, of steady writing. I would turn off the clocks, eat, drink and sleep only when I felt like it and settle down to sixty hours of 'unstructured time' to write. I loved these times. I would sink into the writing and lose myself in what I was saying, however technical or descriptive the material. All this was before the capabilities of the internet came to the fore, of course, so there was no question of looking things up. Everything I wrote had to come from within me and my brain, from what I already knew, had experienced, and learnt.

I continued to run CWI-CHI-s every Monday evening. I offered rebirthing sessions one evening a week, helped by one of the enthusiastic graduates from my CHI workshops.

I had been NSW President of ANTA the Australian Naturopathic Association, for a total of eight years, since I graduated. I thoroughly enjoyed steering our profession through its growth and development stages but, as things got more politically difficult, I decided I was not sufficiently well skilled at the games of politics that that post required, and handed over the reins to others. Thus, I now did less in ANTA and more writing. I read and researched massively, more than ever before, via books, medical journals, and tapes of conferences from overseas, from visits to colleagues and colleagues who visited me. I employed one full time-receptionist, as without the shop and its overflow activities, that was all I needed. I continued to give new graduates a place where they could take their first steps into running their own practice, and I continued to lecture.

Throughout this time I continued, of course, to see clients for naturopathic sessions as well as psychotherapy and personal growth. But I was to have one more interesting experience in relation to rebirthing. After one of the evening sessions with a group of six people in my office, one of them, an excellent amateur opera singer, a large woman with a tiny but beautiful soprano voice, surprised us all. At the end of the session, as we were chatting, she suddenly said, "I feel like singing." "Go ahead," I said without giving it much thought. And she did. Suddenly a loud, strong, and beautiful soprano voice swept around the room. It didn't last, not fully, but from then on, she sang with much greater volume than ever before. "My singing teacher can't believe it," she told me later. "We have tried for years to open my voice up, with no real success. Now just one evening of rebirthing, and it has happened. Amazing".

I now had a wonderful, if tiny, home in London. One friend pointed out that everything in that studio apartment did at least two jobs, if not three. The sofa was a bed and the gate-legged table held four folding chairs hidden beneath it. I had a miniature Victorian chair with a foot stool that lived underneath – so seating two. My two metal army boxes, courtesy of grandfather and great uncle during the first world war, acted as both storage boxes and stools to sit on, and so it went. I had a growing circle of friends and acquaintances, and in a room about fifteen feet by ten, I could serve dinner for twenty from a tiny Belling stove by clever juggling with M&S chicken casseroles, frozen peas and mashed potato. I fell into a pattern of throwing a party on my last evening there, even though I would have to leave for the airport at about five o'clock the following morning. This meant that anyone I knew and ran into during my three or four weeks, even on the last day, could be included in this last- minute party. With Waitrose one minute away and M&S two minutes further, I, or a helpful guest, could rush out and restock the wine during the evening should that be needed.

I was also making annual, and then six-monthly, visits to London, because I was growing to love it more and more, and Ireland because I had loved Aunt for sixty years.

What did I like doing best? Seeing clients, researching and learning, or writing books? Difficult to say. I don't know of any three-legged stool that does not fall over when one leg is removed. I loved them all and they all fed into each other. Somehow and with no real effort on my part, I generally managed to keep a perfect balance.

But things were about to change.

Chapter 15

Personal Growth & Development

After the publication of *Living with Allergies*, and the following year's publication of the segment I wrote called 'Offsetting the side-effects of the pill" for *Love, Sex and Fertility* edited by Barbara McGregor, I was ready, as I have said earlier, to take on the challenge of a second book on my own.

I had wanted for some time to find a book or set of tables that listed the nutrient content of foods on a per calorie basis. I could find plenty that gave the nutrient content per serving, but this was of little use if I wanted to find which food had the most of a particular nutrient as the serving sizes inevitably varied not only from food to food, but from book to book. Earlier I had found a small booklet called Guidebook to Nutritional Factors in Edible Food by David Phillips. It was published by the Pythagorean Press back in 1977 in Sydney, and I still have and treasure it. However, as useful as this had been, it was not what I was looking for. I wanted nutrient levels per 100 calories not per 100 grams.

If I was trying to prepare a diet rich in a specific nutrient it mattered how many calories someone had to eat to get their nutrient intake. Working on the assumption that someone's daily intake should be, on average, about 2,000 calories in order to maintain a steady weight, it would make a great deal of difference if they could get their vitamin A from 100 calories of that food rather than eating 1,000 calories of it. It was easy to prepare a diet that gave you the full Recommended Daily Allowance (RDA) of every nutrient if you gave them 5,000 calories of the food, but they would rapidly gain weight and have created just another problem. They would not be happy. By this time it was clear to me that such a book did not exist and that I would have to prepare it myself. This I set about doing. Fortunately, at this time I found a computer program where you could build up your own nutrient spreadsheet on whatever basis you wanted, per weight, per serving, or per calorie. Bingo. It was a clunky program, clearly restricted by computing limitations around 1987, but nonetheless I managed it and wrote:[i] *What's in My Food: Book of Nutrients,* which was published in 1988.

Car Crash

All was going well until I had a car crash. I was driving to the college in the morning rush hour, ready for a day of lecturing. I was in the left lane of a six-lane motorway humped over the Sydney expressway and moving steadily along the empty left-hand lane with two lanes of stationary cars on my right.

The driver of an approaching car was driving towards me three lanes to my right but hidden from me by the stationary traffic. He was from overseas, used to driving on the right instead of the left. Close to the apex he turned at right angles and at speed directly in front of me and drove across my line of traffic. Due to the arch of the road and my low-slung Mazda RX7 sports car, I couldn't see him until he was immediately in front of my bonnet. He brought me to a sudden and jarring halt, from 80 km an hour to zero in about four feet. The vultures, in the form of the pickup truck standing on this part of the highway just looking for an accident to profit from, were on the spot in seconds.

"You hadn't got a chance, lady." "We saw it coming." "We knew you couldn't see him and he was on the wrong side of the road." "You didn't have a chance". I sat there stunned, but knowing my head had been whipped to and fro several times. Serious whip-lash damage was a given, so was the acute pain across my ribs where my seat belt had held me in place.

Max was called. She came to my rescue and drove me to a chiropractor colleague's office where repairs were started on me. I was somewhat bruised and battered, and in a lot of pain. My sternum had been crushed both against the steering wheel by the deaccelerating forces and the tightening and strain from the seat belt across my chest. I coughed consistently for months afterwards. The severe whiplash had done my neck no good whatsoever, and I could not raise my right arm above my shoulder height. As a result, I could not play tennis, certainly not competitively.

Another friend told me I should blame the culprit, charge him, make him, somehow unspecified, pay for the damage he had done to both me and my lifestyle. I tried thinking that way for a few hours. I didn't like the way that made me feel. Angry and resentful. So I decided to ask myself "what's good about this?" as I was in the habit of doing by then. With each event, I chose to assume that I had had some part in creating the situation. After all, I could have taken at least three different routes from my office to the college where I was due to lecture that day. I could have driven either sooner or later. So, I chose to argue, I could have avoided the accident.

It was not a matter of apportioning blame. I differentiated in my mind between 'at cause' and 'to blame'. I chose to consider that at some higher level I had chosen to have this crash for some higher reason, or benefit. I was sure, by then, that at some level of spirit and more, I had chosen most of the events in my life. I also chose to believe that I had had good reason for making this choice – why would I have chosen to make bad choices? Needless to say, many of my friends laughed at me for this approach, but I knew that it had many benefits. Clearly one possible benefit would be that, without the many hours I spent being coached and playing tennis, I would now have a lot of free time. I wondered what I would eventually choose to do with this. Time was to tell, and to pay dividends, as I soon discovered.

Reiki

Reiki training was just being brought to Australia by Barbara McGregor. Not only was she a good friend, she was also editor of *Australian Wellbeing*, one of the major magazines I wrote for. She was instrumental in bringing Beth Gray to Australia and promoting her training program, and Beth Gray was one of the first non-Japanese people to teach Reiki outside Japan. Barbara did the first training herself, and had been keen that I should do the next one. However, I declined. I knew it involved a lot of exposing one's own emotions, 'opening up' and 'sharing'. I did not do emotions. I did not expose them. I did not hug people. I did not share my inner feelings. And I most certainly did not do that in public. That had all been drilled out of me back in childhood. I did not plan to reverse this now, forty or more years later. Learning to help other people was one thing, admitting that I might need help and going through a public and emotional spring-clean myself, that was another. It was not on.

However, Barbara had other plans. She wanted to help restore my battered upper body. As such she wanted to do Reiki on my chest and shoulders and so reduce the persistent cough. This would involve her laying her hands on my most battered parts. She finally drove a bargain with me to which I agreed, mainly to preserve our friendship: if her Reiki treatment on my chest and my cough cured the problems resulting from the accident, I would trust her enthusiasm for Reiki and agree to train in it. I finally agreed, although I remained reluctant, thinking I was fundamentally a biochemist and a scientist. How could I have confidence in it when there was no scientific mechanism for it? I felt sure I would not feel comfortable sitting with a client with my hands on a specific part of their body for half an hour or more, and charging them for the experience. I would not be using this treatment on my own clients, so there was not much point. Nonetheless, her Reiki on my chest did help. I fulfilled my promise and did the training, though I still wasn't convinced of its efficacy. Then two things occurred.

After the first few years in general naturopathic practice, it had become clear to me that restoring overall health and wellbeing required more than just restoring physical health. Reducing stress levels and restoring or improving emotional health was also important. In parallel with this and following a different line of development, I had decided to study a variety of psychotherapy and related techniques. After my own experience of Reiki, it occurred to me that this training could be a first path along this route.

1987 Reiki training

Very soon Barbara and I both did Levels I and II with Beth Gray. Each level of training took five consecutive and very extended evenings (six hours) and then a full weekend. Barbara went on to do Level III, became a Reiki Master and was acknowledged as such by Beth Gray after extensive training covering about ten years. It was very different to the commonplace Reiki training I have encountered since in London. This is very much shorter and more casual, often less than a day for each level. The extensive trainings were all worth it, though, for the results we both got, and for the countless others that Barbara then trained, and who all achieved amazing results.

MI and Reiki

MI, after his recovery from 'terminal' metastatic lymphatic cancer, had kept in touch with me and referred several of his family, all of them in their seventies, to me. I had another call from him one morning and I was concerned, fearing the return of his cancer. I was only slightly reassured when he limped into my office on one leg, two crutches, and dangling his second foot above the ground. He was clearly in significant pain. He explained that he had what he had initially been told was a sprained ankle. He had been hobbling on it for six weeks, only then to be told it was actually a torn Achilles tendon and not a sprained ankle at all. Could I help? He had also been told that no operation was possible in view of his bad heart and poor vascular system, and that nothing could be done for him. In confirmation of this his seventy-plus physiotherapist sister had also told him it would take at least two years of regular physiotherapy before he could expect to be able to put his foot on the ground again. So he had little reason for hope there either.

I explained that I did not know of any vitamin, mineral, herb, or diet that could re-join the two parts of a tendon that had not only been torn apart, but after six weeks had almost certainly separated and shrunk with a significant gap between the two ends. I told him that all I could offer him was Reiki, this new 'skill' I had just learnt but in which I had little experience or personal confidence (thus destroying any potential placebo effect). Since he had, under my care, lost all sign of what he had been told was terminal systemic lymphatic cancer, a level of possible confidence did remain, however, and he chose to accept my offer. We set to.

He came in once a week and I held his left ankle and heel in my 'hot' Reiki hands. We chatted for half an hour. Each time he left he displayed a modest but definite improvement and he progressively reduced his reliance first on his crutches and then his walking sticks. Gradually he was able to put more and more weight on the ankle. Each time, as he got up to leave, we could both see that we had made a step forward. Two crutches became one crutch and a stick, then two sticks, then one stick until after a couple of months he was walking unaided. We were both delighted. I was interested professionally and now had reason to consider Reiki at least more seriously than had been my initial intention.

Aunt, Ribs and Reiki

With the various changes that had taken place in my life, the increased amount of work I could do now that I was no longer gardening or playing tennis and had completed the re-establishment of the shop and dispensary, my income had gradually increased. One of the first things I had done was to book a flight to Ireland and go to visit Aunt.

This time when visiting Aunt I was to make more use of Reiki. I arrived at Dublin airport to be met at the Arrivals gate by her husband. On his own. Where was Aunt? Where was her enthusiastic rush to a huge bear hug? I looked around and saw her painfully levering herself out of a chair. I went swiftly over to her, ready and hungry for the first hug, only to be held back. "No, no," she said, "don't touch me, I have three cracked ribs. And don't make me laugh. I can't even cough, I am in mortal agony." I had planned and saved for this trip. I was only going to be with her for three weeks. Whenever in the past we had been together we had laughed and joked a lot and had gone for lengthy walks over her Irish bog, where she and her husband lived. Poor Aunt. This was all now apparently out of the question. And this, in turn, was going to put a definite pall on proceedings. I gave it some thought that night as I lay waiting for jet-lagged sleep to catch up with me. I finally decided to try Reiki on her, even though this would be only my second attempt with this technique.

The next morning while we sat round the breakfast table, I asked, and was allowed, before she brushed me off, to put my hands over her cracked ribs for about ten minutes. That was all her trust and impatience would allow. The process was repeated that evening and the next morning. Then I went shopping for them and was somewhat amazed on my return to hear Aunt say, "Listen" as she gave a couple of tentative coughs. She then suggested that I could hug her, but gently. She called a halt at a fifty per cent pressure but admitted by that evening that her ribs were hardly hurting at all, and not at all by the next morning, forty-eight hours after I had started using the Reiki. We were both delighted.

She then surprised me rather by saying, "I suppose a lot depends on what you think, doesn't it?"

"Yes, of course," I said almost without thinking, but then I stopped and considered. There had been something odd about the way she had said it. "What makes you say that?" I asked.

"Well, I knew it would work."

"Really? Why or how? After all, *I* wasn't certain it would work, how come you were so sure?"

"Oh, I knew you wouldn't risk making a fool of yourself."

I hadn't realised that that was a risk I had been taking.

1987 NLP

As part of my new 'post-tennis-playing' plan, I next studied Neurolinguistic Programming, NLP. It was probably the most rounded and 'left-brained' of all the various skills and techniques I was to study in the coming months. I doubt I would have had much in common with right-brained Richard Bandler, one of the two NLP co-founders. I was fortunate in that it was the other co-founder, left-brained John Grinder, who set up Grinder de Lozier & Associates in America, which opened up the training in Australia. A team of two of their members would arrive in Sydney on a Thursday, teach that evening and for the next three very full days, then leave us free to keep in touch with our own responsibilities for the next four days. Or we could have individual sessions with them during the week, then do another three-day training the second weekend of their visit, before they returned to America. This was repeated three times more, with three different pairs of trainers. Thus we had over four periods, each of eight days, or a full thirty-two days of intense training with equally intense application and study in the intervening weekdays. The training was a wonderful, enlightening and enriching experience.

One of the weekends was conducted by Michael Grinder, John Grinder's younger brother and colleague. I found Michael to be a particularly helpful trainer. Then, for the last fortnight John Grinder himself came to Sydney. I found NLP in general, and many of the techniques I learnt during that period, to be of immense value, and have used them since to, I hope, great effect.

Louise Hay

As I got over my inhibitions I did several personal development workshops, all within a short time frame. I was enjoying this, excited by what I was learning, how I was developing personally, and the increased amount of help I could give to clients as I learnt a number of techniques. Louise Hay brought the concept of affirmations to Sydney. As an adult, I have always been of a positive and optimistic frame of mind, and so found myself fully in tune with this concept. I readily forget anything bad, negative, or unpleasant that happens in my life or my daily activities, and almost never dwell on them, normally only remembering the good times. After all, by comparison with my first eighteen years, nothing can really be so bad. Focusing on them and practising her techniques, was an easy extension to this and something I was happy to pass on to my clients in treatment sessions.

Sondra Ray and Rebirthing, 1988

About this time Sondra Ray and her team brought us the practice of Rebirthing. This is an excellent technique for throwing up buried past traumas, unhelpful beliefs, and negative automatic responses, and then releasing them. With the understanding that comes, following the use of this technique, many problems can be unearthed, released, and left behind. The experience itself is also amazing. Rebirthing is a form of connected, deep, intensive and extensive breathing that changes your oxygen levels significantly. In the process of doing this, old and buried problems, memories, and constrictions are released. We were told that past traumas are buried in the energy or etheric fields of the body, and that, when oxygenated by this breathing technique, they can be released as the muscles respond, relax, and let go.

The course lasted twelve very long, intense weekday sessions consisting of afternoon-evenings spread over a term, with time for practising in between. Rebirthing achieves results, in gentle and unchallenging ways, that enable people to move on with their lives. Once trained, I conducted individual sessions integrated with my day-time consultations, and held regular evening group rebirthing sessions in my Sydney practice. I have since done similar sessions in or associated with my practice in London.

Robert Kyosaki

It was time for my next venture into these personal growth workshops, the ones I had sworn I would never do but was now learning to enjoy and benefit from! The next one was called 'Money and You' which I did in 1989. It was followed by a second one 'Creating Wealth' in 1990. Both were presented by Robert Kiyosaki who I found to be an inspiring and helpful trainer. He was clearly using our attitude to money and wealth to unlock some of our inner inhibitions and uncertainties. During a chat with Robert, I shared my idea, newly formed, of taking this further myself.

In our culture of 'stiff upper lip' and all that, it had increasingly become increasingly clear to me that many people, usually unconsciously, developed problems with their physical body as a safe way of getting their emotional needs meet. By that I meant that it was relatively 'safe' to ask for sympathy and understanding when we had a physical health problem as this would normally be met with "Yes, of course, how can I help?" It was less safe to ask for help over emotional issues such as being scared or unhappy. If one expressed statements such as "I am really unhappy", "I don't feel loved and wanted", please make a fuss of me", such a request could well be met with "pull yourself together, just get on with it like everyone else has to", or something similar. I thought that by helping people to explore and uncover the emotional needs that underlay their health problems and releasing some of these inhibitions, they could move ahead with recovering from and even preventing some of their physical health problems. Robert thought my idea was a good one and chided me, "Don't wait until you've studied and learnt more, get on with it, do it now. You already have enough experience and knowledge".

Choosing Health Intentionally

Thus emboldened, I did just that. I set to and wrote the workshop that I then called Choosing Health Intentionally (CHI). This developed out of the ideas that I had been mulling over, that ill health could be considered a safe way to get our emotional needs meet. It isn't always, of course, but the subject is too large to tackle here. A single example will have to suffice.

Deidre's problem was very specific. Her symptoms were focused on serious candida-based vaginal problems with the associated itch, pain, and white discharge. The problem was so bad that sex with her husband was extremely painful, such that he did not enforce it. I advised her as to what I thought she should do to treat and cure her physical problem. She returned to see me several times looking quite happy and unconcerned, but reporting no improvement in any of her physical symptoms. I finally got her to admit that she kept failing to do as I had suggested. She gave several reasons as to why she had not been able to follow the routine, but then admitted that she really didn't mind not being able to have intercourse. When I asked a few more questions, I learnt that the vaginal problem was a perfect excuse for her to avoid intercourse with her husband, something she did not like or want any longer. She was just happy not to have to face up to the problems with her unhappy marriage, one in which sex had even become unpleasant to her. She felt sure that if she and her husband started such a discussion and spoke about it in any depth, the probability of divorce would arise. She was very much afraid of this as, with three very young children and no income of her own, she did not know how she would manage. Having thrush was a lot less painful or frightening,

In fact, the CHI seminar covered a lot of concepts and ran for fifty-five hours over three and a half days, from Thursday afternoon until late Sunday evening. It brought up many surprising and interesting results and helped a lot of people to resolve their problems, both physical and emotional.

Choosing Weight Intentionally

For my next seminar I had taken these ideas and applied them to food issues, weight loss, and weight gain. I called this second seminar Choosing Weight Intentionally. It was based on an underlying suggestion that people's weight is often associated with their beliefs and issues about their weight and looks. This was a two-day seminar and ran for twenty hours. More of this one later.

CHI, the Book

I was very keen to share my ideas with a wider audience than the seminar groups, and in this I was fortunate to meet up with a 'shadow' or 'ghost' writer, MME. MME was a participant in one of the early three-and-a-half day (fifty-five hour) CHI workshops. Every day he sat in the front row, not changing seats as he had been asked to do. From there he asked endless questions and he argued relentlessly against almost every premise I presented. This was wonderful, of course. As usually happened, the fifty-four other students were getting more and more interested in the ideas I was putting forward. They were learning more and more about themselves and the problems and stumbling blocks in their lives that were holding them back. Each time MME raised a question or an objection, the other fifty-four students argued back at him, for they were all in tune with what I was saying and doing. Facing up to and arguing with MME seemed to help them to fully formalise and understand the depth of what they were learning. Finally, on the morning of the Sunday, the last day, I said to MME:

"Michael, for the past two and a half days you have sat in the same seat even though I have asked everyone to swap seats after each hour-long block so that they could gain a different perspective and sit next to different people. You have declined to do this, and I have let you. I have also answered all the points you have raised. How would it be if for this last day you would swap seats each hour, as the others do, and instead of asking questions or challenging all that we are doing, you would be willing to sit quietly and simply listen, take the ideas in, and let your mind process them? He decided to agree – he could hardly do otherwise.

I assumed that for the first two and a half days he had been sitting there formulating his ideas, questions, and objections, just waiting for an opportunity to raise and present them, rather than focusing on what was being said as the subject moved forward. I assumed this was what I was meant to think, particularly as his black cross on a red silk shirt proclaimed him to be part of one of the organised western religions. He certainly had plenty of such questions and objections, which he raised whenever I gave him the opportunity, which was frequently. For instance, the conservative and traditional religion which I assumed he followed, included views that clearly clashed with the possibility of 'other lives' and reincarnation. Such topics came up for discussion from time to time, as many of the other participants raised questions on such matters, or I suggested expanding our horizons, from time to time.

As I had expected, by the end of the last day this had brought about a change in his thinking. By the time they were all leaving, he sought me out and said, "That was really interesting. I realise now that what you are saying really does make a lot of sense. I would like to write a book about it. Could I help you write yours?" I agreed to this and left him to do the writing.

In fact, I had set out several times over the years of presenting this seminar, several times a year, to write a book about the contents, but it had always seemed to be an overwhelmingly vast subject and one that was difficult to explain succinctly, or compress into a single book. Consequently, I had, to this date, given up on the effort. MME certainly condensed the material far better than I had done in any of my attempts – I always wanted to add just one more example or explanation. As a result, I was able to publish *Choosing Health Intentionally*[ii] in 1990. After that I wrote the follow-on seminar *Choosing Weight Intentionally*. Then I was being asked for more, so I wrote the third seminar on further aspects of personal growth and clearing. To keep the naming going, I called it *Choosing Self Intentionally*. This focused people's minds on really concentrating on the type of person they wanted to be, and enabling them to develop in that direction.

Parts Dialogue

By this time, of course, I was on a roll. I had become interested in the idea that we each had our inner child, our inner parent, and our inner adult. I went beyond that and assumed that we each had an inner Critic, an inner Driver and many other Parts. I called this seminar, Parts Dialogue, and ran it over a two-day weekend. The participants worked in pairs as they each took on the various roles as directed. It was probably the most relaxed and enjoyable of the four seminars, though I suspect they learnt more from the other three.

This was also something I could do with clients on an individual basis. I set them up, each one taking on the role of the indicated part and then talking to an imagined version of themselves left back in the empty chair they had just vacated. Using this technique, I was told, felt like a voyage of self-discovery to most of the participants.

After *Choosing Health Intentionally* had been accepted by Simon and Schuster for publishing, they asked if I could write something else. It was then the Thursday before Easter, my last client was late, so I started to play with ideas. In the end the client didn't turn up, but I kept writing. I had by then written and presented the *Choosing Weight Intentionally* (CWI) workshop several times and so I thought I could also turn this into a book.

I chose a few examples to explain the concepts. Two women provided the first ones. They attended the same seminar. Both were attractive. Both were overweight and both claimed to be very keen to be significantly slimmer. They had each dieted or been on diets for years. Neither of them had ever lost a significant amount of weight, and for both of them there had been times when their weight went up. One was a successful advertising executive in an office full of men. She was married to a man who drove a delivery van for the same company. During the workshop she figured out that, deep down, she was afraid to lose weight, the reason being that she thought that if she did, some of the men in the office would invite her out. If they did, she knew she would accept simply for the fun of it, but she loved her husband and didn't want to upset the marriage, so it was safer to stay fat and not be asked out.

The other married woman also worked in an office full of men. During the same seminar, coincidentally, she came to realise that she was afraid that if she lost weight one of the men in her office might find her more attractive and invite her out. If they did, she would have to refuse. Her worry was that if she turned them down, they would not like her. Two very different assumed scenarios for a similar problem. The women had each, unconsciously, found the safest way to get their needs meet: namely, to stay overweight and hide their attractiveness.

I had already presented this two-day seminar a few times. It occurred to me, on this Thursday afternoon, that I could turn this seminar into a book too, and, that it would be a shorter one and easier to write than the CHI book. Suitably inspired, I wrote. Suddenly it was ten o'clock and I had planned an outline and written 2,000 words. It was time to pack up and go home. But I was fired with enthusiasm, and I spent the weekend writing. By the end of the weekend, I had 5,000 words written and I phoned the publisher to let them know. They were hugely enthusiastic and asked if I thought I could write the full book in time for the spring publishing deadline in May, ready for the (Australian) summer sales in October. That gave me only about a month to write a whole book, but the adrenaline was flowing, and I agreed. I was lucky. I had the four days of Easter, and now I had another three weekends. Head down and tail up, I focused fully and let the words flow. I hit my deadline. In the end it took only ten days to complete the book – nine days for the writing and one day to reread and edit it. It was an amazing experience. I suddenly felt I knew what some authors have meant when they say, 'The book wrote me'. CWI was also published by Simon and Schuster, this one in 1992.

CWI-CHI

Having prepared and presented the CHI and CWI workshops several times (bi-monthly for CHI and monthly for CWI), I was encouraged and delighted to find that the growing number of participants wanted more. As a result, I set up a program whereby we met up every Monday evening. Each week I prepared a short set of exercises and we dealt with different emotional issues each time, all along the lines of the two major seminars. Thinking up the name for these Monday evening sessions wasn't difficult. Choosing Weight Intentionally (CWI) and Choosing Health Intentionally (CHI) soon condensed into CWI-CHI which then became 'Quickies'. I ran CWI-CHI evenings every Monday for a long time. I also offered rebirthing sessions one evening a week, helped by one of the enthusiastic graduates from my CHI workshops. All this was in addition to running my naturopathic practice, lecturing at the college, and writing the regular articles that were being requested by the various magazines.

Janet attended one of the CHI workshops that I was presenting. She loved it so much that she managed to persuade her Greek husband to attend the next one, a couple of months later. Her stance was that their marriage was so rocky that if something didn't change soon, they would almost certainly separate. Being Greek, her husband apparently expected his wife to do all the work round the house, plus care for the children, plus do a fulltime job, while he did his fulltime job, but then relaxed and went out in the evenings with his friends. He also felt entitled to shout at her anytime things weren't done to his liking.

During the rebirthing session in which he was the participant, I was called over to his position at one point to help. He was lying on his back, and it was clear from what he was saying that, in his mild 'rebirthing trance', his mind had taken him back to a time when as a foetus he was inside his mother's uterus and experiencing what she experienced – something that occurred frequently in these sessions.

"That's not right, that's not right," he was crying.

"He [his father] is treating her [his mother] badly. It's terrible. He is treating her the same way that I now treat Janet. It's not right. I'm never going to treat Janet like that again."

He continued in this vein until his breathing relaxed and returned to normal. He was true to his word. He never did treat Janet like that again. I didn't see him again either, but a Christmas card later that year assured me that the change in him was wonderful and the marriage was now secure. Janet continued to come to many of the CWI-CHIs.

The first three of these seminars, CHI, CWI, and CSI, each took a lot of preparation and a team of assistants. They involved a number of props, of so-called 'games' and challenges. These in turn required a number of assistants. After the first one the various participants were generally very keen to 'stay involved in the energy' or to repeat the seminars, and they gradually formed a large body of people who were keen to do them again and to help the new participants. It was a wonderful time to be working with these energies.

'Parts Dialogue' was a little different. It was easy to present. It could, and was, done in my office, either in a small group or in solo consultations. It needed no assistants, no special preparation, and no set-up. It has proved to be particularly popular over the years and I have continued to give it from time to time.

Neither CSI nor Parts Dialogue have led to books, though they could readily have done so, as could the CWI-CHIs with all the interesting examples and stories that they produced.

---

[i] Xandria Williams, *What's in My Food: Book of Nutrients*, Nature & Health Books, Oct 1988

[ii] Xandria Williams, *Choosing Health Intentionally: Unlocking Your Subconscious for a Better Emotional and Physical Future,* Simon and Schuster, 1990, Letts Publishing UK, 1992

Chapter 16

Unexpectedly Back to London

I had come back to London a few days earlier and taken possession again of my studio flat in Chelsea. In the preceding few years I had fallen more and more back in love with London, at least with 'my' part of it. This was focused on Chelsea and central London in general, on South Kensington and Sloane Square in particular. This was where I first 'came alive; found happiness, and had a sense of belonging, from the age of eighteen onwards. It was also the part where my relationship with Aunt had germinated, taken root and grown and developed. It was hardly surprising that I felt a strong sense of connection with it.

As always, I was delighted to have this flat (my second in London) already established, my clothes on hangers (no need to iron), toiletries and all else still there in bathroom cupboards, just where I had left them when I had left London a bit more than five months earlier. As I had no need to bring large amounts of luggage with me, it also meant I had only minimal unpacking to do.

After a few days catching up with friends, as usual I took off for Ireland to visit Aunt. Uncle, now seventy-six, was no longer driving and so I was met at Dublin airport by Housekeeper's son, and driven down to Killinagh Lodge where I received the usual amazingly warm reception. Aunt has always been enormously precious to me, for herself above anything else, in the same way I was to her. Effectively, she was the only family I had, so these visits were the only times that I felt 'at home among family'. But boy, did I feel at home. We had little catching-up to do as we had been sending the usual hour-long weekly tapes to each other since my last visit. Nevertheless, we managed to talk non-stop.

On Christmas Day 1995 we had the usual Christmas celebrations with pre-lunch drinks at the house of one family, followed by lunch at the home of another, and then back to Killinagh Lodge with just one or two friends for a relaxed evening round the fire with a bottle of wine and, by common agreement, no more food.

A few days later, Aunt and I were taking the dogs for their usual pre-breakfast walk. There was frost on the ground. It also lay on all the branches and twigs of the trees, now shorn of their leaves. We set off down the Avenue, although 'Avenue' is a rather grand name for a tree-lined lane of only single-car width, that gives way in time to more open land, and then goes on to the bog face where we had cut turf in earlier summers.

The sun, rising only slowly, was still low in the sky. It shone gently through the frost-outlined branches and, as so often, I couldn't help contrasting this with the heat and ruggedness of the Australian bush.

I was thinking of nothing in particular, and certainly had made no plans for the words that were about to pop out of my mouth.

"You know," I mused aloud, "you looked after EJ (Aunt's mother-in-law) and had her living with you for the few years up to her death. Then you had Gran (Aunt's mother and my grandmother) living with you for several years until her death. You looked after them both. But what about you? Who's going to look after you?"… short pause … "*I could, you know.*"

I think it hadn't occurred to me, consciously, that Aunt wasn't immortal. After my awful childhood, that I had simply endured, I had grown to know and to love her more and more, and to depend on, and to trust and rely on her immense affection and support. She had been a constant backbone in my life, a security against which I had faced the world. Now, at eighty-three, she was seemingly fit, healthy, and indomitable, albeit becoming progressively more crippled with arthritis and so slower in her movements. Like me, she was of independent mind, so I was hardly surprised at her response to my question and comment. "Oh nonsense, dear, you couldn't do that ... well, never mind ..." She waved my concern away and we went on walking, calling the dogs, and talking to each other. We mentioned it no further and I thought little more about it, at least consciously, for the next twenty-four hours.

The next morning, back on our walk, I found myself saying, again without much forethought, "I really could, you know, I could come back here and be with you." I had no idea what I expected her response to be. What I was suggesting was, in effect, a move from Sydney back to – what? – UK – London – Ireland.

Her response was immediate and a surprise. "We could build on an extra bedroom ..." Even though I had asked the question, I was stunned. Aunt *never* asked for anything. She did not like to receive presents, to receive anything, to be beholden to other people. She avoided having other people doing things for her. I recalled their fiftieth wedding anniversary, the golden one, when I had, appropriately, given them fifty gold presents. It was no big deal, none of the presents was actually gold, the whole thing was a bit of fun, wrapped up in gold paper. As I gradually ran out of ideas for yet another 'gold' present, I had allowed it to include Golden Syrup, Gold Blend coffee, a chocolate doubloon wrapped in 'gold' metallic paper and, in final desperation, some yellow post-it notes. But by the time she was unwrapping perhaps the twentieth present, she was almost too overwhelmed to continue. I had probably had the more fun, searching out and buying the items – and yes, I did manage to reach fifty.

Her enthusiastic response, then, to my suggestion the second time, told me that she really would absolutely love me to come back to be near her, in some way yet to be determined, and at some future date. (Being eighty myself as I write this, I can understand this all the better. At that time I simply thought she would live forever.)

We more or less left it at that. Back in London, a few days later in my tiny studio flat I played idly with ideas. I decided to check out prices of suitable properties in South Kensington or around Sloane Square, the epicentre of my London life. I did this in a mood of 'it would be fun to see a few London flats'. I played with the idea of having sufficient space for me to work from home, if needed. To this day I have no idea of how serious I was, but clearly something had been building inside me. I was growing progressively more aware that my love for London grew each time I came back, as did my regret at leaving it. And all this in spite of having an excellent set up in Sydney, lots of friends, a successful practice, and all the other professional activities that I valued so highly.

I spoke with Aunt on the phone the next morning. "It won't work, dear, she said, "CR [her husband] is not keen on the idea. Although he thinks more highly of you than anyone else that visits us, including his own niece, he can't contemplate the upheaval of building on another room."

"That's alright. I've already figured that it would work best if I live in London and spend large chunks of time with you."

To this she made no objection, which I took to be relieved acceptance that the plan could go ahead. So somehow it was settled, at least as the start of a plan. Perhaps at eighty-three, with a husband with progressive dementia, she was finding it tough going. They would argue with me for saying so, but they had a rather Victorian marriage where she insisted that he make the decisions. He had been a brilliant engineer. Early in the Second World War, he was even air-lifted out of Singapore just prior to the Japanese marching in, and then on to Ceylon where he was employed on radar and communication research for the rest of the war. However, he also had had a squint when they first married and he had lacked self-confidence. This she had tried to build up to a point where he had finally taken over all the decisions, thus it was a bit unsettling for her as he lost control.

I put the receiver down and gave it some thought. I had only a few days before I was due to fly back to Sydney, so there was no time to waste. One estate agent showed me a delightful apartment in Sloane

Gardens. Perfect. It had a spacious entrance hall that would make an excellent waiting room and reception area, with a large sitting room cum dining room to the right (for private use). To the left, the smaller bedroom would work for me and the very large double bedroom would make the perfect office. I could come here, work, see clients, live comfortably, and make frequent trips to Ireland. Was I dreaming? Was this cloud nine? Maybe, but it was also fantastic. My initial idea of just checking out prices had already, within less than two days, metamorphosed into a definite plan to return, at least very frequently and for longer periods. Perhaps even to commute between the two countries. I was so used to travelling that this did not seem impossible.

Then I found the fly in the ointment. There was a tenant in the flat who I was assured would leave as soon as I purchased it. This would have been possible, even probable, in Sydney, on a month's notice. But I recalled enough of London regulations to suspect this might not be so simple here. I checked up and found I was correct. The flat would not actually be vacant for a couple of years. This was not good. It was already Thursday morning and I was returning to Australia at dawn on Saturday morning.

My Third London Flat

There was an estate agent across the road in Lower Sloane Street. I went in and gave them their brief: a two-bed flat, ground floor, within a hundred yards on either side of the Kings Road, between Sloane Square Underground station and the Chelsea Town Hall – and a garden if possible. They looked glum, said they had nothing. I gathered up my things and prepared to depart, wondering, what next? But then a colleague piped up: "We do have one, what about …? It's a hundred and seventy-five yards down Lower Sloane Street, not one hundred, but would you consider that?" Of course I would.

With no time to spare, they took me through the place and I liked it. It spread over two floors and consisted of a very spacious living room and kitchen on the ground floor and two-en-suite bedrooms on the lower ground floor, arranged round a central outdoor space of about six feet by eight feet, facing southwest and so catching all the sun. Wonderful, I thought, for growing herbs. It had a lengthy shared lawn and garden along the back. I took a friend back the next morning and she liked it too. I put in an offer for very close to the asking price that afternoon. It was accepted. Done. I kept the price in pounds sterling in my mind. I knew that if I translated it into Australia dollars the number would be so vast I would quake and might give up on the idea. More excited calls between Aunt and myself followed.

In Australia, the asking price for a property was pretty much what you paid for it, there was little bargaining. In Australia too, once you paid your deposit or the initial agreement was made, I forget which, the seller couldn't pull out. Accordingly, I felt confident there would be no gazumping or faltering at the last challenge while I was back in Australia. In retrospect, it was probably a good thing that I had agreed so close to the full price as the lawyers took two to three months to finalise the sale, even though the husband of the vendor couple was confident I would go through with the purchase. In fact, all went well. He was probably getting more for the flat than he expected, but I too was happy, even thrilled, with the deal.

Selling My Sydney Home

Back in Australia, I put my lovely sandstone house on the market and got a good sale. During the next few months I packed up all the furniture and belongings I would want in London and sent them on their way. I moved the rest of my possessions into the house where I had my practice close to the centre of Sydney. This, fortunately, also had plenty of room for me to live in. I arranged the rest of the place and my sessions to suit my altered needs. I contemplated a life, at least for a while, where I would 'commute' between Sydney and London in about equal measure and see how things developed. I was determined not to walk out on my Sydney clients, though I was careful not to take on any new ones unless they understood that I could only help them with immediate problems, and that I might well be leaving Sydney altogether in the near future.

I have speculated since about my ability to make decisions, especially around buying properties, changing jobs, and moving to a new country, seemingly on the spur of the moment, and seemingly with success. I suspect it is because, at least subconsciously, I know exactly what I want and I grab it when the opportunity arises.

My furniture was due to arrive there and I would have the subsequent couple of months to unpack, settle in, and start to consider establishing my career there.

A Sydney Naturopath versus ....

Being an ANTA -registered naturopath in Sydney was at that time in many ways similar being a GP. People were as enthusiastic about having 'their' naturopath as they were about having 'their' GP. As naturopaths we could refer our clients to doctors or specialists, the health insurance funds covered our fees, or at least part of them, and we were able to run busy and successful practices. We were part of a well-established career path and healthcare service. I also had my lecturing, and the writing.

.... a London Naturopath

In 1996, when I started to build my bridge to London and develop my career over there, I had without thinking expected to find things similar in London. But twenty-five years ago, naturopathy was not a common term in London and any effort I made to explain my profession was commonly meet with "oh you mean you're a homoeopath like the one the Queen has". I soon realised I was going to find it more difficult to set up in practice and be taken seriously in London than I had anticipated. But there was little time to worry, and in any case, I was having too much fun and certainly wasn't planning to turn round and reverse my plan.

I unpacked, arranged things with enthusiasm, and made tentative attempts to find a few London clients. I offered help to the local health food shop and spoke with a few people I knew via Imperial and the Royal Society of Chemistry, and had a thoroughly good time, enjoying the London life that was opening for me.

Global Commuting

Before long it was time to go back to Sydney and wind down the practice there over the following few months. After that, it was back to London, another two months there, and then a return again to Sydney. By this time, however, I knew without a doubt that I really did want, in the near future, to move totally to London. I knew that by then I would have taken care of all my existing Sydney clients and so would not be leaving anyone in the lurch. As well as a smooth transition for them, I made arrangements for people, in time, to take over my lecturing commitments. Sadly, long-range internet video consultations were not yet possible.

I also spoke with the editors of the various magazines I wrote for and explained that I hoped to go on writing for them. I was pleased to find that they hoped for this too, and did not see any problem with this arrangement. After all, they were already used to my frequent perambulations. They were also keen to have contributions from me in so far as I could bring aspects of my travels and relocations into the articles I would write for them. In addition, I already had commitments in place to start writing for a couple of UK-based magazines.

So it was time to put the Sydney house on the market, close the practice down fully, pack up and be ready to leave. Since I had had two houses in Sydney, each over twelve hundred square feet, and I was moving to only one home in London, it was clear that I would not be able to take everything with me, nor did I want to. I sold a lot and gave a lot away until I was down to a bare minimum. Eventually, I had it all planned and organised.

I gave my usual last-evening party – though this time it was not just the last-evening-before-travelling party, but also the last evening full stop. Mindful that I had thought my move to South Africa had heralded a long-term stay there, and hadn't, I left myself options to return to Sydney should I find this move had been a mistake, even though I doubted that this would ever happen. I had spent nearly twenty-five years in Sydney, a large chunk of my life to date. I had made a large number of friends here, among the students, clients, colleagues, and the various social circles in which I moved. I also found it easier to say good-bye on a wave of "I'll be back" which a lot of people expected anyway, rather than "this is forever".

The final party was huge and the house was packed with people. All the remaining furniture not sent to London, had been given or promised to friends and I had made arrangements with one friend such that the final items in the house would be collected after I left, the next day. Much of it would then go to one of the Rudolf Steiner Homes for people in need of special care, which delighted me.

As I would be flying over America, I would have a generous luggage allowance and could take two large 30 kg suitcases with me, and I had these almost packed and ready. I told the friends that poured into the house for this final party, that everything else except my suitcase and hand luggage could be taken by anyone who wanted it. This worked out well – until, that is, I was about to serve up the evening meal. It was, necessarily, a very simple one of curry, rice, and bowls of condiments. Then I found there were no plates. Odd. I knew I had an extensive set of Poole pottery. Much muttering and questioning followed. Then hilarity. We found that the couple who had asked to have the dinner set had already packed it into their car. This was retrieved and the meal could proceed.

The only missing guest was GF, my third receptionist. She had learnt a month or so earlier that her father, back in England, had been diagnosed with cancer, and she had resigned so that she could go straight back and be with him.

Somehow, and magically, I had managed this amputation without letting anyone down, and had left no threads hanging.

London Landing

The commuting of recent months could have been unsettling, but in fact by the time I had truly left Sydney and settled back in London, I was totally sure that I was right to have made this move. Now it was time to set about establishing my career all over again, and with even greater focus. I wondered where to start. I had no immediate thoughts of working from my home and planned to rent professional rooms. Initially I rented a room on a sessional basis in Harley Street. This impressed me enormously. When I grew up here, around the nineteen fifties, only the very top doctors could get rooms in Harley Street, it was the pinnacle of one's career. At least, that is how I remembered it. Now, suddenly, it seemed I could do the same, as the people practising in Harley Street in 1996 made up a much more eclectic mix than back in the 1960s.

I was fortunate with the location of my new home (which is still my home) in Lower Sloane Street. I have two Underground lines at Sloane Square station and at least nine bus routes that pass within a couple of hundred yards of my house. If I ever did work from home, I thought, people would be able to get to me easily. Getting to Harley Street for me meant just one bus, and it went almost door to door. However, it could take forty minutes and it meant trundling a large number of books, items of equipment, and boxes of supplements with me each time, so very soon I looked for rooms closer to home. I was lucky again, and was able to rent one in a pathology laboratory just off Sloane Square. Finally, I had found my London base.

Daisy Trails

The last time I had lived in England, or thought about the English countryside, was 1968, and now, nearly thirty years later, I could barely remember where towns and villages were. I loved getting out of London from time to time, exploring and travelling, and of course I also liked to be independent. I bought a tiny campervan. It really was tiny, approximately four feet by ten feet, but it contained a bed, chair, table, sink, two-burner stove, small box fridge and even a flush loo. I loved her. As a white Daihatsu it seemed logical to call her Daisy. I joined the Caravan Club and was almost certainly the smallest member of it. This was in the late 1990s when we were not yet dependent on the internet with its necessary cable connections and power source. As long as I took my computer and any books I might need with me, I could travel and work anywhere, and in Daisy I did just that.

Starting my London Practice

As I settled into my consulting room, I found I enjoyed the companionship and intellectual exchanges with the people working in the laboratory there. Until this time I had used my computer, or a sequence of them, merely as glorified word processors. It was now time for me to learn more. One of the scientists at the laboratory was a wonderful teacher and got me started.

Initially I worked there for only one day a week, but gradually that increased. At the start of my time in London I had, of course, very few clients. In Sydney I had built my practice as a result of owning and working in my health food shop Natural Gourmet, and Pharma Natura the dispensary, where I had started. More students had come from the college teaching I had been doing. With all of these pursuits, it had grown organically, and I soon realised that here in London it was going to be a challenge, and one for which I had no real experience.

Working in Sydney in my own health food shop I had rapidly built up a working knowledge of the various supplements and products that were available and had learnt which ones got the best results, and where to buy them. I emulated this, here in London, by talking with local health food shop owners. They were happy for me to 'hang around' in their shops and to learn which suppliers they thought provided the best products. I also talked with a number of their customers and tried to help them too. But this was 1997. Still no one seemed to know what a naturopath was. I might have done better if I had called myself a nutritionist, but in Australia, the top level and most thoroughly trained people were the naturopaths and not the nutritionists.

I went to a number of conferences and Expos, met people there, talked, and more. I already had a few contacts in the UK, mainly via SM my writing agent, and the books I was writing at the time. Early on I was asked to lecture in biochemistry and nutrition at the BCNO, the British College of Nutrition and Osteopathy, as it was called then. This offer I accepted with alacrity.

Lecturing in London

I had anticipated a stable period of lecturing. However, very soon the BCNO told me that the course I had designed and was teaching was 'too difficult' for their students, 'not wanted' by their students and, perhaps more accurately, was above the level of what the college wanted. Would I please lower the standard and set less demanding exam papers. The naturopathic colleges that I knew at the time were those in Australia, where there was one in each state, one in America, the John Bastyr College in Washington state, and the College in Portland, Oregon, now known as the National University of Natural Medicine (NUNM). All of them, at least at the time, seemed to have somewhat similar levels of education. Without having given the matter much thought, I had assumed that the standard in England would be similar.

I thought back to the very early years in Sydney in 1973 when I had started to teach the same two subjects, nutrition and biochemistry, to the students at the Chiropractic College. Those students had had very little interest in either nutrition or biochemistry. This should not have surprised me. They were studying the physics of the body, not its chemistry.

BCNO, despite its name, seemed to be about three percent naturopathic students and over ninety-five per cent osteopathic students. I soon realised that, like the chiropractic students who had been the first students I had lectured to on these subjects back in Sydney, they too were not much interested in the chemistry of the body, preferring instead to focus on the physics of its structure. When I was asked to lower my standards, as happened after about the first set of exams, I did so, although with reluctance. Some months later, at the end of that teaching year, the same request was made again. I gave it some thought and decided that I was not much interested in teaching at the level they required and I dropped it. I was heartened, though, that about a dozen of the students, and/or recent graduates, had asked for an advanced course in therapeutic nutrition. This I was happy to give, and both they (I was told) and I thoroughly enjoyed it.

Soon after that, CNM, the College of Naturopathic Medicine, was fully started, initially at Regents College. Because it was a college that taught nutrition, I had assumed that the Board and the students would want a thorough training in these topics, similar to the standard that we had given in Sydney. In this too I was mistaken. I was soon faced with a similar situation to the one at BCNO, or at least partially so. This time, while half the class was thoroughly enthusiastic about the level at which I was teaching, the other half seemed to be focused on getting a course that was as simple as possible, with easy exams and the chance of a speedy and relatively painless qualification. The only trouble with that sort of training, however, is that once you have qualified and go out into 'the real world' you realise how little you know, and you wish you had been taught more (and listened more).

Thus the time came again that I decided I did not want to teach at the lower level that was requested. I was fortunate in that I was not dependent on earning an immediate income, and so yet again I stopped teaching. However, there was one significant benefit to come from this college. They were able to attract a large number of students and thus they 'spread the word' about nutrition and healthcare, to a large number of people. This probably hastened the general awareness of nutrition as a serious topic of study and professional training. Other courses were then offered by the college such as herbal medicine and homoeopathy, and happily it was to be 'third time lucky' as I was also asked to give some of the lectures at ION, the Institute of Optimum Nutrition. Things here went much better and I enjoyed teaching once more.

In Australia I had been in the habit of putting both my phone and address details, home and office, in each book I published. It was not considered to be unusual. My aim had always been to teach and pass on knowledge as much as I could, and so I had wanted readers to be able to contact me for further information. As NSW state president of the Australian Natural Therapies Association (ANTA) I had been keen to encourage newly graduating students. I was also keen to refer appropriate enquiries to practitioners in other parts of the city for treatment with other modalities such as massage, or physical therapies, modalities that I was not keen to incorporate in my own schedule. I did not consider it unusual or strange to put my contact details in my books, and I had reason now, in London, to be glad of this. Fortunately, I had had time and the wit to put my London as well as my Sydney details in the book that, fortuitously, was to be published at about the time I was setting up my practice in London.

I had suggested this to my English publishers, who were aghast and suggested that I could perhaps put my phone number in each book, but only that, and certainly not my address. In the end we compromised and I was able to add P O Box details as well. However even that was a bit of a challenge. In Sydney there would typically be a P O box system in each post office. All the boxes would generally be built into the wall facing the street to make a bank of post-office boxes that could be accessed both from inside the building and from the pavement outside. In Sydney I had had a key to my box and so could collect mail at any time of the day including weekends and holidays.

To my horror, I found the system in London was much less organised. First of all I had to get a bus or tube from Sloane Square to Victoria, then walk some distance. To collect my mail, I had to queue at a counter for my turn – no accessing the box myself. In fact, there were no actual boxes, just shelves with occasional partitions, and although I had been given a box number no one seemed to know where it was. The 'boxes' were certainly not lined up in numerical order and as I watched people shuffling mail into a variety of these 'boxes', I already anticipated the problem. When my box was finally located and I was given the pile of mail in it, I found half of it was for me – good, thank you – but the other half was for an assortment of people who were obviously missing theirs. Goodness knows how many of my letters had gone into other people's sections. I soon gave up on that system.

There was generally a two-year lag between agreeing and confirming a book, writing it, and getting it into final publishable form. Several books had been requested, negotiated, or agreed on during my last two or three years in Sydney. About this time, the series of four books that my then newly-acquired writing agent Sarah Menguc had organised for me, began publication.

Love Health and Happiness was also published by Hodder and Stoughton in 1995, retitled as *The Four Temperaments* by St Martin's Press, US, 1996, and published by Kabel, in Germany, in 1997. It was subsequently published in Russian and in Greek 1998.

Fatigue, the secret of getting your energy back was published by Reed Consumer Books, Cedar U.K. in 1996 and in Poland two years later. I thus wrote these four books in three years. This, in addition to my clinic and commitments, was a busy time. It was completed while I was still in Australia but published soon after I arrived in London. As a result, almost every client who came to see me complained of fatigue (I learnt to call them 'clients,' not 'patients' as was the norm in Australia). These clients seemed surprised that I could help them with anything other than fatigue. One day a woman phoned, saying her asthma was bad and she'd have to cancel and come another day.

"Come in anyway, and I can help you with your asthma."

"Oh, do you treat asthma too?" was her surprised response.

Fatigue was popular, and conveniently became the core that helped to get my practice off the ground. However, after a year or more of nearly all my clients suffering from fatigue, I was beginning to long for clients with different problems, although I was grateful for this boost to my clinical activity. As if that was not enough, I wrote yet more books. A publishing house had planned to write a series of quick and easily readable books. They planned this as a series that they intended to market at stands at supermarket checkouts. As such they wanted to buy the books and the copyright outright from me. This was unusual. The normal procedure was for the author to be given a financial advance, of sufficient size as to make it worthwhile doing all the work. This was then followed by royalties depending on the volume of sales. However, the outright purchase price I was offered this time was significant and I accepted on that basis. This was a book on herbs and plant preparations, *Herbal Beauty Preparations and Uses.*

I wrote the manuscript, they expressed themselves delighted with it, and paid me. However, the American senior management of the publishing house then apparently pulled the plug on the whole project of a dozen or more books, including those being written by other authors, Nonetheless, I had been congratulated and paid.

As an Australian naturopath, I was used to practising, and being accepted, almost like a GP, but one who used natural remedies instead of drugs, and aimed at restoring health rather than treating disease. I was used to professional acceptance, not the scepticism that faced me in London. After a couple of years in practice here I grew tired of being expected to do no more than help people lose weight or gain energy. This was frustrating and an impediment to building my practice. However, I asked myself my usual question at such times: What's good about this?

The answer was obvious. I had a steady but slow-growing practice and so had plenty of time to think and reformulate rather than go on beating my way down this somewhat blocked pathway. Instead of merely reinventing myself and copying my Sydney working style here in London, I would take a break, I decided. I would take time out altogether, somewhat like a sabbatical, and study something very new – but not quite yet.

Beating the Blues, was published by Reed Consumer Books' Cedar imprint in 1995, at the time of my initial move to London and the plan to make that my permanent base. It was also published by Kabel, Germany, 1997 and by Editora Best Seller, Brazil in 1998. It was a book about depression, and, as a result, for a while I had several clients who were suffering in this way. One of the many clients that this book led to was Valeri G.

"I am depressed," she said as she marched into my office, sat down and firmly placed her bag on the floor beside her. "I'm single, fifty-one and going through the menopause. I have no children and I am suddenly depressed at the thought that I cannot now have any."

"Do you, or did you ever, want children?" This was the obvious question and so I asked it. She seemed unsure.

"Perhaps," I suggested tentatively, "you had decided in a previous life that you wished you had not had them?" I could make that suggestion in Sydney and expect a sort of generalised acceptance. But I was rapidly learning that few people here were open to such ideas. However, she surprised me, although she didn't accept the idea either.

"Oh pooh," she said, "I don't believe in any of that nonsense."

I moved swiftly on. "Not to worry, let's do some work on regression and see if we can discover what has led you to this depression."

She was happy to acquiesce and I did the usual light trance induction. Suddenly she was back as a boy of eighteen in what she said felt like North Africa, working in her father's shop in the bazar selling rugs. She complained of being kept at it all day and never having time for any fun. "Just wait until I have my own shop and can take time off when I want it," she said from her trance state. I thought the session would end there, but suddenly she went in deeper. She was again a male, in fact the same one, but now was nearer to forty than twenty. He was also married, had several children and was again working long hours, but this time at his own shop in the bazaar.

"How do you feel now?" was my next question.

It brought out the immediate and emphatic response, "I'm exhausted, not having any fun, and if I had my life over, I would *never* have children."

With that she sat quietly for a while, gradually came out of her trance and gazed at me. "What was that? Was that a past life?"

It was not for me to decide for her, so I shrugged lightly, paused for a while, and then asked, "How do you feel now, about the depression you came in with?"

"Oh, I feel fine. I never did want children anyway. I don't know why I have made such a fuss." With that she smiled, gathered up her belongings and seemed happy to call it a day. A later card from her assured me that all was well along these lines.

Was it a past life? Or was it a way for her subconscious to bring up her deeper feelings? I am very clear that when working with clients I am being asked to help them resolve emotional issues, not to teach them about esoteric issues. I may or may not believe in reincarnation, but I will certainly use whatever tools I can to improve the happiness and emotional state of my clients, within ethical frameworks of course. Issues such as reincarnation belong, I felt, more properly within the concepts of CHI, CWI, and CWICHIs where they were often requested.

The rest of the books in this group of four were published in quick succession. *Love Health and Happiness* was published in 1995, in Germany in 1995, and in Russia and in Greece in 1998. It was published in the US in 1996, this time under the title *The Four Temperaments,* which I thought a much better title, but I have usually found, as author, that I have little say over either the title or the cover.

The topic of *The Four Temperaments* used to be the opening evening of the CHI workshop, but then developed into the stand-alone seminar workshop that I now run here in London. I have presented this subject, in several forms, as a seminar for practitioners wanting to use the material for their own clients; as workshops for individuals who want to use it for themselves; and as short introductory workshops within other presentations.

So, right from the start in London, and without consciously planning it that way, I was again reinventing myself and building up the three strands of my career: seeing clients, lecturing at colleges, and writing books.

I enjoyed the writing and found that ideas flowed freely and did not occupy a great deal of time. As my practice grew, however, it did demand an increasing amount of my time. In addition, I was making frequent visits of a week each month, to stay with Aunt in Ireland, the prime motive for this upheaval. I had quickly realised that if I did not plan ahead in regard to Irish visits I would never get there, as there would always be other things I had already booked to do, so I got into the habit of booking ahead, a week per month. A very helpful woman in Aer Lingus took over this task. Once I had moved my office rooms in Chelsea, I could rearrange clients around my Irish timetable. Lecture days were less flexible, so during term times I spent slightly less time in Ireland. In August, however, I would go to Ireland for longer periods and include my birthday. Those weeks were wonderful, and I did a lot of writing. I had my own room at Killinagh Lodge and set it up with a comfortable desk so I could work there. As we were still not dependent on the internet, working there created no problem and Aunt got used to answering the phone for me, as appropriate.

I also continued to re-explore England, in Daisy, my tiny but wonderfully practical and convenient, campervan. Initially I could go for four or five days at a time. So I went on *Daisy Trails* and sandwiched them between my commitments to lecturing, helping my clients from my Chelsea office, and my monthly visits to Aunt and Ireland. By avoiding main roads I discovered vast areas of seemingly empty spaces and roads. This version of England is delightful, beautiful, full of interesting and attractive places, and not crowded. In fact, very often it was almost deserted during my roamings. I was in love with the English countryside, the beautiful villages and houses, the historical sites and the various gardens overflowing with flowers from corner to corner. Where I had lived in Australia, rainfall was limited. Gardens had frequently to be watered daily. As a result, many gardens were designed with sprinklers (usually circular) to cope with this, and consequently the corners of gardens frequently became barren spaces. By comparison, the English gardens were bursting with flowers and colour, not only in the centres, but in all the nooks and crannies. I loved all the English flowers, shrubs, and trees, that were such a contrast to the gum trees and eucalypts of Australia (which I had loved in their turn).

There were several self-imposed rules to these Daisy Trails, one an external rule and several I imposed myself. Firstly, I had to be back in London every Wednesday to run my practice in Chelsea, and sometimes on Tuesdays for lecturing. Secondly, I wanted to be free to roam without restraint. This meant that once out of the grip of the M25, I had to take the smallest road at every junction, follow all the brown signs (tourist attractions or places of interest), and not pick my caravan park for the night until five o'clock. In this way I was free to wander until the last practical minute.

One difficulty with being a 'snail' and taking my home with me was that if, in the evening I wanted to take myself out for dinner, Daisy would, of course, come too, and it was perfectly possible that I could drive back and find someone else had put their vehicle in my slot. The safest option seemed to be to spend my evenings in Daisy rather than go out. I would park, push up the roof, set up the table, open the sliding door, and settle down to write. I had my main meal at lunch time, generally in restaurants or other interesting stopping places, and ate a snack in the evening. In the morning I would work until about ten o'clock when all the rush hours were over, and then set off on my explorations. This combination of early morning and evening writing periods gave me a total of about six or seven working and writing hours in the day.

It was all wonderful fun, but it took me many months to adjust back to the size of England, where all the towns and villages are almost adjacent to one another. This was such a contrast to the size of Australia where you can drive for an hour or more before getting to the next township. I recall one time, near the start of my life in London, when I was in Slough for a meeting. I left there at about twelve o'clock. I consulted the map. My route would include Maidenhead, Henley, and more. I recalled Henley as being on the river and decided to head there. I had no idea of the distance but there were several places on the map between me and Henley, and I recall thinking, "It's a pity I'll get there too late for lunch, but at least I can have afternoon tea." I was therefore startled when, only a few minutes later I arrived in Henley. It took a while for me to adjust easily to the truncated English distances.

With the necessary constraint of being in London for Tuesday or Wednesday evenings, each Daisy Trail could only last for five days. Thus, these ramblings were generally kept to the south of England. I did go as far as Cornwall on one occasion, and during two summers I took Daisy over to Aunt and to Ireland where I explored more extensively. In this way I was able to meet all my writing deadlines for several books and two lecture courses for the two different colleges. When the practice grew and extended to two days a week, Daisy Trails were gradually reduced in length.

Associations

I joined the Royal College of Chemistry (RCS) soon after I came back to London. They had regular meetings followed by drinks and a chat. These meetings were hosted by many different people, all of them more or less interested in chemistry, as I am. I say 'more or less', but somewhat to my surprise I found that, as I was to find later in other disciplines too, many people had done a degree in a subject that they were not particularly keen on and had then walked away from it and gone into business, or law, or accounting, or something else entirely. Me? I had studied chemistry just precisely because I loved the subject and found it fascinating, and I have continued to work and think as a chemist ever since, even if it is more theoretical than hands-on practical.

After the Chemical Society I joined the Royal Society of Medicine (RSM). I can't say that I loved medicine. I have very little confidence in medical drugs and procedures, though I do have enormous respect for what it can do for people in emergencies, or who have acute or deeply genetic health problems, or when a variety of surgical procedures are necessary. But as a naturopath who has moved into medicine, I love the blending of the two disciplines and there are always opportunities to fill in some of the medical gaps that were not covered in my naturopathy training. The RSM provides a large number of lectures on specific topics and for those with a technical interest. They also put on more general talks on many different subjects, which again provided the opportunity for mixing and talking for a couple of hours afterwards.

From some of these people I learnt of, and joined, the Worshipful Society of Apothecaries, and the Harveyan Society. These latter two are very much focused on the history of medicine. If I had missed out on the opportunity to study chemistry, I have always thought my second choice would have been history – though I fail to see how I could have made a career at it, certainly not as interesting a career as I have had. I have always taken an interest in the history of chemistry, right back to the phlogiston theory and the life and times of Antoine Lavoisier. I first read about them during my school days and then in the history of healthcare in general, in the centuries from Galen to the present day.

When I discovered the Royal Institution and the laboratory that Humphrey Davey, 1778-1829, had established, I was enthralled. Alumni Societies of both Imperial in London and Otago University with events organised from Dunedin in New Zealand, provided natural homing venues. Through all of these I met and made friends with many people. I loved the talks and thoroughly enjoyed the social life that came associated with them.

One of my favourite London events is the annual Summer Exhibition at the Royal Academy of Arts. The Chemical Society takes over the exhibition for one evening each summer and that is a gem. I can go to that, happily and preferably on my own. I can enjoy all the art. Equally, I can talk to any stranger that I meet there, confident that we are, at least, friends-by-profession, and that I will find an interesting person to talk to. Equally, there is no need on these occasions to get bogged down in what I might think of as tedious, not to say boring, social chatter, about topics I consider to be gossip and time-filling. I can always move on to look at the next picture!

I loved nothing better than a good technical, or scientific debate. I recall one time with JB, a geologist I had known well as far back as my New Zealand days, and then again at the time I went to South Africa. At the time of writing this he was lecturing in Earth Sciences at the Open University and we would meet up every time he came down to London. Like me, he had an open and enquiring mind, and we would have endless and lively discussions and debates every time we met. At one point he said something like "We both have strong views, searching minds and a keen interest in many different subjects. Yet we never seem to argue. I wonder how that comes about?" "Simple," was my quick and almost automatic response. "We are both interested in learning, in getting to the core of the discussion, in learning from each other, not in being right rather than wrong and persuading the other of our own views." Whether or not this is true I am not sure, but we certainly had some wonderful times.

To many people my social life may have seemed limited. To me it was wonderful and exciting. Effectively my family life continued to consist solely of Aunt, and she, as always, provided the emotional warmth that I treasured. I was pleased and satisfied beyond measure that I had come back to England, and was content, in general, with my life here. Even professionally I was content, if not thrilled, by the way my career had developed in the UK. This latter mild dissatisfaction was largely due to the lack of full acceptance of the role and power of naturopathy in the UK and what it could offer, and by the lack of challenge and acceptance of what I could offer, from my clients. My life might have continued like this for a long time – writing books, running a small, but not particularly stimulating practice, lecturing at various colleges to students who were only moderately keen on their studies. As I write this it sounds rather dull. Not a bit of it. I continued to enjoy the research I was doing for all three – the writing, the practice, and the lecturing. However, I knew there could be more.

I little suspected what the next millennium would bring.

Chapter 17

Cancer

O ne morning during one of my visits to Ireland, Aunt said her back was really painful and would I call the doctor. Aunt was eighty-six at the time. She never complained of any health problems, even though she was very stiff with arthritis. I was immediately concerned. The doctor came, they chatted, he drew a blood sample and I drove it to Naas hospital for analysis. That afternoon I was due back in London. I extracted a promise from both of them that they would let me know the results as soon as they were available.

Aunt always seemed invincible to me and somehow it never occurred to me, even then, that at some point she would no longer be there, or that, possibly even right now, there could be a problem. So, later that afternoon, when I drove to the airport and flew back to London with my fingers crossed, I was not unduly worried. A day or two later I phoned Aunt to ask about the results and she said that all was well. Clearly, she had been concerned about bone cancer. Gran, her mother, having had breast cancer, I suspect this had been at the back of her mind for some time as a possibility somewhere in the future. In a similar way, now, I am aware that clients who have had cancer often worry about the smallest symptom elsewhere in their body, thinking it might be a sign that cancer had re-emerged or spread. In their pre-cancer days they would have thought nothing of such symptoms.

A week later, on Saturday, while I was still back in London, I received an unexpected phone call from Aunt's doctor.

"I have your aunt on morphine."

"What? Why? Does she know?"

"No, there is no need to tell her."

I was horrified. Nobody, but nobody, did anything to my indomitable Aunt without consulting her, not even me. She had a mind, a very firm, secure, and stable mind, of her own. I was also confused and not fully thinking straight.

"Why have you given her morphine?"

"Because she has cancer, of course."

I was stunned.

"But she told me you said she didn't have bone cancer."

"No, well, it is spinal cancer, not bone cancer, and I didn't see any need to tell her. In fact, she shouldn't be told, it is much better that she doesn't know."

Incredible. I was shuttling between despair at the thought of cancer, and fury at the way Aunt was being treated.

"She must be told. I will tell her."

"It would be much better if you didn't."

I certainly didn't agree with that, but I had other things to think about than arguing with him.

"What are you doing for her?"

"Nothing. There is nothing to be done."

"How long has she got?"

"Three months."

I hung up. I paced my sitting room, hand over my mouth as if I could put a stop to and block the flow of the thoughts.

Some years earlier Aunt and I had discussed just such a situation. We had promised each other that if any such situation arose, we would keep nothing hidden from the other. We had made our promises. If I said nothing, she would remain relaxed and feeling safe. But would I be letting her down, backing out of the promise I had made? She would learn soon enough anyway. She was far too intelligent to fail to suspect something as the weeks went by. I had to tell her, but not by phone.

I wasn't due to return to Killinagh for two weeks. I thought hard, made plans and phoned her. I claimed that "Australian friends want to visit and stay with me for the next month, over the time I had planned to be at Killinagh with you. Would it be alright with you if I came over this weekend, ahead of their visit, instead?"

"Yes, dear, that will be fine."

No questions. Savvy was my Aunt. I'm pretty sure she suspected. I booked a flight for that Friday evening as usual, and arrived, also as usual, around eleven. Again, as usual, she had a cauliflower cheese in the oven waiting for me. She knew I loved cauliflower cheese, and this had become her habit. I'd never had the heart to tell her, month by month, that by the time that cauliflower cheese, which she had prepared early in the evening and left in the oven before it was finally rescued close to midnight, was well overcooked and a 'mush'. I loved her for it. I didn't dream of telling her. We chatted. I knew I could not tell her about the cancer that night. That would have meant leaving her to go to her bed and lie and think about it on her own. I still wasn't even sure that telling her was the right choice.

The next morning as she and I sat in front of the kitchen window after breakfast, I embarked on my carefully planned gambit. I had thought my words through very carefully, word by word. Depending on what she said, I could pull back from telling her if it seemed that she didn't want to hear any bad news. She, as usual, was in her wheelchair, due to her arthritis, and we sat in the kitchen window looking out over had large garden and the fields beyond.

"You have the doctor coming this morning, don't you?"

"Yes."

"Well, I'm wondering. You know how you don't like to push or question him?"

Aunt was of a generation where a doctor was somewhere 'up there on god's right hand' and not to be questioned or challenged.

"Would you like me to have a talk with him and see if I can learn anything more about your back pain? If there *is* more, would you want to know, or ...?"

"Yes, of course I would." Her response was firm, just what I had expected.

I paused, took a deep breath and said, "In that case, I have to tell you, it is spinal cancer, you do have cancer."

I said nothing more and turned to look out of the window, giving her some private space.

After a bit of silent thought she said, "I don't expect they will let me be in much pain."

With that we got on with the day. A brave woman, my aunt. Very sensibly she never did ask how long, and I certainly wasn't going to tell her, even if she did ask. I abhor the practice of doctors putting a time-limit on someone's life. At best, all they have is averages, and no-one fits the average description. At best, such figures are vague indicators of possibilities. Once given a date or a time limit, it can work on the individual's mind in such a way that there is the danger it becomes a self-fulfilling prophecy.

I set about rearranging my life. I was determined to spend as much time with Aunt as possible. The fact that she didn't protest told me that she was very grateful for that. For the next three and a half months I had a punishing lifestyle. I would spend as much of Monday at Killinagh with her as I could, then leave in the evening for the nine o'clock flight to London, arriving home at around eleven or midnight. I'd settle at my desk, answer the week's mail and get ready for the next day's lectures at the college, going to bed around two or three in the morning. I'd lecture all day Tuesday, do more office work all evening and into the night if necessary. Then I'd see clients all Wednesday, and finally go straight from there to Heathrow for the last flight back to Ireland, arriving back at Killinagh close to midnight.

Aunt had a wonderful support family. 'Old Mrs P' had been her housekeeper when she first returned to Ireland in 1968. Then 'Young Mrs P' had taken over. The latter was a wonderful carer and was delighted to take on the job of helping Aunt, probably more than Aunt wanted but was too tactful to say. Young Mrs P did tell me, soon after I started this regime, that Aunt's spirits sank as soon as I left on

Monday evenings and didn't perk up until she was sure I was on the plane on the way back on Wednesday evenings. So I knew I had to keep going at this routine, even if it was demanding, and in any case I wanted to be with her as much as possible.

In the following weeks we talked our heads off, free from the need for pretence. We also discussed what I would do afterwards, which Aunt liked to focus on.

"Don't let this house be a millstone around your neck," was one of her instructions. We both knew that she had left the house to me.

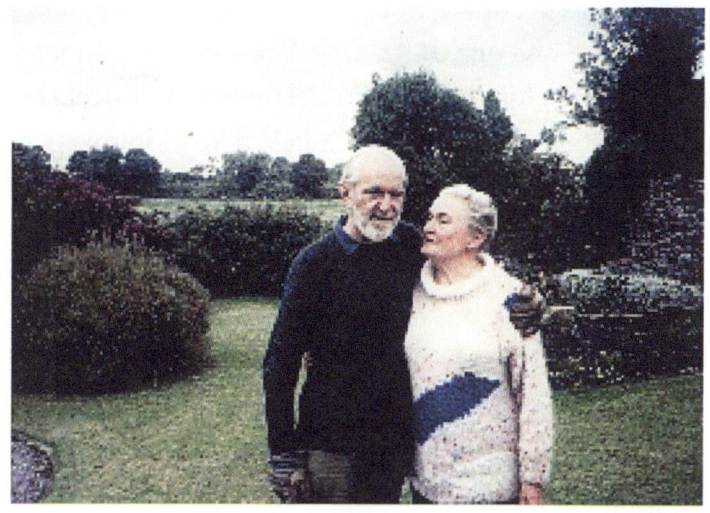

"I will look after Uncle properly, and make sure he can continue to live here and never have to go into a home – with Mrs P's help, of course," I promised her.

We had two weeks more than I had been led to believe, but at least I was able to keep her at home and was with her when she passed. On the last evening we sat together, holding hands, and sharing the occasional sentences. It was devastating. I had made all the necessary arrangements. After the ceremony in the local church, all our friends came back to the house for the party that she and I had planned. It was just like the many parties that we had planned together over the years I had been coming here. From time to time, I would forget that when the party actually took place Aunt would no longer be here and with us. Then it would all come rushing back.

The party, or wake, was, in spite of the circumstances, a great success and she would have enjoyed it and approved. Two days after the cremation I returned to London. I already knew the will. The property and almost everything in it came to me. When I first came back to London from Sydney, they had both given me power of attorney and we had planned everything, the various bequests and donations and more, so there was nothing to learn about or discuss.

I had promised Aunt I would care for Uncle. The plan had been that young Mrs P and one of her five daughters would move into the house and look after him. I would go over to Ireland a weekend a month to pay the bills and sort things out. Uncle, a total introvert, and I had never had any real sort of a relationship. In fact, he had no real sort of a relationship with anyone but himself, and with Aunt upon whom he had depended for his wellbeing. This was born out by the fact that he had declined to come to the crematorium, but had then looked devastated when I left to return to London. Sometime later I realised that by then I had replaced Aunt in his confused mind. He thought that I, looking very much like Aunt and doing many of the things that Aunt did and said, was actually his wife. I suspected that he thought that the person who had died and for whom there had been the funeral, was somehow my mother, but of that I was never sure.

Two days later, back in London, I had another phone call. The doctor again. Uncle had pneumonia and was fading fast. I was told there was no need for me to hurry over, in fact I probably wouldn't be there in time. Naturally I grabbed my bag and flew. He looked startled to see me. This was when it began to occur to me that in his semi-dementia state, he had indeed come to think of me as his wife, and it probably explained why he was devastated when I left and was now sinking further into developing pneumonia.

As Uncle was a complete introvert who lived in a world of his own, hardly talking to anyone, it was soon clear that to keep him alive and in minimum distress, I would have to go over there as much as I could. My plan to go to Ireland once a month, purely to check up on things, pay the bills and such, would obviously not do. I would have to go over every weekend and spend some time with him whenever he was awake. I fell into the routine of going over every Friday evening and coming back to London late on the Sunday. This was a pattern that he soon adapted to, though he never did get the hang of the changed relationship, as he saw it. Some evenings he was angry and confused when I, 'his wife' as he seemed to think I was, refused to go to bed with him. But in time he adapted to it and lived for another year, also passing at home with me sitting on the bed beside him.

My Smallholding

In my distress at the loss of Aunt, and while looking after Uncle-by-marriage who slept through most of each day, I needed something to do during the time I was at Killinagh. I threw myself at my inheritance: two ducks, two dogs, two donkeys, six cats, fourteen acres of Irish 'bog' (not really boggy) and an almost senile Uncle. Mrs P was very keen that I should add goats to my inherited menagerie, and I was easily persuaded, reviving fond memories of Chocolate Drop in West Australia. It seems that Young Mrs P had had goats herself some years earlier for one of her daughters who had been allergic to cow's milk.

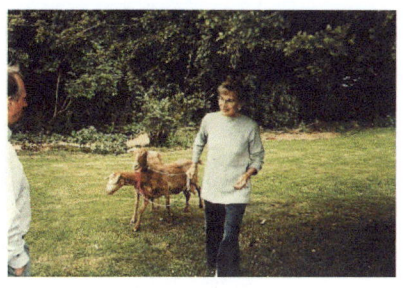

She wasn't, of course, going to stop there, so hens were added to the livestock. None of this could have been done without her help, and it was, to some extent, a way of thanking her for looking after Uncle so well.

In time Uncle passed, but it was to be another two years before probate was granted and I could even consider selling up even if I wished to. I had to continue to look after the property for that time and keep it occupied and safe. I threw myself into this, to assuage my loss.

I reduced my visits to alternate weekends and continued to work on the large and growing vegetable patch.

I was intrigued by alpacas which I had seen in an issue of the Smallholder Magazine. The son of a friend of Aunt's, who was looking for a job that would bring him back to Ireland from Australia, thought that alpaca farming would suit him. I agreed on a herd that he would farm, and we would run a joint business together, breeding and selling them. I linked with a UK herd and, for various reasons, agreed to have about a hundred and thirty of them. This was madness, of course, and so this number was rapidly reduced to about eighty. According to the relevant Irish government authorities and veterinary bodies, I was the first person in the country to have imported these delightful animals.

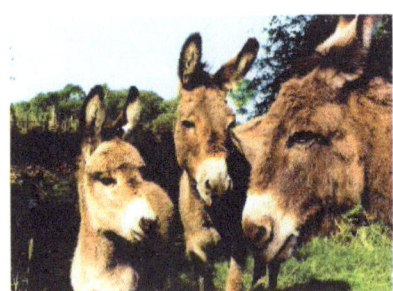
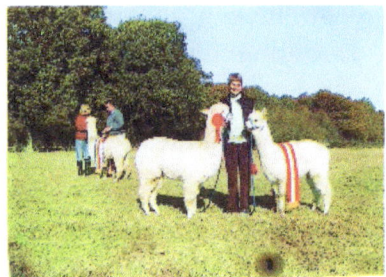

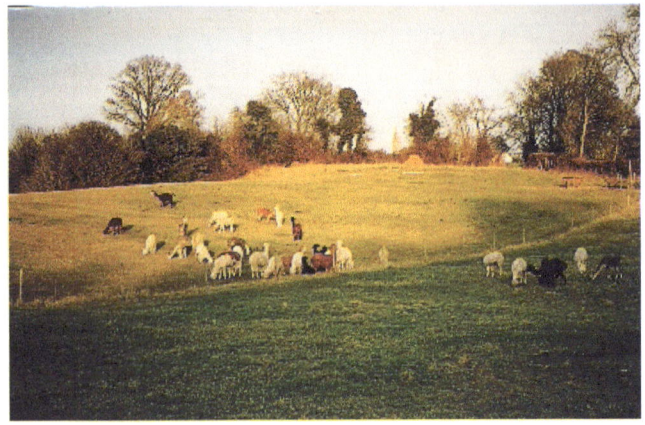

I also gave free rein to my other interest that had surfaced through the preceding decades: I gardened. I gardened so extensively that I was almost heading for a smallholding.

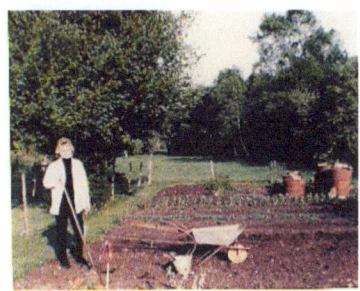 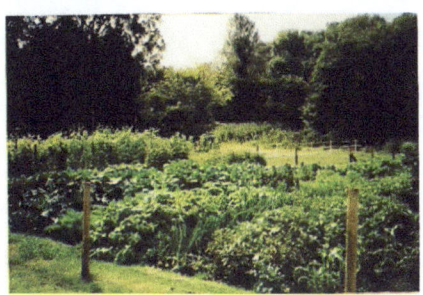

Young Mr P, son of the younger Mrs P, had overseen the outdoor maintenance of the property at Killinagh after I had inherited it. Unfortunately, it had soon became clear that the 'son-of-a-friend-of-my-Aunt' who had claimed to be so keen to work with the alpacas, clear the land and 'improve the place' soon found it was not for him. He was doing a poor job and not even taking very good care of the animals. He was also difficult to work with and known to frequently 'gild the lily' as to what had been done in my absence. I found this enormously stressful. Worse still, I stopped enjoying my weekends at Killinagh. Eventually, I had to offer an ultimatum: either he would have to change his ways or I would have to take over. The result, as I suspected, meant I was left 'holding the baby'. I could have gone back to looking after the land on my own, if that was all there was, but I could not manage the alpacas by myself. Nor could they readily be sold, as I had about ninety percent of the alpacas in the country. Again, young Mr P took over. He found a local assistant to do the daily feeding and take care of the alpacas in my absence. Fortunately, they are very self-sufficient animals and need little maintenance.

Equally helpful, there were three people who simply fell in love with the animals and visited whenever they could. They soon became known as the 'alpacaholics' and even came with the animals to some of the shows we attended. Eventually, the more serious of them began to join me regularly on the alternate Sundays when I was there and the alpacas needed mating and checking for pregnancy status. This was a two-person job for which I definitely did need help. I loved the animals and thoroughly enjoyed the whole smallholding experience. A new routine developed. For three days a fortnight I played at 'smallholding'. For the other eleven days I worked in my practice in London.

At the same time, I continued to see clients in London, but for most of them their problems continued to be about either fatigue, weight loss, or vague forms of 'general health', so I still did not have the busy fully accepted practice I had known in Sydney. I continued to lecture at various colleges, and to write: the three ever-present threads to my professional life. This continued to be somewhat frustrating as the lack of recognition for naturopathy was ongoing. There were few of the challenging cases I had had in Australia, and relatively few conferences, although I still continued to enjoy it.

One woman was keen to lose weight. I gave her a diet plan that, she said, fitted in with her food preferences. Two weeks later she assured me she had stuck to it but hadn't lost a single ounce. I asked her to complete the diary form that I used. She did this, filled in a week's worth of meals and posted it back to me. I was dismayed but not surprised.

"Have you eaten only what I suggested?"

"Yes, absolutely"

"What is this chocolate eclair I see on Tuesday afternoon?"

"Oh, yes, but that was only one. I was out having coffee with a friend and we had one each."

"But I see another one here on Friday afternoon. Did you have anything else, a sausage roll, or something?"

"No, absolutely not."

"But here it is, at the bottom of the page …"

There are none so blind as those who will not see. Only I didn't say that aloud to her.

This and similar episodes convinced me that I had to look further afield if I was going to develop my practice to anything remotely as interesting as the one I had had in Sydney.

In time this all settled down into a routine. I then came to realise that I was ready for a further challenge. I needed a new avenue of information and research. Now in my early sixties, not totally dependent on a practice income, I was certainly not willing to even contemplate retiring. What would I do if I retired? According to many of my friends I would have time to relax and do what I loved and enjoy my hobbies. But I was already doing exactly that, and to the fullest extent, so retirement was definitely uninteresting and out of the question.

Investigating Cancer

In spite of the constant travelling and the physical activity, I had energy and curiosity to spare and I had become quietly interested in cancer. Throughout the previous two decades I had had some general glancing relationships with people with cancer:

One of these was the woman I had spent a couple of days with when our plane had been grounded in Newfoundland one winter. She had terminal cancer and was just hoping she could enjoy her short stay in England and get back to Sydney before she passed. She had been happy to talk about her experience. Her interest in new clothes and makeup and her determination to look her best for this trip and her last few weeks, was an inspiration.

MI had probably been my first client with cancer, and following what limited help I could give him, had lived on for many years past his medical prognosis of four months.

One friend, MC, had died of cancer in Sydney without me knowing what to do, or without any authority that she would accept.

For several years I had taught a module on cancer when lecturing at a couple of naturopathic colleges.

Then Aunt of course. I knew for certain that she would not have followed any suggestions I might have made as to changes in her diet, or a pattern of supplements, never mind detoxing or any other step. Besides, at eighty-six she was stiff with arthritis and, denied her one enduring hobby, that of gardening, she had few interests left. With a husband she adored but who by then had little idea who she was, she was tired of life and finding it all a great struggle, although she remained cheerful, fun, and positive until the end.

I love to study. I began to put increasing amounts of time and effort into reading and learning more about cancer, and more particularly into what I, as a nutritional biochemist and naturopath, could learn and do about it, and doing this in ever greater depth. Medicine had been working on it for more than a century with little apparent or significant success. Medical proponents might argue with this, but the numbers were hardly encouraging and the suggested treatments were painful and rarely impressive. In fact, it could even be said that the statistics and outcomes had become progressively worse. As a biochemist, the naturopathic approach to cancer appealed to me as a unique topic on which to work, and research. Gradually my enthusiasm grew

Cancer is unique in that it is not a disease *of* a particular organ or tissue, instead it occurs *at, in* or *on* a particular organ or tissue, or else more systemically. Nor is it caused by specific pathogens. It appears to be more affected by a deficiency of nutrients, the presence or damage caused by toxins or poor lifestyle choices. And like many health problems, it was aggravated or worsened by stress. That is how it appeared to me at that time. As such it was a health topic particularly appropriate for study from a naturopathic perspective, especially to one keen on restoring homoeostasis. I started to read, while at the same time developing and nurturing my London practice.

I combined this with travelling. My fortnightly trips to Ireland were beginning to feel more like local commuting trips. They hardly counted as the travelling that I so much enjoyed. I had started my move over from Australia in early 1995 and settled here later in 1996. Aunt passed at the start of 1999 and Uncle at the end of that year. I didn't go on the lengthy Daisy Trails as Aunt and I had planned. That was not feasible with all the commitments that I had in London and Ireland. However, after Aunt had passed, I developed the habit of going on shorter trips by plane to various parts of Europe and close by. Some trips were more targeted, such as Christmas trips that were generally built around seeing one or more operas, or some other such event. I also found river cruises appealing. Sitting in a comfortable cabin, researching and writing all day followed by sociable dinners, was a life that suited me perfectly. What could be better? At least for a while? All the catering, shopping, cooking, general housework, and more were done for me. I had nothing to do all day but read what I had brought with me, and write, then dance the evenings away.

I did one much longer cruise round South America from Santiago to Tiera del Fuego, out to the Falkland Islands and up to Rio de Janeiro where I meet up with TM and his wife. Odd though it may sound, the three of us were destined to become good friends, and sometime later they both came to Killinagh on a visit. In all the quiet times on these trips I continued to work, delving into the books I had brought with me, or what I could research online. One Christmas I hired an apartment in Funchal, Madeira, for a couple of weeks and read and wrote intensely. I went on more river cruises through Europe … and I wrote.

Cancer Research

By now my developing interest in cancer had become a serious pursuit. I decided to take it a step further, to study, do more research, and focus almost entirely on cancer as a major career move. Like a tumour that could be detached from the surrounding tissues, it seemed to me that cancer was a subject that was not only interesting but discrete in itself. It was also one that I suspected few naturopaths in England were exploring at that time.

To check this out I used the fact that I had not been back in the UK for long, and I assumed, correctly, that no one would know me or recognise my voice. I contacted a number of people who I was told could help me with information on cancer. I received answers such as, 'Oh yes, I can help you, I have a number of herbs that can help with cancer', or, 'Massage is really helpful. If you care to book in, I can give you a healing massage'. All I learnt was either that no one here could provide in-depth help for someone who had cancer – or that if there were any practitioners who *could* help, they were extraordinarily difficult to find.

I set about studying cancer in a more structured way. I had always thought that if I were to work with cancer, I would have to have done a significant amount of prior research and study and be well prepared. Cancer is a huge topic. I would have to learn all I could about its cause, development, and progression, and how these processes could be reversed by naturopathic means, and without using dangerous radiation, toxic chemicals, or destructive surgery. If, ultimately, I was not able to come up with a solid, evidenced basis and clear concepts of what I could do, at the very least I would have had an enjoyable time doing the research. If, on the other hand, I took it on within my clinic, and as my speciality, I would almost certainly find myself running against the medical/allopathic approach. I had better be prepared for that too.

When taking on MI as a client in Sydney, I had come across plenty of anecdotes and personal case histories, of people enthusing over the many different protocols they had tried: this herb or that herb, red clover or echinacea, this diet or that, veganism or macrobiotics, these nutrients or those, selenium or intravenous vitamin C. Massage could help, or it could spread the disease. Meditation and relaxation were good, or one should simply get on with one's life.

I was determined, as I had been throughout my career, that everything should be on a sound biochemical and scientific basis. This was easier now as it was the start of the 21st century, the internet was in full swing and almost anything could be researched. I didn't have any particular expectation of growing a practice on this basis, however. I assumed that if people in the UK were so reluctant to put confidence in naturopathy for general health problems, they were highly unlikely to do so when they had cancer.

Nonetheless, at about this time I stopped endeavouring to develop a general naturopathic practice. I stopped hiring a consulting room and planned to work entirely from home instead, focused fully on researching and writing. It was 'unstructured time', that phrase again, that often came to mind, and it was wonderful. Huge swathes of my time up to then had been spent fitting in the writing and research around client appointments and fixed lecturing hours. That had all meant that I could be called at any time and have to drop what I was doing and attend to the matter in front of me. All my time was now unstructured. Other than the two trips to Ireland each month, I was free to read and explore cancer to my heart and brain's content.

I studied, I read, I used the internet, garnering everything I could find on cancer. Yet again Robert and Marie Erdman in Seattle were mines of information. They were always happy to share and I had lengthy conversations with Robert on the subject. They deluged me with names and addresses of people in the US who were active in the field, worldwide but particularly in America and among our nutritional colleagues. They supplied me with details of conferences, and sent lengthy copies and reports – it was clear that I would have to become a lot more computer savvy and rely further on it. I also continued to travel, of course, but now focused these trips on venues, clinics, and events related to cancer, and I visited clinics and laboratories in many different countries.

Clinical Visits

In Switzerland I particularly recall the Lucas clinic in Arlesheim, where Rudolf Steiner had lived and worked. I was keen to learn more of his spiritual science approach to an understanding of cancer, and its implications both physical and spiritual.

In the UK, the Park Attwood Clinic in Worcestershire was open. I visited there, talked with the wonderful doctors, particularly Dr

Maurice Orange. I was impressed with so many aspects of their approach to cancer that I am tempted to write about it now, but I must stick to my plan and save that for the next book otherwise this one will be too large and too long and in danger of never being finished.

Suffice to say that I sent several clients to Park Attwood during the many years before its untimely closure, due largely to an excess of generosity and a resultant lack of adequate funding. They integrated both naturopathic and drug/medicine approaches and incorporated physical and natural remedies such as herbs, nutrients, and diet, along with rhythmical massage therapy, eurythmy, hydrotherapy, and artistic therapies. This integrated approach was collected under the one title of anthroposophical medicine. I was delighted to see the ways in which they catered for the needs of the individuals in their care.

One client I recommended to go there was advised to attend some of the artistic opportunities during his two-week stay. He insisted he was no artist and could not draw, paint, or sketch. However, after some discussion and experimenting they found common ground in sculpture. He was then questioned as to whether he preferred 'additive' sculpture where you add more and more clay (or whatever material you are using) to what you are building, or 'subtractive' sculpture, where you cut away and remove what you don't need. Suddenly, by the end of his visit, he was becoming really enthused. He loved the additive idea and could not understand how people could figure out what to remove and not suddenly find there was no material left in the place where he wanted to put a hand, or whatever. He said that when he learnt that, he suddenly fell in love with clay modelling. When he got home, he started with plastic and then found a local pottery group he could join and where he could use their kiln. Enthused, excited, and happy with this new hobby, he produced some delightful results, and his health improved.

I was reminded of MI in NSW who had found gardening, even organic gardening, frustrating, but then fell in love with hydroponics. I had suggested to him many things to the point when he said to me one day, "I will do these things you suggest, reading and meditations, but right now I am too busy learning about hydroponics and building what I need, to have time to have cancer." It's no wonder he lived so far beyond his prognosis.

Cancer Conferences

In America there were cancer conferences in many different parts of the country, but mostly on the West Coast. I visited many of them. In fact, I met up with people at conferences from so many different countries that I lost track. I met Frank Wiewall from 'People against Cancer' at a conference in London. He was interested in what I was doing and invited me to visit him in Iowa. I did, and for a while we considered working together. His approach was to work with individuals at the basic level, then refer them on to someone in the large network he had built of individuals who specialised in specific types (locations) of cancer. But in time I realised (a) that I did not have, or know of, a network of specialists in the UK and (b) that I myself was the practitioner, whereas ultimately Frank was not. Nevertheless, he had a very impressive setup and I learnt a lot from him and his way of working, even though I didn't follow it.

At the start of this phase I went twice to the Cancer Control Society's annual convention in Southern California. This has been a regular event since 1973. Speakers at the convention include medical doctors, nutritionists, naturopaths, herbalists, and many others, plus researchers, writers, and reporters, as well as many people with cancer, all focused on the disease in its various forms and manifestations.

These conventions are an excellent 'showground' to inform people about the amazing number of therapies and options that are available. They are excellent for the clients as they have the opportunity to mingle and talk with both practitioners and other patients like themselves, and hear their stories. It is a great introduction to someone who wants to learn more about just what is available, and to do so fast. It is also great for the practitioners, particularly those in

America, as I'm sure many of the participants eventually became their clients.

For me this was an amazing foundation for what I was building. I talked with and questioned hundreds of people with cancer, learned their stories, what they had been through, the practical problems they faced and their solutions, how they had discovered what they needed to know, what protocols had worked, and what hadn't. It became very obvious that strategies that worked for one person did not necessarily work for another. Instead of arguing about which method was the best, I focused more and more on the variety of strategies that different people had used and that *had* worked *for them.* I talked with professionals working with cancer, who had been doing so for a while. I became very excited by it all. I discovered the work that had been done in America, as well as Australia, which was well ahead of what was being done in the UK.

On both occasions, these Cancer Conferences were followed by a well-planned coach trip to several clinics and hospitals in Tijuana, just inside the Mexican border. Tijuana had by then, the early 2,000s, become a focal point for many practitioners and the people running the clinics and hospitals who have been forced out of America by the US's antagonism to any approaches to cancer that went beyond conventional surgery, chemotherapy and radiation. I was interested in the very different approaches taken by the various institutions and practitioners, many of which combined a medical approach with alternative ones, some following an entirely alternative approach. This was nearly twenty years ago as I write this, and much has changed since then. Likewise, the use of computers and the internet has also mushroomed.

I visited Pamela McDougal in Idaho. She had worked with William Kelly for five years just prior to his death. During the previous several decades, Kelly had developed his own unique protocols for cancer and had helped many thousands of clients. He had died only a few months prior to my last visit. As a result, Pamela had a lot of interesting and up-to-date information to share about his ideas, his experiences, and the way he worked.

I met and visited Dr Emil Schandl of American Metabolic Laboratories in Florida and learnt of the tests that his laboratory offered for the very early detection of cancer. These are tests that I have advised many clients to use ever since. They include blood and urine test for the earliest biochemical signs of cancer, detecting it even before the presence of a detectable tumour could be made, possibly five years before. It can be used for both early detection and for prevention, and thus for the start of health-generating strategies. It can be used to monitor the results obtained by the strategies people are following. In addition, it can be used to ensure that someone is continuing in a full remission and not just closing their eyes and hoping a tumour does not return.

I am frequently asked why doctors don't use this test. The answer is simple. Doctors are tumour focused. They need the presence of a tumour large enough to be 'seen' so that they can either cut it out or direct their radiation onto it or be justified in prescribing highly toxic chemotherapy. However, cancer does not just suddenly reach that size and then appear. A tumour is the end result of a lengthy oncological process. During most of this time it escapes detection by the conventional medical tests. By the time it is detected it is often too late to offer a successful and painless treatment. Certainly, an opportunity has been lost or delayed.

About this time, I read the following in *the Lancet* (a leading British medical journal) that opened my eyes to what I considered to be a grossly inadequate approach.

Dr A: "We know that CEA (Cancer Embryonic Antigen) is frequently but not always indicative of colon cancer. Should we not be testing people who have already been treated for colon cancer for CEA at intervals after their initial treatment, to be sure that it has not returned?"

Dr B. "There is little point in doing that as even if the CEA result is raised, it will not tell us the location of the problem. It's better to wait until a tumour has formed and is large enough to be detected. Once we know that we will know where to operate."

I was appalled by this. Cancer is a systemic disease. The subtle systemic signs and symptoms can be detected biochemically, by this test long before a tumour is large enough to be identified by other more sensitive means. This early indication of an active cancer process allows for energetic and efficient, as well as harmless, prevention or reversal strategies to be implemented.

On one visit to America I had planned to visit Robert and Marie Erdmann again. They had been living in England while I was still in Sydney, but had moved to north of Seattle during my first few years in London. This trip would be the first time I had seen them for a while. I was saddened to be told that Robert had died a few days ahead of my arrival and while I had been travelling. Nonetheless, I had an interesting time with Marie, who had insisted that I visit her as planned. She was as enthusiastic and generous as ever with photocopied articles and recommendations as to people I should meet, and more, and we had an enjoyable few days together.

I then went north to the Wolfe clinic in Canada and gained more ideas. I was interested to see how Wolfe worked. He seemed to spend his whole time on the phone, perambulating around his office and warehouse, talking to customers about their cancer and writing out orders for the products that he recommended and that in turn, were parcelled out by his team of waiting staff and sent off to the clients.

I Don't Treat Cancer ... I Treat People

Back in London, when I finally settled down, my practice came alive again, but with a difference. It was developing a new focus. By this time, it was entirely devoted to people with, or concerned about, cancer. I did not encourage clients with other health problems. The practice grew largely by word of mouth. People began to talk more about what I was doing and call for help with cancer. In the past few years I had learnt a lot about the naturopathic approach to cancer and, moreover, I had delved deeply into the metabolic and biochemical theory of cancer, rather than the genetic view, the view and belief held by most people in the medical profession. Clearly there were two main theories, two approaches running side by side and not readily compatible. These led to two different strategies and tactics.

The medical, genetic theory is not readily compatible or consistent with either the genetic evidence around cancer or with a scientific approach. Worse, it does not lead to a logical or therapeutic program or an effective prevention strategy or recovery plan. Once the genetic makeup of tumours began to be examined, it was found that a tumour did not have merely one or two genetic lines, as would be expected if it started from a single, or even only a few genetic faults such as is predicted by the genetic mutation theory of cancer. Instead, it was found that a tumour could have in excess of one or two hundred thousand faulty genetic lines. This leads to the high probability that each tumour starts with a large number of different faults. It would also seem to indicate that, to be successful, any drug treatment would have to address each of the mutations that were discovered. In addition, all of this would have to be discovered and developed in the short time between detection and the possible end of life of the patient. Furthermore, each treatment would almost certainly be unique to each patient and so at vast cost.

The metabolic theory of cancer, on the other hand, actually predicts the possibility of this number of genetically damaged cells and cell lines, all starting with the altered structure and function of the mitochondria, and following a widespread set of situations that adversely affected the mitochondria. It also suggests and leads to a simple, straightforward, and non-toxic protocol of prevention and recovery. All this, however, is for the next book. I gradually set up my office at home in London and started to see clients there. Because of my history of working in several different parts of the world, and because of the referrals this led to, many of my clients were coming from different locations and countries. As a result, clients were making contact first by phone, and then as soon as they were available, by Skype and Zoom. Almost without any effort from me, the practice both grew and spread geographically. It made sense to work from where I lived rather than rent rooms in a formal clinic or office, and to avoid spending time commuting. This was also helpful as I was often having consultations at 'international' times, convenient to the client's time clocks, but possibly not mine, and I could best schedule these appointments from home.

I was soon writing books on cancer, based both on what I had been learning and on my own experiences.

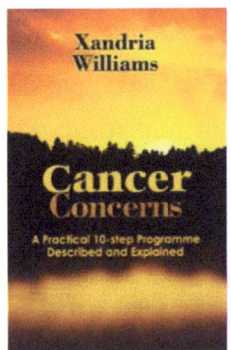

Cancer Concerns describes the many treatments and protocols that key professionals have developed that can help you move out of the cancer process if you are already concerned about it. It was published by Xtra Health Publications and Writersworld in the UK in 2011.

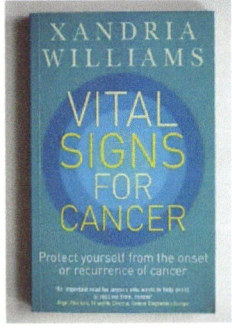

Vital Signs covers the many lifestyle changes and symptom clusters that might warn you of changes you should be making in your lifestyle to help to prevent cancer, or to establish a working platform on which you could build the start of a recovery. It was published initially in 2008, by Piatkus in the UK. It was followed by the American version, *Vital Signs for Cancer: how to prevent, reverse and monitor the cancer process,* published by North Atlantic Books in 2012.

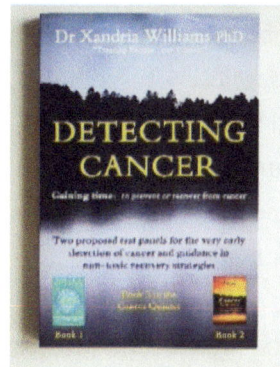

Detecting Cancer describes the test for the very early detection of cancer before there is even any sign of a detectable tumour, and then puts this into context with suggestions as to strategies to follow. It was published by Xtra Health Publications and Writersworld in 2013.

In parallel with this I was asked, yet again and for the third time, to teach at the College of Naturopathic Medicine. Each 'lecture' was to last for a full day and be on a specific topic. Thus, I continued to lecture once more in many aspects of nutrition, but as my practice got ever busier, I reduced this to giving lectures only on cancer. This consisted of about six days a year to six different groups of students. These I thoroughly enjoyed. I was highly encouraged by the enormous amount of interest and enthusiasm shown by the students.

From the start in my cancer-based practice, I frequently worked long distance, making use of skype or zoom. This was possible with much of cancer treatment as so much is based on changing people's diets and lifestyle and for me, working long-distance, this could have been an especially wonderful way of working in Ireland and could have meant I spent a lot more time working from my base there as well as from my home in London. However, while phone and internet connections were possible in Ireland, they were not good enough for an effective and efficient IT office from my home there, so my time in that country remained largely limited to people who lived within travelling distance. Others I continued to consult with from my London office. Between these consultations I continued to care for my fourteen acres of land and for my alpacas, all eighty or so of them.

Right from the start it had been obvious to me that people with cancer were often left out on a limb by standard medicine. They would have a surgeon, an oncologist, a radiologist, a variety of specialist nurses, but not one person who masterminded their overall care. Frequently they didn't know which specialist to turn to for advice on a particular problem. Worse, they rarely met other people with the same problem with whom they could share their experiences.

As a result of these reflections, I set up the *CanSurvive Resource Centre*. In addition to consultations for people who wanted support in whatever they were doing, I encouraged attendance at the weekly Free Friday evening 'Open House' meetings. People would come, bring a plate of raw, organic, low carbohydrate food to share, and swap recipes, stories, and experiences. Then students wanted to join and it developed further. This carried on the tradition I had had in Sydney in the 1980s when I had offered a free Open House evening once a week. Initially that had been for students at the Naturopathic College where I taught. Then it had become the setting for the CWI-CHIs that followed on from the Personal Growth workshops that I ran until the mid-1990s. After that they had been focused on rebirthing sessions.

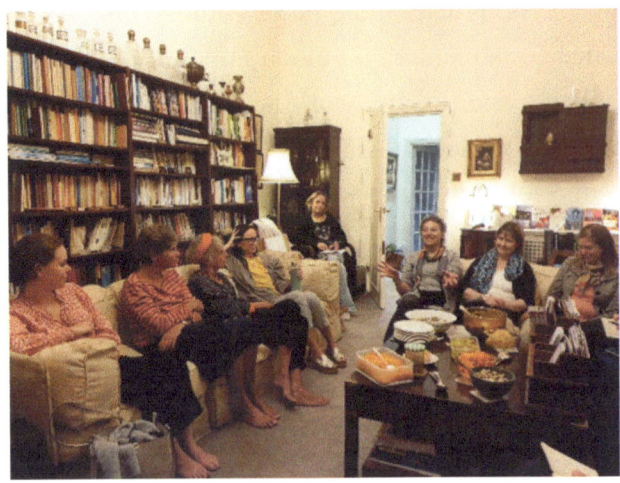

In London, these evenings were aimed first at meeting requests from the students who wanted to learn more than the college course gave them, first about biochemistry, then nutritional questions, and then to cancer-concerned clients. I had chosen Friday evenings because by this time all the various associations to which I belonged gave interesting, stimulating, and not-to-be-missed talks and discussions on several of the other four weekday evenings.

I realised just how much that, in spite of moving halfway round the world, from Sydney to London, I had in many ways merely reinvented myself here in London. The Natural Gourmet in Sydney had been replaced by Xtra Health Ltd in London, the dispensary I had built up in my London premises. My extensive college lecturing in Sydney had been replaced by intermittent periods of lecturing in different colleges in London. My practice in London, the CanSurvive Resource Centre, had simply become more internet-based and cancer-focused than in Sydney. My forays into gardening in Australia had now morphed into my fifteen acres in Ireland and the alpacas. This was, in effect, the smallholding that I had always hankered after when I had first moved to Pennant Hills in Sydney. The psychotherapy that I did in Australia almost as a separate practice, had now become an integral part of many of the consultations I gave as I supported people through cancer.

I wrote and organised a series of teaching seminars on cancer. These grew into the Advanced Cancer Care course. I ran workshops on stress, destressing, and restoring emotional balance. This is a vital part of any healthcare program and should certainly be part of cancer prevention or recovery. I ran seminars on the 'Four Temperaments', or the four emotional types. By helping people to better understand both themselves and other people, a number of potentially stressful situations can be reduced or resolved.

I ran seminars on the various metabolic types. Understanding these enables us to advise on the diets, supplements, and related programs that suit and are helpful for specific people, rather than focus on programs for different health problems or diseases. This understanding should form the basis of any healthcare practice, and none of what we do should be a 'one approach fits all'. Each person is unique and should be cared for and supported on a foundation of this understanding.

I started our Coffee Club program of daily zoom talks and discussions at the beginning of the COVID lockdown in 2021. I realised that many of my clients lived alone and relied for company on the many small social interactions provided by shopping trips, excursions out for a social cup of coffee, and casual meetings. None of these would be possible within the restrictions of lockdown and many people could be lonely. Initially we ran these Coffee Club meetings twice a day (morning and evening), seven days a week, (cancer does not stop over the weekends) as a sort of mobile IT meeting venue.

My 80th birthday was provided by the many members of our Coffee Club and was a wonderful celebration of all that had led me to this point. I floated through that day, outdoors and in glorious sunshine, on a sea of love and warmth from amazing clients, students, and friends. Working with people with cancer, realising how much positivity there is in such a group, being able to help people with this disease when we now have such a positive foundation to the understanding of it, is an incredible privilege and pleasure.

Everything I write and have written throughout my clinical life comes from my conviction that it is much healthier, safer, less toxic, and more effective to *restore homoeostasis* than to try to manipulate the body and its physiology and biochemistry in ways that you *hope* you understand. The body is made up of thousands of interactive metabolic pathways and is infinitely more complex than we imagine.

~ ~ ~

Friends and students have tried for several years to persuade me to write my autobiography. I declined for a long time. I insisted I was not a public figure and few people would be interested. These same friends then focused their persuasions on the anecdotes and stories about the people and situations I have worked with for the past few decades, and have described in my lectures as a way of bringing the information to light. Eventually I have succumbed, but have insisted that the main focus is my professional autobiography and everything leading up to it.

Almost all my more recent cases involve cancer, of course. They all involve real life experiences. Other people's. But I have presented them in such a way that I have, I hope, made them nearly anonymous.

So, I end this retrospective here. I have, so far, had a wonderful life. My enthusiasm for and pleasure in all that I have done has never waned. I also love what I do now and hope to keep doing it.

I have found great joy in looking back over those years, which is what this book is about, and have loved writing it. I hope you have enjoyed reading it as much and have found it both interesting, and something you can learn from.

It is fortunate that one of the class of 1958 (to 61) has kept up with most of us, and we now manage to have occasional meetings when a few of us are in London.

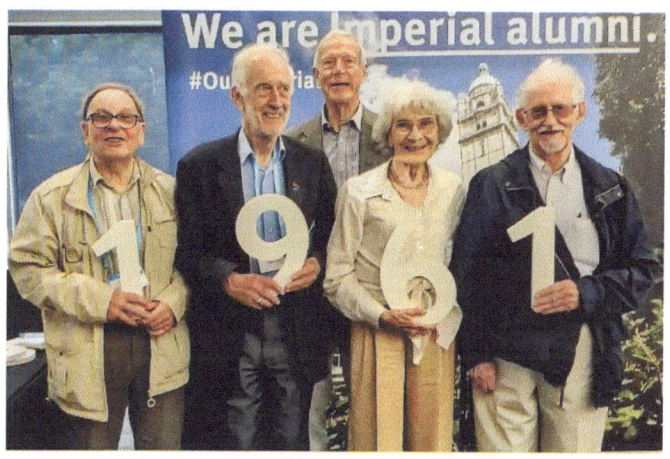

Workshops, seminars, books, practice (and life) strategies

You will have read, in Chapter 15, of my exploration of mind-body health care in the 1980s and 90s under the umbrella title of 'Choosing Health Intentionally', and the other seminars and workshops this encompassed. When I first returned to London in the 1980s there was little appetite for naturopathy and arguably even less for this approach to health care. In the decades since then we have learnt a lot about the power of the mind and how to harness it. We have developed the skills we already have and have acquired new ones. We have started to learn how to reduce 'self-sabotage' and are beginning to develop ways of measuring what we are doing and the results that are being achieved. These results show up experientially of course. Have we done it all, already? I suggest not.

At the start of the twentieth century physicists thought they knew it all. They fully understood atoms, how molecules were made, how the physical world was built, and how it worked at the chemical level. They thought that perhaps in the future there would be no more to discover. Then someone split the atom and an entire new world of science opened.

Perhaps we are at or close to such a turning point now. We are gradually developing tests we can do and measurements we can make, and how to carry this exploration forward with a deeper understanding. It will be important that we encompass not only the mind and the body, but all the senses, emotional, spiritual, and more, and learn ever more about them. It will be important to be inclusive, not exclusive, to open our minds to what, for now, may be undreamt of possibilities.

We are at the start, and we don't even have a comprehensive name for the totality of what the current research is, or could be leading to. Much has been learnt and given many names: 'energy medicine', 'mind-body healing', 'quantum healing', and so on.

I plan to move ahead in this direction, and to do this in several ways – by personal research and development, by having regular 'Open' Zoom-type meetings and discussions, by running seminars and workshops, and, most importantly, by sharing all we come to know.

Appendix

Publications

1986: *Living with Allergies*

Recognize and understand individual food allergens, family food groups, how to avoid your allergens and how to create alternative recipes, including optional and safer recipe alternatives. Includes 4-day and 8-day rotations and others if needed.

1988: *What's in My Food?*

The quantity of each nutrient in individual food on a per-calorie basis, rather than on a per-weight or per serving basis. This has many beneficial uses, particularly when planning the most nutrient-dense and beneficial diets.

1992: *Choosing Health Intentionally*

Unlocking your subconscious for a better emotional and physical future. A discussion of the ways in which your thoughts can give you control of your life, how to change them, and how to use and benefit from this practice. This can help you reduce stress, increase the smooth flow of your life, improve relationships, and reduce tension smoothly and without struggle.

1992: *Choosing Weight intentionally*

How to lose and/or gain weight (depending on your goal) without dieting. Our workshops have shown that many people self-sabotage their progress on a diet for subconscious reasons. This book and the workshops have helped to expose these buried energies.

1993: *Stress, Recognise and Resolve*

Out of print

1993: *From Stress to Success*

Ten steps to a relaxed and happy life. Incorporates a combination of psychological approaches and nutritional and dietary considerations.

1995: *Love Health and Happiness*

Understanding yourself and your relationships through identifying your balance of the four temperaments. Four questions that will indicate which of the sixteen sub-temperaments best describes you.

1997: *Eating Right*
    Out of print

1997: *Natural Cures for Common Ailments*
    Out of print

1995: *Beating the Blues*
    A guide to avoiding and lifting depression. Provides a number of ways of reframing pessimistic moods.

1996: *Fatigue*
    The secrets of getting your energy back. An explanation of what your body needs to ensure optimal energy, enthusiasm, and wellbeing.

1996: *The Four Temperaments*
    How to achieve love, health and happiness by understanding yourself and the people around you (similar to *Love, Health and Happiness)*

1996: *Ideal Weight Ideal Shape*
    How to lose and gain weight without dieting.

1997: *You're Not Alone*
    A guide to understanding and overcoming feelings of isolation. Includes emotional and psychological guidance and practical strategies.

1997: *Natural Cures*

1998: *Overcoming Candida*
    The ultimate cookery book. How to eat well and enjoyably while avoiding the associated problems.

1998: *Liver Detox Plan*
    The revolutionary way to cleanse and revive your body. A description of the huge importance of the liver, the functions it performs and the nutrients that it needs. These are also available as a nutritional supplement complex: 'Liver Support'.

1998: *Building Stronger Bones Naturally*
    The osteoporosis diet and exercise plan to reduce your risk of developing this degenerative disease.

2002: *Fighting Osteoporosis*

A concise handbook of practical strategies.

2003: *The Herbal Detox Plan*

The revolutionary way to cleanse and revive your body with plants and foods that can also add pleasure to your diet.

2005: *Food for Life*

Recipes and food suggestions for people suffering from, or wanting to reduce, the risk of cancer.

2010: *Vital Signs for Cancer*

How to prevent, monitor, and reverse the cancer process.

2011: *Cancer Concerns*

A practical 10-step programme described and explained. Non-toxic strategies for supporting people with cancer and restoring homoeostasis and good health. Includes a description of tests for monitoring progress.

2013: *Detecting Cancer*

Gaining time to prevent or recover from cancer. Two proposed test panels for the very early detection of cancer and guidance in non-toxic recovery strategies. Includes tests that are arguably the earliest test for detecting cancer anywhere in the body, and ways of monitoring recovery and progress.

2022: *Fifty Years a Naturopath*

An autobiography of the professional life of this author.

~ ~ ~

To learn more, Dr Xandria Williams can be contacted

By phone: (44) 020-7824-8153

By mobile: (44) 07474-108-208

By email: xandria@xandriawilliams.co.uk

For more details and *Ongoing Naturopathic Notes*, see her website:
www.xandriawilliams.co.uk

Printed by: Copytech (UK) Limited trading as
Printondemand-worldwide.com
9 Culley Court, Bakewell Road, Orton Southgate,
Peterborough, PE2 6XD

BV - #0005 - 031022 - C42 - 234/156/20 - PB - 9780956855244 - Gloss Lamination